Child Behavioral Health in Sub

Fred M. Ssewamala • Ozge Sensoy Bahar
Mary M. McKay

Editors

Child Behavioral Health in Sub-Saharan Africa

Towards Evidence Generation and Policy Development

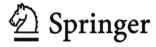 Springer

Editors
Fred M. Ssewamala
Brown School
Washington University in St. Louis
St. Louis, MO, USA

Ozge Sensoy Bahar
Brown School
Washington University in St. Louis
St. Louis, MO, USA

Mary M. McKay
Brown School
Washington University in St. Louis
St. Louis, MO, USA

ISBN 978-3-030-83709-9   ISBN 978-3-030-83707-5   (eBook)
https://doi.org/10.1007/978-3-030-83707-5

Cover image: Two Zimbabwean girl students walking, village east of Mutare, Manicaland Province, Zimbabwe, Africa. © Robert Fried / Alamy Stock Photo

This Springer imprint is published by the registered company Springer Nature Switzerland AG
The registered company address is: Gewerbestrasse 11, 6330 Cham, Switzerland

Preface

Introduction

Children in sub-Saharan Africa (SSA) comprise half of the total regional population, yet behavioral health support and services are severely under-equipped to meet their needs. In fact, recent estimates suggest that one in seven children in SSA struggle with a mental health challenge. On the African continent, poverty, violence, and child-serving resource scarcity may exacerbate the burden on children and impede the allocation of needed support. As African children and adolescents advance in age and soon emerge as the primary drivers of educational, economic, and health well-being of nations across the continent, more attention is being paid to meeting the behavioral health needs of the population, particularly young people.

To date, behavioral health policy is at an early stage across SSA and primarily focuses on the development of guidelines or identification of workforce shortages. At this stage, there is an opportunity to give serious consideration to the context-specific influences in SSA for the purpose of enhancing individual- and population-level childhood behavioral health. Chapters in this volume elevate sensitive issues in SSA, such as high levels of stigma associated with mental illness, skepticism of professionalized responses in contrast to community or religious solutions (e.g., mental health advice sought from prayer camps, religious leaders, or healers), large number of youth orphaned by HIV and other health epidemics, and lack of economic opportunities for African youth.

This edited volume is organized into five parts: 1) Child Mental Health in Sub-Saharan Africa; 2) Current Efforts in Policy, Research, and Practice in Child Behavioral Health: Case Examples; 3) Violence and Child Mental Health in Sub-Saharan Africa: Case Examples; 4) Poverty and Child Mental Health: Case Examples; and 5) Interventions Focused on Child Behavioral Health in Sub-Saharan Africa: Case Examples. The first two parts were intentionally created to highlight foundational issues and summarize existing knowledge related to factors, which uniquely affected the behavioral health of children in Sub-Saharan Africa, as well as influences on policy, research, and practice on the continent. The remaining three parts offer specific examples of efforts to understand and address issues across an expanded set of African countries in order to highlight opportunities and evidence-based innovations.

More specifically, Part I, Child Mental Health in Sub-Saharan Africa, consists of four chapters. First, in "Children at the Intersection of HIV, Poverty, and Mental Health in Sub-Saharan Africa," authors Ssewamala and Sensoy Bahar describe the numerous and compounding threats to childhood behavioral health and emotional well-being across SSA. Not only the burden experienced by children and their families historically and in the present day highlights the need for investment in support and service systems for children, but also given the high burden on large numbers of children, group-, community-, and population-level support is indicated, including combination and multilevel approaches to improve childhood behavioral well-being.

Further, in "Poverty and Children's Mental, Emotional, and Behavioral Health in Sub-Saharan Africa," authors Nyoni, Ahmed, and Dvalishvili apply two frameworks to understanding mechanisms by which poverty exposure may impact childhood behavioral health. More specifically, this chapter focuses on the impact of food insecurity, housing conditions, socioeconomic status (SES), household assets, parents/caregivers' employment status/family disadvantage, number of people living together/overcrowding, and exposure to poverty or economic interventions on youth mental health.

Next, Chapter 3, "Improving Child and Adolescent Mental Health in Africa: A Review of the Economic Evidence," addresses three critical issues in SSA: (1) the extent, nature, and risk factors of childhood and adolescent mental disorders, as well as the economic consequences for the individual, family, and society as a whole; (2) the state of the economic evidence base on mental health programs and interventions for children and adolescents in low-resource settings; and 3) the most immediate economic considerations relevant to introduction, integration, and scale-up of evidence-based programs and interventions to improve child and adolescent mental health and well-being in such settings.

Finally, rounding out Part I, the chapter "Child Maltreatment and Mental Health in Sub-Saharan Africa," written by Bauta and Huang, highlights the need to attend to child maltreatment in order to support child behavioral health. The authors offer a contemporary summary of knowledge on basic science, practice, and policy related to child maltreatment in African settings. The prevalence and epidemiological research on maltreatment and child health (including physical and mental health) are documented. Based on existing knowledge, recommendations for a global agenda for child maltreatment prevention and control, resources, systems, policies in Africa, as well as the challenges in integrating violence prevention services and child mental health care in African settings are outlined. Specific frameworks and strategies to address child violence, abuse, neglect, and mental health needs are made.

Next, in Part II, Chapter 5, "Child Behavioral Health in Ghana: Current Efforts in Policy, Research, and Practice," Asampong and Ibrahim discuss the current investment in child mental health, as well as map out ways to strengthen the country response, including highlighting the need for appropriate measurement and screening tools, incorporating behavioral health services in all regional and district hospitals, and supporting advanced research into childhood behavioral health problems, promotion, and prevention.

In "Children and Child Behavioral Health in Nigeria: Current Efforts in Policy, Research, and Practice," Madu and Osuji emphasize that even though Nigeria is the most populous country in Africa, there is a critical need to bolster the number of trained mental health personnel and elevate official attention to child and adolescent mental health services and policies within the country. In particular, the lack of current and representative epidemiological data on the mental health of Nigerian children is a serious barrier to advocacy and planning policy initiatives. Thus, there is the need to focus on capacity building and training. In addition, the need for widespread education of the Nigerian public on the recognition of mental health disorders burdening children and adolescents in order to reduce stigma is emphasized.

Chapter 7, "Child and Adolescent Mental Health in Kenya: Do We Need a Child and Adolescent Mental Health Policy?", emphasizes significant progress that has been made, particularly that the mental well-being of children is recognized and extensively covered through several acts of parliaments, policies, and both global and regional conventions of which Kenya is a signatory. However, the authors identify additional steps needed to advance childhood behavioral health, including the need for a single platform dedicated to child and adolescent mental health as a policy document. Addressing this need is described as key to guide implementation of additional mental health strategies for children and adolescents.

Finally, the chapter "Towards Entrapment: An Escalating Reality for Children and Adolescents Living with HIV/AIDS in Uganda" completes Part II. This chapter draws on existing materials from previous studies and interviews in order to understand contemporary influences on children's mental health in Uganda, namely changing family systems, transient families, and financial schemes related to HIV and "revolving door experiences" of vulnerable children. Implications for interventions anchored in salutogenesis could create new pathways to address the adversities of children in Uganda.

Part III, Violence and Child Mental Health in Sub-Saharan Africa: Case Examples, consists of three chapters. The first, "The Role of Social Norms: A Case Study of Intimate Partner Violence Among Adolescent Girls in Nigeria," focuses on intimate partner violence (IPV) and its particular threat to girls and women in sub-Saharan Africa. This chapter presents findings from a study, which examines the relationships between community contextual influences, alignment with gendered expectations, and IPV. The findings underscore the importance of identifying and considering the social and gender norms in a given setting before implementing programs and policies aiming to empower women and girls. Policies and programs that promote behavior counter to the contextual norms run the risk of generating unintended consequences for the very individuals these policies aim to help. Such

programs and policies should work to simultaneously address broader gender inequitable norms in order to ensure positive impacts for women and girls in all arenas.

Chapter 10, "Current State of Child Behavioral Health: Focus on Violence
Against Children in Uganda," describes the progress made related to children's
rights in Uganda. In particular, the Violence Against Children Act has fueled
advancement, but there are still critical gaps in both policy and practice. The authors
clearly identify opportunities for improvement and recommend improved coordination, evidence generation and utilization as well as increased investments in preventive and response services for violence against children.

Finally, the last chapter in this part, "Determinants of Intergenerational Trauma
Transmission: A Case of the Survivors of the 1994 Genocide Against Tutsi in
Rwanda," explores the transmission of trauma, models of transmission, intersection
of PTSD in parents and parent-infant attachment, determinants of the PTSD transmission within the Rwandan context, as well as possible pathways of child traumatization in post-genocide Rwanda.

Part IV, "Poverty and Child Mental Health: Case Examples," includes three
chapters with the first, "Food Insecurity, Malnutrition, and Child Developmental
and Behavioral Outcomes in Ghana," authored by Aryee, Gyimah, Chapnick, and
Iannotti. In this chapter, the authors provide an overview of the food insecurity in
Ghana, including determinants and consequences on child health, development, and
behavioral outcomes. In particular, the chapter focuses on 1) defining food insecurity
and malnutrition and describing the situation and trends globally and in Ghana; 2)
identifying key consequences of food insecurity and malnutrition on child health,
development, and behavioral outcomes globally and in Ghana; and 3) characterizing
policy, program, and research solutions that have been applied in Ghana for achieving food security and reducing malnutrition.

Next, "Child Labor in Ghana: Current Policy, Research, and Practice Efforts"
focuses on the behavioral health needs of children engaged in productive economic
activities, work that deprives them of their childhood, potential, and dignity and that
is harmful to their physical and mental development. Again, there is an emphasis on
existing and new policy, research, and practices to curb the current observable child
labor trends in Ghana.

Finally, in the last chapter in this part, "Children Living on the Street: Current
Efforts in Policy Research and Practice in Ghana," the authors focus on the Greater
Accra region of Ghana, where nearly 61,492 persons under 18 years of age are living
and working on the streets. Findings from a qualitative study are presented with
methods exploring the existing efforts targeted towards addressing the situation of
children living on the street. Results revealed that there is no common platform that
brings these institutions together to leverage their unique strengths to advocate for
comprehensive/multi-sectoral government policy. Forging of multilevel and
multifunctional partnerships to achieve both their common and unique goals in
order to advance child behavioral health and safety is recommended.

The volume concludes with Part V, "Interventions Focused on Child Behavioral
Health in Sub-Saharan Africa: Case Examples. Two chapters complete the book,
with the first being "Caregiver-Child Communication: The Case for Engaging

South African Caregivers in Family-Based Interventions." In this chapter, Parchment, Small, and Bhana explore the historical legacy of apartheid on Black South African families, particularly related to parenting and parent-child communication. Findings from their study examining the relationship between contextual challenges and frequency of caregiver-child communication among a sample of South African families are presented. Results support the notion that the family, in particular Black South African adult caregivers, is integral in potentially preventing youth from engaging in risky situations. It also reinforces the need for policies to strengthen family stability and relationships.

Finally, Chapter 16, "Social Enterprises for Child and Adolescent Health in Sub-Saharan Africa: A Realist Evaluation," presents findings on social enterprises as a means to improve the behavioral health and well-being of children and families. The authors present the results of an evaluation of social enterprises appraised by the Schwab Foundation for Social Entrepreneurship, one of the world's most influential social entrepreneurship organizations in sub-Saharan Africa. Nine social enterprise interventions were assessed with findings supporting the use of social enterprises to address the unmet health needs of children and adolescents in sub-Saharan Africa. The chapter ends by suggesting avenues for future research to advance sustainable social enterprises aimed at improving the health and well-being of children and adolescents in the region.

The intent of this volume is to pull together existing knowledge on the specific needs of young people in SSA, particularly emphasizing their behavioral health challenges, contextually specific influences on their well-being, and recommendations to advance support, resources, policies, and practices on the continent. The range of authors rely on data to highlight unique and too often compounding challenges facing children and their families, as well as highlight approaches and strategies worth investment and scaling. The behavioral health of children in SSA is of vital importance given the large proportion of the population still quite young in age. As these children grow and develop, their wellness could be vitally important to the overall health and economic vitality of many countries within SSA.

St. Louis, MO, USA   Fred M. Ssewamala
                                                               Ozge Sensoy Bahar
                                                               Mary M. McKay

Contents

Contributors

Rabab Ahmed, MD, MPH Ministry of Health and Population, Cairo, Egypt

Collins Airhihenbuwa, PhD Georgia State University, School of Public Health, Atlanta, GA, USA

Lois Aryee Brown School, Washington University in St. Louis, St. Louis, MO, USA

Emmanuel Asampong, PhD Department of Social and Behavioural Sciences, School of Public Health, University of Ghana, Legon, Ghana

Clare Ahabwe Bangirana, MME The AfriChild Centre, Kampala, Uganda

Besa Bauta, PhD Silver School of Social Work, New York University, New York, NY, USA

Arvin Bhana, PhD Department of Psychology, School of Applied Human Sciences, University of KwaZulu-Natal, Durban, South Africa

Sarah Blackstone, PhD University of Virginia School of Medicine, Charlottesville, VA, USA

Alice Boateng, PhD Department of Social Work, University of Ghana, Legon, Accra, Ghana

David Bukusi, PhD Kenyatta National Hospital, Nairobi, Kenya

William Byansi, MSW Brown School, Washington University in St. Louis, St. Louis, MO, USA

Ariadna Capasso, MFA School of Global Public Health, New York University, New York, NY, USA

Cindi Cassady, PhD Department of Clinical Psychology, University of Kibungo, Kibungo, Rwanda

Melissa Chapnick, MPH Brown School, Washington University in St. Louis, St. Louis, MO, USA

Mavis Dako-Gyeke, PhD Department of Social Work, University of Ghana, Legon, Accra, Ghana

Ernestina Korleki Dankyi, PhD Centre for Social Policy Studies, College of Humanities, University of Ghana, Legon, Ghana

Daji Dvalishvili, MD, MSW Brown School, Washington University in St. Louis, St. Louis, MO, USA

Oliver Ezechi, MBBS, PhD Nigerian Institute of Medical Research, Clinical Sciences Division, Yaba, Lagos, Nigeria

Titilola Gbaja-Biamila, MBBS, MSc Nigerian Institute of Medical Research, Clinical Sciences Division, Yaba, Lagos, Nigeria

Emmanuel A. Gyimah, MPH Brown School, Washington University in St. Louis, St. Louis, MO, USA

Keng-Yen Huang, PhD Department of Population Health, School of Medicine, NYU Langone Health, New York, NY, USA

Lora Iannotti, PhD Brown School, Washington University in St. Louis, St. Louis, MO, USA

Abdallah Ibrahim, DrPH Department of Health Policy, Planning and Management, School of Public Health, University of Ghana, Legon, Ghana

Juliet Iwelunmor, PhD Saint Louis University, College for Public Health and Social Justice, Department of Behavioral Science and Health Education, St. Louis, MO, USA

Agatha Kafuko, MA Department of Social Work and Social Administration, Makerere University, Kampala, Uganda

Ednah Ndidi Madu, PhD College of Nursing and Public Health, Adelphi University, Garden City, NY, USA

Stacey Mason, MPH Saint Louis University, College for Public Health and Social Justice, Department of Behavioral Science and Health Education, St. Louis, MO, USA

Muthoni Mathai, PhD Department of Psychiatry, University of Nairobi, Nairobi, Kenya

Anne Wanjiru Mbwayo, PhD Department of Psychiatry, University of Nairobi, Nairobi, Kenya

James Mugisha, PhD Department of Sociology and Social Administration, Kyambogo University, Kampala, Uganda

Teresia Mutavi, PhD Department of Psychiatry, University of Nairobi, Nairobi, Kenya

Célestin Mutuyimana, MSc Center for Mental Health, College of Medicine and Health Sciences, University of Rwanda, Kigali, Rwanda

Ucheoma Nwaozuru, PhD Saint Louis University, College for Public Health and Social Justice, Department of Behavioral Science and Health Education, St. Louis, MO, USA

Thabani Nyoni, MSW Brown School, Washington University in St. Louis, St. Louis, MO, USA

Chisom Obiezu-Umeh, MPH Saint Louis University, College for Public Health and Social Justice, Department of Behavioral Science and Health Education, St. Louis, MO, USA

David Oladele, MBBS, MPH Nigerian Institute of Medical Research, Clinical Sciences Division, Yaba, Lagos, Nigeria

Timothy Opobo, MSc The AfriChild Centre, Kampala, Uganda

Hadiza Osuji, PhD Silver School of Social Work, New York University, New York, NY, USA

Tyrone M. Parchment, PhD School of Social Work, Boston College, Boston, MA, USA

Ilana Seff, DrPH Brown School, Washington University in St. Louis, St. Louis, MO, USA

Ozge Sensoy Bahar, PhD Brown School, Washington University in St. Louis, St. Louis, MO, USA

Vincent Sezibera, PhD Center for Mental Health, College of Medicine and Health Sciences, University of Rwanda, Kigali, Rwanda

Latoya Small, PhD Luskin School of Public Affairs, University of California Los Angeles, Los Angeles, CA, USA

Fred M. Ssewamala, PhD Brown School, Washington University in St. Louis, St. Louis, MO, USA

Lindsay Stark, DrPH Brown School, Washington University in St. Louis, St. Louis, MO, USA

Yesim Tozan, PhD School of Global Public Health, New York University, New York, NY, USA

Florida Uzoaru, MSc Saint Louis University, College for Public Health and Social Justice, Department of Behavioral Science and Health Education, St. Louis, MO, USA

About the Editors

Fred M. Ssewamala, PhD is William E. Gordon Distinguished Professor at the Brown School at Washington University in St. Louis, Missouri. Dr. Ssewamala leads innovative, interdisciplinary research that informs, develops and tests economic empowerment and social protection interventions aimed at improving life chances and long-term developmental impacts for children and adolescent youth impacted by poverty and health disparities in low-resource communities. He holds a joint appointment in the Washington University School of Medicine, and directs the International Center for Child Health and Development (ICHAD) and SMART Africa Center.

Currently, Dr. Ssewamala is conducting five large-scale longitudinal randomized control trials across sub-Saharan Africa funded by the National Institutes of Health: Kyaterekera Project, Suubi+Adherence-R2, Suubi4Her, SMART Africa and Suubi4Stigma. Another project, Suubi4Cancer, explores care for children living with HIV with suspected cancers. In addition, he is a co-principal investigator on several NIH-funded training projects that focus on training early-career researchers committed to careers in child behavioral health.

Dr. Ssewamala has over 100 peer-reviewed articles in high-impact journals on family economic empowerment and related health and mental health outcomes as well as HIV prevention. He serves on the editorial board of the *Journal of Adolescent Health* and co-edits the *Global Social Welfare* journal. He is a member of the Society for Social Work and Research, American Public Health Association, and the Siteman Cancer Center. Ssewamala is also a fellow of the American Academy of Social Work and Social Welfare.

Ozge Sensoy Bahar, PhD is Research Assistant Professor at the Brown School at Washington University in St. Louis, Missouri. Sensoy Bahar's research focuses on child and family well-being in global contexts characterized by poverty and associated stressors. Her current research program focuses on youth experiences of child work and labor, as well as the individual, family, and contextual factors leading to child labor in two country contexts, Turkey and Ghana. Dr. Sensoy Bahar has led two research studies funded by the National Institutes of Health focused on the unaccompanied migration of adolescent girls for labor in Ghana. The goal of her work is to develop culturally and contextually relevant interventions to reduce risk factors associated with child labor. As a qualitative methodology expert, she also leads the qualitative components of multiple NIH-funded studies.

Sensoy Bahar completed a three-year, externally funded post-doctoral fellowship at the McSilver Institute for Poverty Policy and Research at New York University Silver School of Social Work. Currently, she serves as one of the co-directors for the International Center for Child Health and Development at the Brown School. She also serves on the editorial board of the *Global Social Welfare* journal.

Mary M. McKay, PhD is Neidorff Family and Centene Corporation Dean of the Brown School at Washington University in St. Louis, Missouri. Dean McKay joined the Brown School as dean in 2016. Dean McKay's academic experience connects deeply to both social work and public health. She has received substantial federal funding for research focused on meeting the mental health and health prevention needs of youth and families impacted by poverty both in the US and globally, specifically in Sub-Saharan Africa. She also has significant expertise in child mental health services and implementation research methods, as well as over 20 years of experience conducting HIV prevention and care-oriented studies, supported by the National Institutes of Health.

She has authored more than 150 publications on mental and behavioral health, HIV/AIDS prevention and urban poverty, and more.

Prior to joining the Brown School, Dean McKay was the McSilver Professor of Social Work and the inaugural director of the McSilver Institute for Poverty Policy and Research at New York University's Silver School of Social Work. She previously served as the head of the Division of Mental Health Services Research at Mount Sinai School of Medicine. Her prior academic appointments include Columbia University and University of Illinois at Chicago.

Part I
Child Mental Health in Sub-Saharan Africa

Children at the Intersection of HIV, Poverty, and Mental Health in Sub-Saharan Africa (SSA)

Fred M. Ssewamala and Ozge Sensoy Bahar

Introduction

Sub-Saharan Africa (SSA) remains the world's most affected region in the HIV epidemic, home to 71% of people living with HIV worldwide (UNAIDS, 2014). Notably, HIV/AIDS epidemic continues to spread in young people, with adolescents being reported as the only age group where HIV prevalence appears to be rising (UNAIDS, 2013). Many countries in the region also report limited child and adolescent mental health (CAMH) services, community violence, and pervasive poverty (Bruckner et al., 2011; Fulton et al., 2011; Kleintjes et al., 2010; WHO, 2005, 2011a, 2011b, 2011c, 2011d). When combined, these characteristics negatively impact communities' responses to mental health functioning and HIV, among children and adolescents (Bruckner et al., 2011; Fulton et al., 2011; Ssewamala et al., 2009). Studies indicate that AIDS-affected communities and family members often suffer recurrent mental health complications including trauma and depression (Atwine et al., 2005; Cluver & Gardner, 2006, 2007; Rotheram-Borus & Stein, 1999; Sengendo & Nambi, 1997). This is exceptionally worrisome because (1) it negatively impacts the overall HIV care and prevention efforts, and (2) specific to children and adolescents, it may severely undermine their future development, social functioning, and reproductive health choices (Patel et al., 2007) negatively impacting the overall growth and development of SSA for generations.

HIV/AIDS and co-occurring mental health problems are further exacerbated by pervasive poverty (Costello et al., 2003; Duncan & Brooks-Gunn, 2000; Lipman et al., 1996; McLeod & Shanahan, 1996; Pollitt, 1994). Poverty not only affects a community's ability to care for its members' physical and mental health, including children, but also impacts individual members' functioning and psychosocial well-

F. M. Ssewamala (✉) · O. Sensoy Bahar
Brown School, Washington University in St. Louis, St. Louis, MO, USA
e-mail: fms1@wustl.edu

© Springer Nature Switzerland AG 2022
F. M. Ssewamala et al. (eds.), *Child Behavioral Health in Sub-Saharan Africa*,
https://doi.org/10.1007/978-3-030-83707-5_1

being (Case et al., 2004; Foster, 2006). Thus, persistent poverty, by adversely affecting individual and community functioning, constitutes a critically important risk factor for chronic poor mental health functioning. Specifically, children and adolescents in communities with persistent poverty, disease (including HIV/AIDS), and violence are more likely to suffer from chronic mental health challenges (Sengendo & Nambi, 1997).

To date, few efforts in SSA have explored interventions capable of targeting the root causes and consequences of persistent poverty, violence, and co-occurring mental health problems, particularly depression and trauma. In addition, few studies aimed at enhancing mental health functioning of communities and families have addressed critical, culturally congruent, and scientifically documented risk factors of persistent family poverty, community violence, and impact of HIV/AIDS. Most investigators in SSA target their intervention studies primarily on personal/individual trait models, emphasizing generic psychosocial counseling (Bajos & Marquet, 2000). Such interventions often fall short of fielding and testing contextually grounded, multidisciplinary, combined approaches necessary to break the vicious cycle of persistent poverty, community violence, HIV risk, and co-occurring mental health problems that affect children, adolescents, and their families. Moreover, it is critical that mental health and HIV prevention interventions in SSA countries are guided by contextually relevant methods and conceptual models developed and tested in SSA. An important step in this direction is research studies targeted at examining combination interventions addressing persistent poverty, co-occurring mental health problems, and HIV infection in the SSA region.

Burden of HIV/AIDS Among Youth and Families in SSA

The HIV/AIDS pandemic in SSA continues to devastate families and to spread among young people, with adolescents being reported as one of the vulnerable groups where HIV prevalence appears to be rising (UNAIDS, 2013). Adolescence is a particularly vulnerable developmental stage with high risk for HIV, sexually transmitted infections (STIs), and poor mental health functioning. Higher depression among young people has been associated with cofactors of HIV risk (Barhafumwa et al., 2016). Adolescents facing adversity, particularly poverty, exhibit high rates of early and risky sexual behavior, pregnancy, and drug abuse (Fergus, & M., A., 2005; Gregson et al., 2005; McLoyd, 1998; MOH Uganda & ORC Macro, 2006; WHO, 2014). Simultaneously, adolescents face serious challenges to mental health functioning with trends varying by age. Moreover, adolescents affected by AIDS experience even more severe mental health problems than other at-risk groups (Cluver et al., 2008; Cluver et al., 2012; Han et al., 2013; Karimli & Ssewamala, 2015). Studies of AIDS-affected adolescents living in poverty in some SSA countries show high rates of depression (Han et al., 2013; Karimli & Ssewamala, 2015; Ssewamala et al., 2012), anxiety, learning problems (Curley et al., 2010; Ssewamala & Curley, 2006), and risky sexual behaviors (Ssewamala et al., 2010b, 2010c; Jennings et al.,

2016). Compounded by poverty, the lack of self-esteem and hope for the future can influence sexual risk taking and increase HIV risk.

Education is critical to adolescents' future life chances. However, adolescents and youth orphaned by AIDS are considerably less likely to attend and engage in school, primarily due to lack of economic and familial support (Hall et al., 2008; Garmezy, 1994; Rutherford, 2000; Ssewamala et al., 2009). To illustrate, in Uganda, the proportion of orphaned primary school pupils missing a term was almost twice as high (27%) compared to non-orphan pupils (14%) (Garmezy, 1994). Children and adolescents who obtain more schooling are likely to have improved behavioral and health outcomes. For instance, in most SSA countries, young people who complete secondary school have a lower risk of HIV infection and are more likely to practice safe sex compared to their counterparts who only complete the primary level (Ssewamala et al., 2010d). When young people drop out of school, they become more susceptible to poverty and risk-taking behaviors, further exposing them to the possibility of contracting HIV.

Children and adolescents living with HIV and experiencing poverty also face unique challenges related to their HIV treatment and care. Specifically in SSA, individual- and family-level financial instability, including lack of assets, monetary income, and material resources, deters people living with HIV/AIDS from adhering to their prescribed regimen. Furthermore, people often cease taking their prescribed HIV medications due to the inability to address a significant side effect (Au et al., 2006; Faber et al., 2011; Mukherjee et al., 2006). An increased appetite is a side effect of ART, and ART requires greater caloric consumption, especially when patients initiate ART. An increased appetite can have serious implications for people in SSA (Au et al., 2006; Faber et al., 2011; Polisset et al., 2009). For impoverished families, there will be an increased burden on limited resources when families cannot meet this demand. Studies in SSA report fear of increased appetite and not having sufficient food as barriers to ART adherence (Au et al., 2006; Gusdal et al., 2009; Weiser et al., 2003). Further, financial instability impacts ART adherence through transportation costs to health clinics. Studies from SSA, including Uganda, show that the costs of transportation to health clinics impeded individuals from attending their scheduled follow-up appointments and obtaining refills of antiretrovirals (ARVs) (Tuller et al., 2010; Weiser et al., 2003). As a result, many patients have gaps in their treatment regimens and often cease taking ARVs for long periods of time. Gaps in treatment increase the risk of virologic failure and resistance to first-line HIV drugs (WHO HIV/AIDS, 2011a), yet second-line drugs are expensive and unavailable in many resource-constrained settings. In low-resource settings, YLHIV sacrifice healthcare, including adherence to treatment and other basic needs (e.g., food, clothing, and school fees) (Biadgilign et al., 2009; Gusdal et al., 2009; Hardon et al., 2007; Ramadhani et al., 2007; Weiser et al., 2003).

These heightened risks indicate the urgent need for culturally relevant interventions and a training infrastructure for a new cadre of researchers to address the complex and multilayered issues facing young people and their families in SSA.

Limitations of Individually Oriented Theoretical Models

The HIV/AIDS pandemic continues to spread among young people, with adolescents being cited as the only group where HIV prevalence continues to rise (UNAIDS, 2013). Innovative culturally congruent theoretically guided approaches are needed to address the important cultural and contextual factors, which significantly affect prevention and intervention responses. To date, most HIV intervention programs have been based on theories that are typically social cognitive in orientation: Health Beliefs Model (Becker & Mainman, 1975; Becker et al., 1977; Rosenstock, 1966), Theory of Reasoned Action (Montano & Kasprzyk, 2002) and Planned Behavior (Ajzen, 1991; Fishbein, 1967; Montano & Kasprzyk, 2002), Self-efficacy theory (Bandura, 1986), and Social Psychological Model (Fisher & Fisher, 1992). *These theories emphasize a deficit in individuals that must be changed (knowledge, attitudes, beliefs, or behaviors). Few simultaneously attempt to address co-occurring mental health challenges.* These traditional, individually oriented theoretical models fail to account for the contextual and structural specific issues that influence HIV risk, and that may explain the limited success of HIV interventions in a poverty-impacted region like SSA dominated by structural challenges such as poverty, community violence, and high HIV infection rates each year. In such communities, applying CHP approaches rooted within structural level theories, such as ecological perspective (Bastard et al., 1997; Bronfenbrenner, 1977), institutional theory (Ssewamala & Sherraden, 2004), empowerment theory (Rappaport, 1981), and an Afro-centric paradigm (Kambon, 1992; Karenga, 2003), emphasizing structural and culturally specific factors in establishing and maintaining protective behaviors may be needed.

Thus, to optimize the effectiveness of interventions for HIV prevention and care, and to address co-occurring mental health issues in the context of HIV/AIDS, researchers should utilize both individual trait-focused and structural level theoretical approaches, augmented with theories that are culturally and contextually relevant to SSA in order to develop effective HIV interventions. These combined and contextually specific approaches to HIV risk reduction and co-occurring mental health problems consider the individual backgrounds, relationship context, immediate social context, and broader cultural values and beliefs in which HIV risk behavior and poor mental health functioning occur.

Role of Combination Interventions in Addressing the Burden of HIV/AIDS and Mental Health

Studies and theory (Sherraden, 1990; Sherraden, 1991) suggest causal pathways between family economic resources, education, mental health, and HIV risk. Single interventions are often useful but insufficient to address problems as complex and multidimensional as child and adolescent mental health (CAMH) and HIV risk for young people. Given the failure of most single interventions to significantly decrease these rates, investments in combination interventions are critical to provide an interdisciplinary, multilevel response needed to reduce new HIV and STI infections in a way that single interventions alone have not yet been able. UNAIDS and others in the HIV research community have observed an urgent need for strategies to shift towards combination HIV prevention (CHP) (Kurth et al., 2011; Hankins & de Zalduondo, 2010; UNAIDS, 2010). UNAIDS defines CHP as: "The strategic, simultaneous use of different classes of prevention activities that operate on multiple levels (individual, family relationships, community, societal), to respond to the specific needs of particular audiences and modes of HIV transmission, and to make efficient use of resources through prioritizing, partnership, and engagement of affected communities (UNAIDS, 2010)." CHP seeks to realign program components for maximum effect, to tailor prevention efforts to local epidemics, and to ensure that components are delivered with the intensity, quality, and scale necessary to achieve intended effects (Hankins & de Zalduondo, 2010).

In alignment with the UNAIDS call for combination HIV prevention interventions and the National Institutes of Health (NIH) priority area of health disparities (NIH, 2015), this chapter recognizes the need for researchers working in countries heavily impacted by HIV/AIDS to conduct child and adolescent mental health research in the context of HIV/AIDS using rigorous culturally congruent research methods, and testing combination HIV prevention interventions. This will ultimately provide a solid foundation for the development and implementation of evidence-based HIV prevention and mental health interventions for youth and families impacted by HIV/AIDS in SSA.

Although advances have been made in the science of child and adolescent mental health, and HIV intervention and prevention research, the application of scientifically based, culturally congruent prevention intervention models tailored to the worldviews and life contexts of communities heavily affected by poor mental health and HIV remains limited (Wyatt et al., 2002). Most HIV prevention interventions for SSA are still guided by theoretical models originated in the global north and lack cultural congruency, and sometimes contextual relevancy (Wyatt et al., 2004). The continued spread of HIV within SSA (24.7 million in SSA are living with HIV) (UNAIDS, 2015) suggests a scientific, moral, and ethical imperative for culturally congruent prevention and intervention models that expand upon and/or augment the current western-focused interventions and incorporate SSA culturally specific interventions.

In the absence of a cure, research in HIV prevention remains of critical importance to generate evidence that may save lives, especially in low- and middle-income countries (LMICs), including the poor SSA countries with the biggest disease burden. Testing and applying innovative interventions that promote sustainable behavioral change among young people, their families, and communities are needed. This chapter acknowledges that single interventions are often useful but insufficient to address problems as complex and multidimensional as *co-occurring mental health and HIV risk* challenge.

An Evidence-Based Combination Intervention in the Context of Poverty, HIV/AIDS, and Mental Health

The International Center for Child Health and Development (ICHAD) at the Brown School at Washington University in St. Louis, Missouri, is already engaged in work that uses combination interventions to address HIV and CAMH in poverty-impacted communities in the SSA region. ICHAD contributes to the reduction of poverty and improvement of public health outcomes for children, adolescents, and families in low-resource communities, particularly those in sub-Saharan Africa and other developing nations, through innovative applied intervention research; raising public awareness and support for economic empowerment interventions; and informing public policy and programming. ICHAD houses several ongoing and completed NIH-funded studies focused on HIV and CAMH using combination interventions in the SSA region (see Table 1).

All these studies use an evidence-based combination intervention informed by synergetic models that aim to build human and financial capital concurrently and operate at the individual, family, and community levels, where financial, nongovernmental, and, sometimes, state governance institutions are involved (Ssewamala et al., 2010c). These synergetic models utilize a combination strategy in which a single program or policy seeks to intervene in the reproduction of poverty with impacts registered across a variety of social indicators, such as health, literacy, social functioning, gender empowerment, and educational outcomes. Such approaches epitomize a bottom-up, threshold model of development. The threshold model does not wait to address one adverse condition at a time but instead seeks to address the interrelated dimensions of poverty in an integrated and collaborative framework. Such a model provides for potentially compound benefits produced by combined initiatives, particularly those that encourage context-specific saving up, such as savings programs targeting HIV-impacted youth in SSA. This is in contrast to the limitations of single-focused asset-based development programs, particularly those that involve higher risk saving down.

More specifically, the combination intervention, known as Suubi (Hope in Luganda—local language in the region where the studies are conducted), uses a combination of the components described in Table 2, depending on the specific population and aims of that particular study.

Data from our studies have shown the positive impact of this evidence-based combination intervention on several health, mental health, and developmental outcomes among adolescents impacted by HIV/AIDS. For example, in our Bridges study, adolescents in our treatment groups had increased economic stability. Moreover, at 24-months post-intervention initiation we found a significant unmediated effect of the intervention on children's mental health as measured by the Child Depression Inventory, the Beck Hopelessness Scale (Zimet et al., 1988), and the Tennessee Self-Concept Scale (NIDA, 1993). In the short run, controlling for socioeconomic characteristics, adolescents in the intervention arms were more likely than participants in the control arm to report increased scores on HIV knowledge,

Table 1 ICHAD studies

Suubi (2005–2007; R21MH076475)	Suubi tested the efficacy of a family economic empowerment intervention which includes opportunities for asset ownership, development of future planning skills, enhancement of mental health, and reduction of risk-taking behaviors for children orphaned due to AIDS in Uganda
Suubi-MAKA (2008–2012; R34MH081763)	Suubi-MAKA further developed and preliminarily examined a family economic empowerment intervention that created economic opportunities (specifically children development accounts) for families in Uganda who are caring for children orphaned due to the AIDS pandemic
Bridges to the Future (2011–2018; R01HD070727)	*Bridges to the Future study* focused on evaluating the efficacy and cost-effectiveness of our family-based economic empowerment intervention for orphaned and vulnerable children affected by HIV in Uganda. It comprised a total of 1383 participants from 48 government-aided primary schools in Uganda. Participants were followed for 5 years. Participants in this study were randomly assigned to one of the three intervention groups (usual care, treatment 1 with a 1:1 matching rate, and treatment 2 with a 2:1 matching rate) of the child development accounts (CDA). Participants received mentorship to help them make better life decisions and reduce sexual risk-taking behaviors, and IGA sessions to help them select a better IGA for asset accumulation
Suubi + Adherence (2012–2018; R01HD074949)	*Suubi + Adherence study* examined the impact and cost associated with an innovative economic empowerment intervention to increase adherence to HIV treatment among HIV-positive adolescents on antiretroviral therapy (ART) in Uganda. This study included 710 participants from 39 clinics that dispensed ART medications to HIV-positive adolescents. Participants were followed for 5 years and it is one of the few studies with the lowest attrition rates. Participants in this study were assigned to either control (usual care) or treatment (with a bank account and cartoon sessions). Adherence to ART was measured by the use of a wise pill device, pill counts, clinic records data, and biomarkers (CD4 and viral load tests)
Suubi4Her study (2017–2022; R01MH113486)	The *Suubi4Her study* examines the impact and cost associated with Suubi4Her, an innovative combination intervention that aims to prevent HIV risk behaviors among 14–17-year-old girls living in communities heavily affected by poverty and HIV/AIDS in Uganda. This study follows 1260 adolescent girls from 46 secondary schools in south western Uganda and is in its third year. Adolescent girls are randomly assigned to one of the three study arms. The interventions include financial literacy training (FLT), income-generating activities (IGA), and a bank account and the multiple family group sessions (MFG)

Source: Adapted from Tumwesige et al. (2021), with permission from AME Publishing Company.

Table 2 Description of intervention components

Intervention component	Description
Financial literacy training workshops	Participating children/adolescents and their caregivers receive six 1–2-h workshop sessions that cover components on saving and financial management. The sessions introduce participants to the notion of saving and saving strategies; discuss career planning; and help participants begin utilizing financial institutions, including saving in banks
Mentorship	Each child/adolescent has a mentor who would visit with them monthly for the duration of the intervention. The one-to-one mentorship program is intended to help children/adolescents overcome a variety of challenges they face in daily life by fostering meaningful and lasting relationships with near-peer/adult role models. Mentors are high school and university students trained by the schools or NGO staff depending on study conditions
Income generation activities	Participants are trained on investing in income-generating activities (IGA) during the FLT workshops and are allowed to use up to 30% of their matched savings to invest in an IGA intended to benefit children/adolescents and their caregiving families. The IGA portion is intended to promote economic stability
Youth/child development accounts	Each child/adolescent in the treatment arm receives a youth development account (YDA), which is a matched savings account held in the child/adolescent's name in a financial institution under the Central Bank (Bank of Uganda). ICHAD partners with four national banks operating in the study area: Centenary Bank, DFCU Bank, DTB, and Stanbic to host the YDAs. Any of the AY's family members, relatives, or friends are allowed and indeed encouraged to contribute towards the YDA. The account is then matched with money from the program (at 1:1 or 1:2 match rate), with a cap. A savings account statement is generated monthly for every AY. Each AY, with his or her primary caregiver as a cosigner, has access to the money in his or her account (excluding the matching funds) for emergency purposes. When an AY is ready to pay for school fees, the check for the matching funds is written in the name of "the school" which the AY is attending. The AY then contributes his or her portion of the total cost for the academic term. The approximated matched amounts should be enough to pay for about 4 years of adolescents' secondary education in a public school under universal secondary education. AY's access to the matching funds is conditional on an AY having completed the six sessions required for FLT workshops within 24 months of enrolment in the program
Multiple family group (Amaka Amasanyufu)*	Multiple family group (MFG) intervention is a 16-session manualized evidence-based intervention for families of children with disruptive behaviors and focuses on family strengthening. The targeted skills and processes are referred to in the curriculum as the 4Rs (rules, responsibility, relationships, and respectful communication) and 2Ss (stress and social support).

(continued)

Table 2 (continued)

Intervention component	Description
	The MFG involves up to 20 families. At least two generations (child/adolescent and caregiver-parent, aunt, grandparent) of a family are present in each session. Content and practice activities foster learning and interaction both within the family and between families

Source: Reused from Tumwesige et al. (2021), with permission from AME Publishing Company.
aHappy Families in Luganda—the local language in the study area.

better scores on desired HIV-related beliefs, and better scores on HIV prevention attitudes, pointing to the potential role of family economic empowerment in promoting the much-desired HIV knowledge, beliefs, and prevention attitudes among children and adolescents orphaned by HIV/AIDS. In regard to educational outcomes, on average, children and adolescents receiving the intervention showed lower dropout rates and higher scores on their primary leaving examinations (Hamilton et al., 2011).

In our Suubi + Adherence study focused on perinatally infected adolescents in Uganda, we found that the proportion of virally suppressed participants in the intervention condition steadily increased. For example, we found significantly lower odds of youth in the intervention condition having a detectable viral load at both 12 and 24 months. Specific to financial savings, the mean savings for participants in the intervention arm increased from USD equivalent of $2.15 at baseline to $19.34 at 24 months, while the control arm participants' mean savings increased from $1.78 to $4.44 over the same time period. Overall, the findings indicate that in the short term, combination interventions with an economic empowerment component have the potential to bolster finance, mental health, HIV prevention, and ART-related health outcomes such as HIV viral suppression by improving ART adherence among vulnerable adolescents living in low-resource environments (Ssewamala et al., 2020).

Conclusion and Future Directions

The nexus between mental health, poverty, and HIV risk has been overlooked in studies focused exclusively on economic security, potentially explaining the mixed results of exclusively poverty-focused interventions, such as conditional cash transfers (Baird et al., 2012; De Walque et al., 2012; Pettifor et al., 2016). Indeed, as emphasized in the *Lancet* series on the science of HIV prevention, there is an important role for "combined" interventions to address multiple dimensions of preventive health (Hankins & de Zalduondo, 2010; Kurth et al., 2011). To date, HIV prevention, care, and support intervention efforts in SSA communities have primarily been "transported" from outside the region, mainly from the global north. Hence, it is critical to know how combination interventions aimed at vulnerable groups like children and adolescents affected by HIV/AIDS would fare in low-resource contexts as we begin to build and implement a policy agenda for this population. Therefore, it is critical to identify efficacious and potentially replicable intervention strategies developed and tested within the global south's existing institutions and infrastructure and proven to have longer term effects.

AIDS-affected children are prone to poor health and mental health and may be ill equipped to become productive adult members of society. Yet, there is inadequate longitudinal data to fully understand the developmental trajectories of AIDS-impacted adolescents in low-resource settings. Longitudinal research on children and adolescents impacted by HIV has mainly taken place in developed countries, representative of only ~15% of the world's population (Karimili et al., 2015; Ssewamala et al., 2010a). The little we know about their health and mental health in low-resource countries comes primarily from short-term research studies (Baird et al., 2012; Curley & Ssewamala, 2006; Fulton et al., 2011; Karimli et al., 2014, 2015; Kleintjes et al., 2010; Nabunya et al., 2014; Ssewamala et al., 2010a; Ssewamala & Sherraden, 2004). Although valuable, these studies provide only snapshots and do not offer a holistic view of the various factors that shape the trajectories of this vulnerable group. As we think about next steps in research, we should consider longitudinal research with rigorous methodology and repeated measures are needed to determine how early small investments impact vulnerable youth as they transition from adolescence to young adulthood and adulthood. Given the intersection of HIV/AIDS, mental health, and poverty, training young researchers working in countries heavily impacted by HIV/AIDS on the science of implementing combination interventions will enable the mental health and HIV prevention and intervention field to generate knowledge on culturally congruent multisectoral/interdisciplinary responses in the HIV care continuum. Building research capacity that is culturally and contextually responsive to the geopolitical context of SSA in addressing HIV prevention/intervention and co-occurring mental health problems in SSA countries heavily impacted by HIV/AIDS, especially in the HIV "hot spots" including urban centers, and poor CAMH services, is also an urgent priority.

References

Ajzen, I. (1991). The theory of planned behavior. *Organizational Behavior and Human Decision Processes, 50*(2), 179–211.

Atwine, B., Cantor-Graae, E., & Bajunirwe, F. (2005). Psychological distress among AIDS orphans in rural Uganda. *Social Science & Medicine, 61*(3), 555–564.

Au, J. T., Kayitenkore, K., Shutes, E., Karita, E., Peters, P. J., Tichacek, A., et al. (2006). Access to adequate nutrition is a major potential obstacle to antiretroviral adherence among HIV-infected individuals in Rwanda. *AIDS, 20*(16), 2116–2118.

Baird, S. J., Garfein, R. S., McIntosh, C. T., & Özler, B. (2012). Effect of a cash transfer programme for schooling on prevalence of HIV and herpes simplex type 2 in Malawi: A cluster randomised trial. *The Lancet, 379*(9823), 1320–1329.

Bajos, N., & Marquet, J. (2000). Research on HIV sexual risk: Social relations-based approach in a cross-cultural perspective. *Social Science & Medicine, 50*(11), 1533–1546.

Bandura, A. (1986). *Social foundations of thought and action: A social and cognitive theory.* Prentice-Hall.

Barhafumwa, B., Dietrich, J., Closson, K., Samji, H., Cescon, A., Nkala, B., & Gray, G. (2016). High prevalence of depression symptomology among adolescents in Soweto, South Africa associated with being female and cofactors relating to HIV transmission. *Vulnerable Children and Youth Studies, 3*(11), 1–11.

Bastard, B., Cardia-Voneche, L., Peto, D., & Van Campenhoudt, L. (1997). Relationships between sexual partners and ways of adapting to the risk of AIDS: Landmarks for a relationship-oriented conceptual framework. In L. Van Campenhoudt, M. Cohen, G. Guizzardi, & D. Hausser (Eds.), *Sexual interactions and HIV risk* (pp. 44–58). Taylor & Francis.

Becker, M. H., Haefner, D. P., Kasl, S. V., Kirscht, J. P., Mainman, L. A., & Rosenstock, I. A. (1977). Selected psychosocial models and correlates of individual health-related behaviors. *Medical Care, 15*(5 Suppl), 24–46.

Becker, M. H., & Mainman, L. A. (1975). Sociobehavioral determinants of compliance with health and medical care recommendations. *Medical Care, 13*(1), 10–24.

Biadgilign, S., Deribew, A., Amberbir, A., & Deribe, K. (2009). Barriers and facilitators to antiretroviral medication adherence among HIV-infected paediatric patients in Ethiopia: A qualitative study. *Sahara Journal, 4*, 148–154.

Bronfenbrenner, U. (1977). Toward an experimental ecology of human development. *American Psychologist, 37*(7), 513–531.

Bruckner, T. A., Scheffler, R. M., Shen, G., Yoon, J., Chisholm, D., Morris, J., & Saxena, S. (2011). The mental health workforce gap in low-and middle-income countries: A needs-based approach. *Bulletin of the World Health Organization, 89*(3), 184–194.

Case, A., Paxson, C., & Ableidinger, J. (2004). Orphans in Africa: Parental death, poverty, and school enrollment. *Demography, 41*(3), 483–508.

Cluver, L., & Gardner, F. (2006). The psychological well-being of children orphaned by AIDS in Cape Town, South Africa. *Annals of General Psychiatry, 5*(1), 8.

Cluver, L., & Gardner, F. (2007). The mental health of children orphaned by AIDS: A review of international and southern African research. *Journal of Child and Adolescent Mental Health, 19*(1), 1–17.

Cluver, L. D., Gardner, F., & Operario, D. (2008). Effects of stigma on the mental health of adolescents orphaned by AIDS. *Journal of Adolescent Health, 42*(4), 410–417.

Cluver, L. D., Orkin, M., Gardner, F., & Boyes, M. E. (2012). Persisting mental health problems among AIDS-orphaned children in South Africa. *Journal of Child Psychology and Psychiatry, 53*(4), 363–370.

Costello, E. J., Compton, S. N., Keeler, G., & Angold, A. (2003). Relationships between poverty and psychopathology: A natural experiment. *JAMA, 290*(15), 2023–2029.

Curley, J., Ssewamala, F., & Han, C.-K. (2010). Assets and educational outcomes: Child development accounts (CDAs) for orphaned children in Uganda. *Children and Youth Services Review, 32*(11), 1585–1590.

Curley, J., & Ssewamala, F. M. (2006). School attendance of orphaned children in sub-Saharan Africa: The role of family assets. *Social Development Issues, 28*(2), 84.

De Walque, D., Dow, W. H., Nathan, R., Abdul, R., Abilahi, F., Gong, E., & Rishnan, S. (2012). Incentivising safe sex: a randomized trial of conditional cash transfers for HIV and sexually transmitted infection prevention in rural Tanzania. *BMJ Open, 2*(1), e000747.

Duncan, G. J., & Brooks-Gunn, J. (2000). Family poverty, welfare reform, and child development. *Child Development, 71*(1), 188–196.

Faber, M., Witten, C., & Drimie, S. (2011). Community-based agricultural interventions in the context of food and nutrition security in South Africa. *South African Journal of Clinical Nutrition, 24*(1), 21–30.

Fergus, S. Z., & M., A. (2005). Adolescent resilience: A framework for understanding healthy development in the face of risk. *Annual Review of Public Health, 26*, 399–419.

Fishbein, M. (1967). *Readings in attitude theory and measurement.* Wiley.

Fisher, J. D., & Fisher, W. A. (1992). Changing AIDS risk behavior. *Psychological Bulletin, 111*(3), 455–474.

Foster, G. (2006). Children who live in communities affected by AIDS. *The Lancet, 367*(9511), 700–701.

Fulton, B. D., Scheffler, R. M., Sparkes, S. P., Auh, E. Y., Vujicic, M., & Soucat, A. (2011). Health workforce skill mix and task shifting in low income countries: A review of recent evidence. *Human Resources for Health, 9*(1), 1.

Garmezy, N. (1994). Reflections and commentary on risk, resilience and development. In H. Rea (Ed.), *Stress, risk and resilience in children and adolescents: Processes, mechanisms and interventions.* Cambridge University Press.

Gregson, S., Nyamukapa, C. A., Garnett, G. P., Wambe, M., Lewis, J. J. C., Mason, P. R., & Anderson, R. M. (2005). HIV infection and reproductive health in teenage women orphaned and made vulnerable by AIDS in Zimbabwe. *AIDS Care, 17*(7), 785–794.

Gusdal, A. K., Obua, C., Andualem, T., Wahlström, R., Tomson, G., Peterson, S., et al. (2009). Voices on adherence to ART in Ethiopia and Uganda: A matter of choice or simply not an option? *AIDS Care, 21*(11), 1381–1387.

Hall, H. I., Song, R., Rhodes, P., Prejean, J., An, Q., Lee, L. M., et al. (2008). Estimation of HIV incidence in the United States. *JAMA, 300*(5), 520–529.

Hamilton, C. M., Strader, L. C., Pratt, J. G., Maiese, D., Hendershot, T., Kwok, R. K., et al. (2011). The PhenX toolkit: Get the most from your measures. *American Journal of Epidemiology, 174*(3), 253–260.

Han, C.-K., Ssewamala, F. M., & Wang, J. S.-H. (2013). Family economic empowerment and mental health among AIDS-affected children living in AIDS-impacted communities: Evidence from a randomized evaluation in southwestern Uganda. *Journal of Epidemiology and Community Health, 67*(3), 225–230.

Hankins, C. A., & de Zalduondo, B. O. (2010). Combination prevention: A deeper understanding of effective HIV prevention. *AIDS, 24*, S70–S80.

Hardon, A. P., Akurut, D., Comoro, C., Ekezie, C., Irunde, H. F., Gerrits, T., et al. (2007). Hunger, waiting time and transport costs: Time to confront challenges to ART adherence in Africa. *AIDS Care, 19*(5), 658–665.

Jennings, L., Ssewamala, F. M., & Nabunya, P. (2016). Effect of savings-led economic empowerment on HIV preventive practices among orphaned adolescents in rural Uganda: Results from the Suubi-Maka randomized experiment. *AIDS Care, 28*(3), 273–282.

Kambon, K. (1992). *The African personality in America: An African-centered framework.* Nubian Nation Publications.

Karenga, M. (2003). *Maat, the moral ideal in ancient Egypt; A study in classical African ethics.* Routledge.

Karimili, L., Ssewamala, F. M., Neliands, T. B., & McKay, M. M. (2015). Matched savings accounts in low-resource communities: Who saves? *Global Social Welfare, 2*(2), 53–64.

Karimli, L., & Ssewamala, F. M. (2015). Do savings mediate changes in adolescents' future orientation and health-related outcomes? Findings from randomized experiment in Uganda. *Journal of Adolescent Health, 57*(4), 425–432.

Karimli, L., Ssewamala, F. M., & Neilands, T. B. (2014). Poor families striving to save in matched children's savings accounts: Findings from a randomized experimental design in Uganda. *The Social Service Review, 88*(4), 658–694.

Kleintjes, S., Lund, C., & Flisher, A. (2010). A situational analysis of child and adolescent mental health services in Ghana, Uganda, South Africa and Zambia. *African Journal of Psychiatry, 13*, 2.

Kurth, A. E., Celum, C., Baeten, J. M., Vermund, S. H., & Wasserheit, J. N. (2011). Combination HIV prevention: Significance, challenges, and opportunities. *Current HIV/AIDS Reports, 8*(1), 62–72.

Lipman, E., Offord, D., & Boyle, M. (1996). What if we could eliminate child poverty? *Social Psychiatry and Psychiatric Epidemiology, 31*(5), 303–307.

McLeod, J. D., & Shanahan, M. J. (1996). Trajectories of poverty and children's mental health. *Journal of Health and Social Behavior, 37*(3), 207–220.

McLoyd, V. C. (1998). Socioeconomic disadvantage and child development. *American Psychologist, 53*(2), 185–204.

Ministry of Health (MOH) Uganda and ORC Macro. (2006). *HIV/AIDS sero-behavioural survey 2004–05*. Ministry of Health and ORC Macro.

Montano, D. E., & Kasprzyk, D. (2002). The theory of reasoned action and the theory of planned behavior. In K. Glanz, B. K. Rimer, & F. M. Lewis (Eds.), *Health behavior and health education* (pp. 67–98). Josey-Bass.

Mukherjee, J. S., Ivers, L., Leandre, F., Farmer, P., & Behforouz, H. (2006). Antiretroviral therapy in resource-poor settings. Decreasing barriers to access and promoting adherence. *JAIDS, 43*(Suppl 1), S123–S126.

Nabunya, P., Ssewamala, F. M., & Ilic, V. (2014). Family economic strengthening and parenting stress among caregivers of AIDS-orphaned children: Results from a cluster randomized clinical trial in Uganda. *Children and Youth Services Review, 44*, 417–421.

National Institute on Drug Abuse (NIDA). (1993). *Risk behavior assessment* (3rd ed.). NIDA.

National Institutes of Health (NIH). (2015). *NIH HIV/AIDS Research Priorities and Guidelines for Determining AIDS Funding*. Retrieved from http://grants.nih.gov/grants/guide/notice-files/NOT-OD-15-137.html

Patel, V., Flisher, A. J., Hetrick, S., & McGorry, P. (2007). Mental health of young people: A global public-health challenge. *The Lancet, 369*(9569), 1302–1313.

Pettifor, A., MacPhail, C., Selin, A., Gómez-Olivé, F. X., Rosenberg, M., Wagner, R. G., & Piwowar-Manning, E. (2016). HPTN 068: A randomized control trial of a conditional cash transfer to reduce HIV Infection in young women in South Africa—Study design and baseline results. *AIDS and Behavior, 5*, 1–20.

Polisset, J., Ametonou, F., Arrive, E., Aho, A., & Perez, F. (2009). Correlates of adherence to antiretroviral therapy in HIV-infected children in Lomé, Togo, West Africa. *AIDS and Behavior, 13*(1), 23–32.

Pollitt, E. (1994). Poverty and child development: Relevance of research in developing countries to the United States. *Child Development, 65*(2), 283–295.

Ramadhani, H. O., Thielman, N. M., Landman, K. Z., Ndosi, E. M., Gao, F., Kirchherr, J. L., et al. (2007). Predictors of incomplete adherence, virologic failure, and antiviral drug resistance among HIV-infected adults receiving antiretroviral therapy in Tanzania. *Clinical Infectious Diseases, 45*(11), 1492–1498.

Rappaport, J. (1981). In praise of paradox: A social policy of empowerment over prevention. *American Journal of Community Psychology, 9*(1), 1–25.

Rosenstock, I. M. (1966). Why people use health services. *The Milbank Memorial Fund Quarterly, 44*(3), 94–127.

Rotheram-Borus, M. J., & Stein, J. A. (1999). Problem behavior of adolescents whose parents are living with AIDS. *American Journal of Orthopsychiatry, 69*(2), 228.

Rutherford, S. (2000). *The poor and their money*. Oxford University Press.

Sengendo, J., & Nambi, J. (1997). The psychological effect of orphanhood: A study of orphans in Rakai district. *Health Transition Review, 7*, 105–124.

Sherraden, M. (1990). Stakeholding: Notes on a theory of welfare based on assets. *Social Service Review, 64*(4), 580–601.

Sherraden, M. (1991). *Assets and the poor: A new American welfare policy*. ME Sharpe.

Ssewamala, F. M., Chang-Keun, H., & Neilands, T. (2009). Asset ownership and health and mental health functioning among AIDS-orphaned adolescents: Findings from a randomized clinical trial in rural Uganda. *Social Science and Medicine, 69*(2), 191–198.

Ssewamala, F. M., Chang-Keun, H., Neilands, T., Ismayilova, L., & Sperber, E. (2010a). The effect of economic assets on sexual risk taking intentions among orphaned adolescents in Uganda. *American Journal of Public Health, 100*(3), 483–489.

Ssewamala, F. M., & Curley, J. (2006). School attendance of orphaned children in sub-Saharan Africa: The role of family assets. *Social Development Issues: Alternative Approaches to Global Human Needs, 28*(2), 84–105.

Ssewamala, F. M., Dvalishvili, D., Mellins, C., Geng, E. H., Makumbi, F., Neilands, T., et al. (2020). The long-term effects of a family based economic empowerment intervention (Suubi +Adherence) on suppression of HIV viral loads among adolescents living with HIV in southern Uganda: Findings from 5-year cluster randomized trial. *PLoS One, 15*(2), e0228370.

Ssewamala, F. M., Ismayilova, L., McKay, M., Sperber, E., Bannon, W., Jr., & Alicea, S. (2010b). Gender and the effects of an economic empowerment program on attitudes toward sexual risk-taking among AIDS-orphaned adolescent youth in Uganda. *Journal of Adolescent Health, 46*(4), 372–378.

Ssewamala, F. M., Keun, H. C., Neilands, T. B., Ismayilova, L., & Sperber, E. (2010c). The effect of economic assets on sexual risk taking intentions among orphaned adolescents in Uganda. *American Journal of Public Health, 100*(3), 483.

Ssewamala, F. M., Neilands, T. B., Waldfogel, J., & Ismayilova, L. (2012). The impact of a comprehensive microfinance intervention on depression levels of AIDS-orphaned children in Uganda. *Journal of Adolescent Health, 50*(4), 346–352.

Ssewamala, F. M., & Sherraden, M. (2004). Integrating saving into microenterprise programs for the poor: Do institutions matter? *Social Service Review, 78*(3), 404–428.

Ssewamala, F. M., Sperber, E., Zimmerman, J. M., & Karimli, L. (2010d). The potential of asset-based development strategies for poverty alleviation in sub-Saharan Africa. *International Journal of Social Welfare, 19*(4), 433–443.

Tuller, D. M., Bangsberg, D. R., Senkungu, J., Ware, N. C., Emenyonu, N., & Weiser, S. D. (2010). Transportation costs impede sustained adherence and access to HAART in a clinic population in southwestern Uganda: A qualitative study. *AIDS and Behavior, 14*(4), 778–784.

Tumwesige, W., Namatovu, P., Sensoy Bahar, O., Byansi, W., McKay, M. M., & Ssewamala, F. M. (2021). Engaging community and governmental partners in improving health and mental health outcomes for children and adolescents impacted by HIV/AIDS in Uganda. *Pediatric Medicine, 4*, 2. https://doi.org/10.21037/pm-20-86

UNAIDS. (2010). *The global AIDS epidemic 2010*. Joint United Nations Programme on HIV/AIDS.

UNAIDS. (2013). *Global report: UNAIDS report on the global AIDS epidemic 2013*. Joint United Nations Programme on HIV/AIDS.

UNAIDS. (2014). *Gap report*. Joint United Nations Programme on HIV/AIDS.

UNAIDS. (2015). *HIV and AIDS Estimates; Uganda*. http://www.unaids.org/en/regionscountries/countries/uganda/

Weiser, S., Wolfe, W., Bangsberg, D., Thior, I., Gilbert, P., Makhema, J., et al. (2003). Barriers to antiretroviral adherence for patients living with HIV infection and AIDS in Botswana. *Journal of Acquired Immune Deficiency Syndromes, 34*(3), 281–288.

World Health Organization (WHO). (2005). *Atlas: Child and adolescent mental health resources: Global concerns, implications for the future*. World Health Organization.

World Health Organization (WHO). (2011a). *Mental atlas 2011*. Retrieved from http://apps.who.int/iris/bitstream/10665/44697/1/9799241564359_eng.pdf

World Health Organization (WHO). (2011b). *Mental Atlas 2011*: Ghana. Retrieved from http://www.who.int/mental_health/evidence/atlas/profiles/gha_mh_profile.pdf?ua=1

World Health Organization (WHO). (2011c). *Mental Atlas 2011: Uganda.* WHO Department of Mental Health and Substance Abuse. Retrieved from http://www.who.int/mental_health/evidence/atlas/profiles/uga_mh_profile.pdf?ua=1

World Health Organization (WHO). (2011d). *The treatment 2.0 framework for action: Catalysing the next phase of treatment, care and support.* World Health Organization.

World Health Organization (WHO). (2014). *Health for the world's adolescents: A second chance in the second decade.* http://apps.who.int/adolescent/second-decade/

Wyatt, G. E., Longshore, D., Chin, D., Carmona, J. V., Loeb, T. B., Myers, H. F., & Rivkin, I. (2004). The efficacy of an integrated risk reduction intervention for HIV-positive women with child sexual abuse histories. *AIDS and Behavior, 8*(4), 453–462.

Wyatt, G. E., Myers, H. F., Williams, J. K., Kitchen, C. R., Loeb, T., Carmona, J. V., & Presley, N. (2002). Does a history of trauma contribute to HIV risk for women of color? Implications for prevention and policy. *American Journal of Public Health, 92*(4), 660–665.

Zimet, G. D., Dahlem, N. W., Zimet, S. G., & Farley, G. K. (1988). The multidimensional scale of perceived social support. *Journal of Personality Assessment, 52*(1), 30–41.

Poverty and Children's Mental, Emotional, and Behavioral Health in Sub-Saharan Africa

Thabani Nyoni, Rabab Ahmed, and Daji Dvalishvili

Introduction

The mental, emotional, and behavioral disorders (MEBDs) in children in sub-Saharan Africa (SSA) can lead to significant impairment and disability, and high social and financial costs for the children, their family, and society as a whole (Baranne & Falissard, 2018; Charlson et al., 2014). Thus, it is important to understand the predisposing, precipitating, and perpetuating factors of MEBD in children in SSA. For the objective of this chapter, we address the complex effects of poverty in the development of many MEBDs in children and adolescents in SSA.

In high-income countries, the association between poverty and the mental, emotional, and behavioral health (MEBH) of children across their life span is well established (Roos et al., 2019; Chaudry & Wimer, 2016; Yoshikawa et al., 2012). Studies show that poverty and MEBH are inextricably linked and can be considered as bidirectional. While children growing up in poverty are subjected to different mental, emotional, and behavioral disorders (Yoshikawa et al., 2012; Walker et al., 2007; Pascoe et al., 2016), it is also true that mental illness can drag children and their family down into a nearly inescapable cycle of poverty (Yoshikawa et al., 2012; Pascoe et al., 2016). Yet little is known about children in sub-Saharan Africa (SSA) despite the high burden of both poverty and MEBD among children such as depression, anxiety, and somatoform disorders (Cortina et al., 2012; Gentz et al., 2018; Hadley & Patil, 2008).

Thabani Nyoni, Rabab Ahmed and Daji Dvalishvili contributed equally with all other contributors.

T. Nyoni (✉) · D. Dvalishvili
Brown School, Washington University in St. Louis, St. Louis, MO, USA
e-mail: tnyoni@wustl.edu

R. Ahmed
Ministry of Health and Population, Cairo, Egypt

© Springer Nature Switzerland AG 2022   19
F. M. Ssewamala et al. (eds.), *Child Behavioral Health in Sub-Saharan Africa*,
https://doi.org/10.1007/978-3-030-83707-5_2

To address the knowledge gap, the purpose of this chapter is to examine the association between several dimensions of poverty and measures of MEBD among children in studies conducted specifically in SSA taking into account the unique characteristics and experiences of poverty in the region. Based on the findings, this chapter provides some recommendations to guide future research, policy, and practice.

Addressing this identified knowledge gap is vital for two main reasons. First, it strengthens the case for the inclusion of children's mental health into the African development agenda and health interventions (Miranda & Patel, 2005; Sachs & Sachs, 2007). Second, it strengthens efforts that are directed towards promoting children's mental well-being, as well as protecting children from adverse effects of poverty on their MEBH (Das et al., 2007; Lund et al., 2011).

For purposes of this chapter, children are defined as any person under 18 years old using a definition of a child from the Convention on the Rights of the Child (United Nations, 1989). This chapter reviews peer-reviewed journal articles published from 2000 to 2020 in English that examine the relationship between different dimensions and measures of poverty and MEBD in children. In this chapter we define MEBD using both categorical and dimensional measures of mental and behavioral disorders of children defined by *Diagnostic and Statistical Manual of Mental Disorders* (DSM) and International Classification of Mental and Behavioral Disorders (ICD). In the review, we include positive dimensions of mental health such as psychological well-being and negative aspects such as psychiatric disorders (Slade 2010; Slade & Longden, 2015). Although the terms mental and behavioral ill health, mental and behavioral disorders, or psychiatric disorders are used interchangeably, this chapter uses mental, emotional, and behavioral disorders (Slade, 2010; Slade & Longden, 2015).

Understanding the Context of Poverty and MEBH in SSA

In defining poverty, scholars use several different dimensions of it. These dimensions include lack of resources needed to meet basic needs (Townsend, 1979, 1987), income level based on the poverty threshold (Toye & Downing, 2006), and indices of multiple deprivations such as low levels of education and lack of housing (Barnes et al., 2007; Toye & Infanti, 2004). However, this chapter defines poverty in terms of the global Multidimensional Poverty Index (MPI). The MPI developed using Sen's capability approach is an international measure of acute multidimensional poverty that has been used in over 100 developing countries, including those in SSA (Alkire & Housseini, 2014; Alkire et al., 2017). According to the recent MPI report, more than 1.3 billion people in 105 developing countries (77% of the global population) live in acute multidimensional poverty (UNDP, 2018). Around 50% of them are children under 18 years of age, and 43% of these children live in SSA (Alkire et al., 2017). SSA also has the highest rate of children (49%) living in extreme poverty (Gill et al., 2016).

Children experiencing poverty are a particular concern because they are dependent on their families and caregivers for basic needs (Roelen, 2017). The specific nature of children's needs, such as education, nutrition, and care, signifies that children's experiences of poverty may differ from the experiences of other household members (De Milliano & Plavgo, 2018). In SSA, household poverty is worsened by the burden of HIV/AIDS that adds more financial stresses (Andrews et al., 2005; Betancourt et al., 2012; Wood et al., 2006). The financial stresses of HIV/AIDS include increased medical expenses, lack of productivity, or income due to illness as well as the additional costs for feeding and clothing more orphaned and dependent children (Kidman & Heymann, 2016; Kidman & Thurman, 2014; Kuo & Operario, 2010). Families that deal with financial and HIV-related stressors also struggle with social and emotional issues that undermine positive parenting resulting in adverse mental health outcomes for both parents and children (Andrews et al., 2005; Wood et al., 2006; Cole & Tembo, 2011; Maes et al., 2010). Moreover, poverty undermines family support and functioning, which is associated with MEB disorders among children (Kidman & Heymann, 2016; Nöstlinger et al., 2006).

Although numbers and statistical data do not reflect the varied experiences and contexts of children, they do give some insight into the depth and breadth of the impact of poverty on the mental and behavioral well-being of children and their families. Studies reported that poverty plays a central role in shaping epidemiological profiles of their mental and behavioral disorders (Kidman & Heymann, 2016; Nöstlinger et al., 2006).

MEB Disorders Among Children and Adolescents in SSA

The coverage of prevalence data in mental and behavioral disorders for children and adolescents in SSA is low or nonexistent. No region in SSA has more than 2% coverage for any mental illness of this target population (Erskine et al., 2017). Specifically, the mean coverage ranges from 0% in central Africa to 0.1% in west Africa, 0.3% in east Africa, and 1.3% in southern Africa (Erskine et al., 2017). However, the global mean coverage across epidemiological studies for children and adolescents for mental and behavioral disorders is about 6.7% (Erskine et al., 2017). Furthermore, as Erskine et al. (2017) emphasized, no studies were reflecting the difference in prevalence of African child mental disorders related to the phenotype, genetics, environmental risk factors, and gene-environmental interactions of mental disorders. The lack of data results in uncertainty surrounding the prevalence and burden of mental disorders in children in SSA and reduces the visibility of mental disorders in comparison with communicable diseases, such as HIV/AIDS, and noncommunicable diseases, such as diabetes (Erskine et al., 2015; WHO, 2016).

The most recent systematic review of community-based studies in SSA estimated that MEB disorders in children are common, with a prevalence of about 2.7–27.0% (Cortina et al., 2012). These rates seem to be comparable with those extrapolated from similar studies in other low- and middle-income countries, which range from 12% to 29% (Kieling et al., 2011). According to Cortina and her colleagues, the most commonly identified mental, emotional, and behavioral disorders among children were depression; anxiety disorders; conduct, disruptive, and reactive behavior disorders; and post-traumatic stress disorder (Cortina et al., 2012). Yet, the prevalence varies widely from country to country in SSA. For example, the prevalence of depression ranged from 8.6% in Uganda and 10.7–21.1% in Malawi to 41% in South Africa (Stewart et al., 2014; Kinyanda et al., 2013; Das-Munshi et al., 2016).

The prevalence data also provides some clues about the context of children's mental health. The data show that demographic data and socioeconomic factors, including gender, ethnicity, and availability and accessibility of mental health services, may be associated with an increasing risk of mental disorders among children in SSA. Specifically, the emerging data highlighted that girls in SSA are more vulnerable to mental disorders compared to boys (Greene & Patton, 2020). Also, data indicates that there are some socioeconomic biases related to the racial categorization and cultural identity in SSA that determine the sets of social and economic opportunities such as housing, education, and health care for children and their families (Ilorah, 2009). Thus, it is not surprising that the proportion of children and adolescents who have access to and utilize mental health services is deficient (WHO, 2018). For example, in Sierra Leone, only 1.2% of children in need of mental health services receive it (Yoder et al., 2016). These biases result in a complex array of negative emotional responses that may be linked to high rates of mental illness such as depression and anxiety among children and adolescents (Franke, 2014).

The Burden of MEB Disorders Among Children in SSA

Evidence on the burden of child and adolescent MEB disorders in developing countries, including SSA, remains limited (Patel et al., 2008). However, the data extrapolated from developed countries shows that depression is the most common psychiatric condition among children and adolescents and a leading cause of disability, as it accounts for 40.5% of disability-adjusted life years (DALYs). Ranking below depression is anxiety disorders (14.6%), pervasive developmental disorders (4.2%), childhood behavioral disorders (3.4%), and eating disorders (1.2%) (Whiteford et al., 2013). However, the burden of mental and behavioral disorders among children in SSA appears marginal compared to the challenge of communicable diseases, such as lower respiratory tract infection, malaria, and HIV/AIDS, and intentional and non-intentional injuries (WHO, 2016). Even though MEBDs among 5- to 14-year-old children have an important impact on the years lived with disability (YLDs), MEBDs were not in the top 20 causes of losses of DALYs in 2000–2015 in SSA (Baranne & Falissard, 2018). It is also worth mentioning that SSA policymakers prioritize reporting YLDs as the allocation of healthcare resources is based on YLDs (Baranne & Falissard, 2018).

The extraordinary burden of managing cases with infectious diseases in SSA interferes with calculating the associated cost with handling cases with mental illness (Erskine et al., 2015; WHO, 2016) making it difficult to estimate the real costs associated with mental illness among children. Yet, a review estimated that mental illness-imposed high direct cost includes mental care costs (Kessler, 2012; Trautmann et al., 2016), and high indirect costs include deterioration of children's family-, social-, and school-related environments (Jack et al., 2014).

Children's Mental Health Care in SSA

The progress in mental health care in most African countries is affected by lack of political will and absence of an overall strategy that regulates resource prioritization and capacity (Alem et al., 2008; WHO, 2018). Only half of SSA countries have policies or plans to improve mental well-being (WHO, 2018). Moreover, almost all SSA countries face shortages of trained mental health professionals and virtually no social service (Alem et al., 2008). In terms of hospital-based services, a median of 0.34 bed is available per 10,000 population, and only a small number is designated for child mental health (WHO, 2018).

The Mental Health Atlas also reports that African countries allocate less than 1% of their total health budget to mental health services. A shortage of trained psychiatrists critically compounds the mental health problem (WHO, 2018). One psychiatrist per country is available to provide psychiatric services across all ages in populations of 9.0, 4.2, and 3.5 million in Chad, Eritrea, and Liberia, respectively (WHO, 2018). Furthermore, half of SSA countries provide any community-based mental health services across all age groups (WHO, 2018; Alem et al., 2008).

Even though the previously listed indicators for mental health services vary between countries in SSA, the relatively low numbers of available services indicate an elevated risk of clinical deterioration among children with mental health problems.

Conceptualizing the Link Between Poverty and Mental Health Among Children

This chapter employs two conceptual frameworks, one by Walker et al. (2007) and another by Yoshikawa et al. (2012), to understand different mechanisms through which poverty impacts children's mental health in low-resource settings. This section describes the main features, strengths, and limitations of these two conceptual frameworks.

In developing countries, including SSA, there are three pathways through which poverty is linked to the MEBH of children under age 5 (Walker et al., 2007). Walker et al. (2007) framework describes (a) biological risk factors such as malnutrition, nutrient deficiencies, and exposure to environmental toxins; (b) psychosocial risks such as parenting including maternal depression and exposure to violence; and

(c) sociocultural risk factors such as gender inequality, mothers' education, and lack of access to services.

Although Walker and colleagues' theoretical framework provides a comprehensive understanding of the different pathways between poverty and children's mental health in SSA, it has several limitations. First, this framework is designed for children below the age of 5. As a result, it may not adequately capture how poverty is linked to the MEBH of older children. Nor does this framework capture how different dimensions of poverty are directly linked to children's MEBH (Alkire & Housseini, 2014; Alkire et al., 2017).

Yoshikawa et al. (2012) addressed gaps identified in Walker's conceptual model and proposed a conceptual framework with both direct and mediated effects of poverty on children's MEBH. Their conceptual model proposes several mechanisms through which the multilevel and types of poverty are linked to the mental health of children in adolescence. Yoshikawa, Aber, and Beardslee's conceptual framework argues that in developed countries poverty has both direct and mediated effects on children's MEBH through (a) parent- and family-level factors (i.e., parent education and marital status); (b) low family income and other dimensions of poverty (i.e., asset poverty, social exclusion); (c) individual, relational, and institutional mechanisms as mediators (i.e., child stress, parenting behaviors, and neighborhood resources); and (d) various child outcomes (i.e., physical health and academic/cognitive outcomes). This conceptual framework provides a more comprehensive conceptualization of the various dimensions of poverty and how they uniquely and collectively (via several pathways) contribute to children and adolescent's MEBH (Yoshikawa et al., 2012). However, Yoshikawa and colleagues' theoretical framework is designed for children living in developed countries and may not adequately capture how poverty is linked to the MEBH of children in developing countries.

To explore the nature of the possible associations between poverty and children's MEBH in SSA, we organized empirical evidence based on how poverty was measured in the context of SSA. Studies conducted in SSA operationalized poverty as food insecurity, housing condition, SES, household assets, parents'/caregivers' employment status/family disadvantage, number of people living together/overcrowding, and exposure to poverty or economic intervention. On the other hand, MEB disorders commonly linked to dimensions of poverty include anxiety, depression, behavioral and post-traumatic stress disorders, internalizing problems, and delinquency. The next sections will discuss in detail how poverty using different measures are linked to children and adolescents' MEBH in SSA as well as the pathways.

Poverty and Children's MEBH in SSA: Empirical Evidence and Possible Pathways

Food Insecurity

Several correlational studies conducted across many different countries in SSA found a significant association between food insecurity and children's MEB disorders. Specifically, around 10% and 15.7% of infants and babies in SSA are born with low birth weight and are malnourished due to a mother's malnutrition (He et al., 2018). Those babies cannot maintain adequate developmental and bodily performance to start life at mentally optimal levels (Bain et al., 2013; He et al., 2018). A review of the relationship between malnutrition and neurodevelopmental disability reported that children (below the age of 5 years) in SSA who suffered from different forms of malnutrition, including stunted growth and wasting, were more prone to cognitive, behavioral, and developmental deficits (Kerac et al., 2014). In Ethiopia, South Africa, and Zanzibari, studies reported that children, aged between 5 months and 12 years, who suffered from micronutrient deficiencies related to food insecurity also exhibited poor psychosocial and cognitive performance (Mabasa et al., 2019; Muktar et al., 2018; Olney et al., 2007).

In studies conducted across SSA among older children, evidence consistently suggests that household-level food insecurity is a risk factor for mental disorders among children and adolescents (Gupte et al., 2014). Studies conducted in Ethiopia, Zimbabwe, Namibia, Tanzania, and Uganda reported that household-level food insecurity was correlated with mental and behavioral illness among older children and adolescents such as somatic disorders as well as internalizing and externalizing behavioral disorders (Jebena et al., 2016; Rochat et al., 2018; Gentz et al., 2018; Huang et al., 2017; Makame et al., 2002).

In Ethiopia and Zimbabwe findings show that food insecurity was associated with MEB disorders among children and adolescents (Jebena et al., 2016; Rochat et al., 2018). In Namibia, Tanzania, and Uganda findings show that food insecurity was correlated with somatic disorders as well as internalizing and externalizing behavioral problems among children and adolescents (Rochat et al., 2018; Gentz et al., 2018; Huang et al., 2017; Makame et al. 2002). In South Africa, food insecurity was a risk factor for post-traumatic disorder among adolescents in general (Closson et al., 2016), and a risk factor for depression, anxiety, and post-traumatic stress among AIDS-orphaned adolescents (Cluver & Orkin, 2009). Conversely, among orphans in general, food security was a protective factor for improved emotional and behavioral well-being of orphans (Pappin et al., 2015).

While several studies conducted in SSA link food insecurity to mental disorders, scant evidence exists that explains pathways through which food insecurity negatively impacts children's MEBH. Although a longitudinal study conducted in Ethiopia found that food insecurity was linked to common mental disorders via physical health, most (91%) of the effects were direct (Jebena et al., 2016). In Uganda, food insecurity was linked to children's MEB disorders through parental depression and inadequate parenting practices (Huang et al., 2017). A qualitative study from Malawi suggested that food-insecure adolescents would have anxiety and symptoms of depression because adolescents worry about food nonavailability (Rock et al., 2016).

Housing (Inadequate Conditions and Overcrowding)

Evidence from SSA suggests that housing (availability, quality, and conditions) is a significant predictor of children's MEBH. For instance, in Uganda and South Africa, inadequate housing (i.e., overcrowding) was associated with depression, low self-esteem, and suicidal thoughts, internalizing and externalizing behavioral disorders among children (Kinyanda et al., 2011; Kinyanda et al., 2013; Marais et al., 2013; Rochat et al., 2018). Also, adverse mental and behavioral health outcomes among children were associated with poor-quality housing, scarcity of neighborhood resources, and neighborhood violence (Marais et al., 2013; Rochat et al., 2018). In South Africa, living in neighborhoods with concentrated poverty that isolate children from the resources increased the likelihood of emotional and behavioral distress, affective disorders, and exposure to potentially traumatic experiences (Bireda & Pillay, 2017; Closson et al., 2016; Langhaug et al., 2010). Children exposed to neighborhood and community violence reported aggression, depression, hyperactivity and attention problems, and post-traumatic stress disorder (Barbarin et al., 2001; Foster & Brooks-Gunn, 2015; Liddell et al., 1994; Magwaza et al., 1993; Ventevogel, 2015).

However, one study conducted in Zimbabwe among orphaned children experiencing multiple changes in residence and living in poorer households did not exhibit higher psychological distress compared to non-orphans (Nyamukapa et al., 2010). This finding suggests that the unstable living arrangements of orphans may not have been perceived by orphans to be as bad as non-orphans. Another possible explanation could be that orphaned children may have developed resiliency and adapted to their living conditions over time (Wright et al., 2013).

Socioeconomic Status (SES)

In SSA, evidence suggests that SES has directly or indirectly affected several types of children's MEB disorders. A study conducted in Uganda found that low SES was directly associated with an increased risk of severe mental disorders (Kinyanda et al., 2011). Other studies conducted in Nigeria, Rwanda, and South Africa found a direct link between low SES, family disruption, and inadequate parenting and social support with higher rates of depression, suicidal ideation, and suicidal attempts (Adewuya & Ologun, 2006; Ng et al., 2015). Evidence from Ethiopia, Rwanda, South Africa, and Uganda suggests that living in disadvantaged communities and low-income households was indirectly linked to children's mental health through parental mental health. Living in disadvantaged communities and low-income households resulted in parental psychological distress, anxiety, poor child-caregiver relationship, harsh and inconsistent discipline, and inconsistent parenting practices which in turn was associated with mental and behavioral health challenges among children (Bhargava, 2005; Huang et al., 2017; Ng et al., 2015; Richter et al., 2000). A combination of low SES and lack of caregiver emotional support for children and adolescent mental health predicted mental health problems among orphans in Ethiopia (Bhargava, 2005).

However, the study conducted in Uganda by Mpango et al. (2017) found that an increase in parental SES was significantly related to an increased risk of attention-deficit/hyperactivity disorder (ADHD) among children. This finding is inconsistent with results from prior studies, which show that lower SES was associated with mental and behavioral disorders. Previous studies conducted in the developed countries reported a correlation between financial difficulty or socioeconomic disadvantage and ADHD (Hjern et al., 2010; Russell, Ford & Russell, 2015). In explaining this inconsistency, Mpango and his colleagues suggested that families with higher SES are usually more sensitive to the child's behavior and academic success, and thus, they might ask more frequently for ADHD testing for their children. In a nutshell, an increase or decrease in the parent's SES status coupled with problematic parenting practices was a risk factor for MEB disorders.

In addition, studies found an association between low SES and poor mental and behavioral well-being of children in SSA related to poverty-related infectious diseases such as HIV/AIDS and malaria (Boutayeb, 2010), as the studies showed children living with HIV/AIDS are at a high risk of mental and behavioral illness due to the malignant course of the disease and the associated stigma (Parcesepe et al., 2018; Gamarel et al., 2017; Betancourt et al., 2014). Specifically, children with HIV/AIDS in SSA demonstrated higher levels of depression (Kamau et al., 2012; Kim et al., 2014; Binagwaho et al., 2016), anxiety (Kamau et al., 2012), and conduct disorders (Salisbury et al., 2020). Also, similar neurological and behavioral deficits were reported among children infected with malaria in SSA (Nankabirwa et al., 2014; Boivin, 2002; Carter et al., 2005, 2006).

Beyond the infections, poverty is linked to children's chronic toxic exposure to lead, arsenic, and pesticide in different areas in SSA (Ahoulé et al., 2015; WHO, 2015; Silberberg, 2006). However, it is still not possible to cover the association between toxin exposure and children's MEBH as most studies carried out on environmental toxins in SSA are dedicated to the quantification and characterization of the toxins and did not assess the MEH environmental toxin-associated risk (Silberberg, 2006).

Household Assets and Resources

Evidence from empirical studies in SSA suggests that the amount of material goods or resources a family has access to could predict children's and adolescent's MEBH.

In Malawi, South Africa, and Zimbabwe, children and adolescents from households with low amounts of assets, who live in vulnerable urban settings, and who face economic hardships had high levels of exposure to traumatic experiences (Closson et al., 2016; Langhaug et al., 2010; Nyamukapa et al., 2010; Rock et al., 2016). The same studies also linked a lack of household assets and resources with higher rates of affective disorders, depression, anxiety, and external behavioral disorders. In Zimbabwe, an association was found between higher levels of daily stressors due to lack of basic needs among orphans and levels of hopelessness, feelings of social isolation, guilty feelings, irritability, depressive symptoms, and emotional distress (Gilborn et al., 2006). In Rwanda, orphans who live in low-resource households reported high levels of depression and social isolation (Boris et al., 2008). Another study conducted in Rwanda showed that impoverished conditions resulted in the marginalization of orphans and affected their mental and behavioral health (Thurman et al., 2008).

Rock et al. (2016) explained that the burden of responsibility to provide basic household needs and the shame associated with the lack of necessities like soap and clothing often led to anxiety and depression among children and adolescents in Malawi. Bireda and Pillay (2017) conducted a qualitative study among South African adolescents orphaned by HIV/AIDS. They found that living in material and relational poverty increased children's and adolescents' sense of emotional distress. Two other studies conducted in South Africa explained that material deprivation might diminish children's sense of drive, and make them less defiant and show less impulsively driven behavior (Barbarin et al., 2001; Marais et al., 2013). A study conducted in Malawi indicated that household hardships could, in some instances, foster the development of social ties that mitigate the effect of stressors (Das et al., 2007; Rock et al., 2016).

In conclusion, the evidence from SSA showed that living in families with limited access to resources was not necessarily correlated with worse MEBH outcomes among children and adolescents (Barbarin et al., 2001; Marais et al., 2013; Pappin et al., 2015). To explain the lack of association, researchers argue that some coping skills and resilience mechanisms, including social networks, helped children and adolescents to mitigate the vulnerability and stressors associated with unemployment or economic hardships (Das et al., 2007; Rock et al., 2016).

Parents/Caregivers' Employment Status and Family Disadvantage

In SSA, parents' employment status and family disadvantage are significant predictors of MEB disorders. One study found that low-quality jobs, low wages, few benefits, high injury rates, and little opportunity for advancement predict family disadvantage, which is a risk factor for children's MEBH (Perry-Jenkins et al., 2000). More specifically, the measure of family disadvantage was a risk factor for children's exposure to numerous types of traumatic events in South Africa (Closson et al., 2016). In Uganda and Zimbabwe, studies found that children living in low-income households with unemployed parents reported experiencing intense feelings of despair, hopelessness, suicidal thoughts, and internalizing and external-izing behavioral symptoms (Closson et al., 2016; Huang et al., 2017; Nyamukapa et al., 2010).

Studies have established two pathways or mechanisms by which parents' employment status and family disadvantage predict MEBH. Firstly, loss of the sole breadwinner limits families' economic resources and hence their ability to purchase resources including educational supplies, food, and housing; access high-quality education; and provide safe environments necessary for a child's development (Nyamukapa et al., 2010). Secondly, the family disadvantage and, by extension, economic hardship increase psychological distress among parents, which negatively impacts the parenting practices/beliefs, resulting in poor child mental and behavioral health (Huang et al., 2017; Meinck et al., 2017).

Economic Empowerment and Poverty Alleviation Interventions

Several economic empowerments and poverty alleviation interventions have been implemented and evaluated to reduce the burden of family poverty and mitigate its impact on children and adolescents' MEBH in SSA. In Burkina Faso, an integrated psychosocial intervention addressing both material and relational poverty was conducted by Ismayilova and colleagues in 2018. This intervention found that combining parental financial assets, such as savings, with the psychosocial inter-vention was associated with better social, emotional, and behavioral outcomes. Similarly, that was implemented in Uganda targeting adolescents orphaned due to AIDS resulted in improved levels of self-esteem and reduced levels of depression (Ssewamala et al., 2009, 2012). This intervention combined several components, including (1) workshops on asset and future planning, (2) peer mentorship on life options, and (3) savings accounts for secondary schooling or family businesses. As a result, the authors were unable to firmly determine which component of the inter-vention was associated with better outcomes. The other economic empowerment intervention conducted in Uganda found positive effects of the intervention on mental health: one was a comprehensive microfinance intervention, which resulted in a significant decrease in depression among adolescents in the treatment group (Ssewamala et al., 2012). This study evaluated an integrated matched savings account intervention that included financial management workshops and family-level income-generating projects to enhance economic stability and reduce poverty and adult mentorship to children. The authors found that children receiving microfinance intervention reported a significant reduction in hopelessness and depression (Ssewamala et al., 2009).

Cash transfer programs have been effective in poverty alleviation including conditional and unconditional cash transfers (Daidone et al., 2019). Conditional cash transfer programs provide money to households on the condition that they comply with specific pre-defined requirements of the program (Handa et al., 2018). Unconditional cash transfers are cash transfer programs that provide cash grants to low-income households without any strings attached (Handa et al., 2018). A conditional cash transfer program implemented in Malawi resulted in a substantially beneficial impact on school-age girls' mental health during the 2-year intervention (Baird et al., 2013). Similarly, in Kenya, unconditional monthly cash transfers of US $20 significantly reduced the odds of depressive symptoms by 24% among orphaned and vulnerable male adolescents, but not for female adolescents (Kilburn et al., 2016).

Although there is strong evidence of the beneficial effects of cash transfers, a review study by Samuels and Stavropoulou (2016) found that cash transfers, whether conditional or unconditional, may trigger or worsen preexisting intra-household distress and community tensions. Baird et al. (2013) also found that the beneficial effects of cash transfers were limited to the intervention period and quickly disappeared after the intervention ended in Malawi.

As the evidence indicates, social protection programs such as social grants could provide a psychological safety net and reduce the odds of common mental disorders (Plagerson et al., 2011). However, Plagerson et al. (2011) emphasized that the negative stereotyping about who receives financial grants leads to social stigma and discrimination from others and could detract from the positive mental health outcomes of the intervention. In South Africa, the Child Support Grant (CSG), a positive impact on the psychosocial needs of adolescents, was partial. The partial effect was due to nonmaterial factors that affect adolescents, such as shame related to poverty and the "social cost" of school, where a premium must often be paid for fashionable clothes or accessories. Additionally, Clossan and his colleagues (2016) found that children whose families received a household social grant in South Africa had higher traumatic experience scores, and the receipt of assistance was not associated with reduced psychological distress in Zimbabwe (Nyamukapa et al., 2010).

Conclusion

Evidence from this chapter suggests that although a wide range of poverty dimensions are used in literature, the most common dimensions include food insecurity, inadequate housing, low socioeconomic status, household assets (and material resources), parents'/caregivers' employment status, and family disadvantage. The most common mental and behavioral disorders discussed were internalizing and externalizing disorders. Although these disorders were measured using several different psychometric tools, evidence shows a relatively consistent trend in which a range of poverty dimensions are risk factors to a variety of mental disorders among children and adolescents in SSA.

The identified studies showed that children living in poverty are at higher risk of developing MEB disorders in general. The individual, family, neighborhoods, and environmental factors might shape the process and outcomes in children. Evidence suggests that poverty is also indirectly linked to children's MEB disorders through social exclusion, high stressors, reduced social capital, and increased risk of violence and trauma, all of which increase the risk for a higher prevalence of MEBH. Specifically, as the review shows, the risks for MEBD increase dramatically if children are exposed to harsh parenting practices, parental stress, social isolation, stressful family living, low material resources and assets, and stigmatization. Still, it is difficult to draw definite conclusions regarding the causality and direction of the poverty-MEB disorder relationship as the vast majority of studies are cross-sectional.

Nevertheless, few studies conducted in SSA show that economic empowerment and poverty alleviation interventions, including cash transfers, savings accounts, and social protection grants, effectively reduce material and relational poverty as well as MEB disorders. The use of integrated approaches to poverty alleviation intervention suggests a recognition of the multidimensional nature of poverty as well as the vulnerability and the role of psychosocial dimensions in achieving well-being (Samuels & Stavropoulou, 2016). However, when cash transfers are provided as part of social protection programs, there is a tendency to overlook their impact of mental well-being. This chapter and another review by Samuels and Stavropoulou (2016) note that since cash transfers can improve psychosocial well-being at the individual level and in relationships, psychosocial dimensions need to be considered in the design, implementation, and evaluation of cash transfer programs.

Furthermore, poverty alleviation interventions must track both positive and unintended adverse social and health effects. For example, there is a need to qualitatively evaluate ways in which the cash transfers may trigger or worsen preexisting intra-household and community tensions. Also, qualitative research is needed to understand ways through which the interactions with staff members hurt beneficiaries' dignity and self-respect—two crucial issues that may increase beneficiaries' distress. Cash transfer programs should consider linking beneficiaries with complementary services that can target specific vulnerabilities of beneficiary subpopulations.

Despite some strength of our findings, there are several limitations to this review that should be mentioned. First, the review was based on peer-reviewed journal articles; grey literature was not included. Second, studies in this review are taken from mostly English-speaking SSA countries, and there are limits to which these findings can be generalized to the whole region. Third, although we examined the link between different poverty dimensions and MEB disorders, we were not able to explore variation between outcomes such as those between depression and anxiety. Fourth, several of the reviewed studies had multiple and diffuse associations and aggregate variables that tend to yield higher associations than more specific variables. Therefore, we, the reviewers, acknowledge the fact that, in some instances, the strength of the associations may have been overstated or understated. Fifth, due to the nature of our studies, this review was not able to explore the impact of macroeconomic factors on the relationship between poverty and MEB disorders in these countries. Sixth, except for a few RCTs or interventions, a vast majority of studies were cross-sectional. Finally, to date in SSA, there have been few studies that cover the impact of poverty on MEBH of preschool age (0–3 years) or neurodevelopmental disorders such as autism spectrum disorder (Kariuki et al., 2016; Erskine et al., 2017).

Future Research

We identified several significant gaps in the literature for future research. First, future studies need to explore disaggregated patterns of comorbidity between different children's MEB disorders. Also, a more detailed exploration of the interrelationships between biological, personal, social, and economic factors that impact children and adolescent mental health in poor communities of SSA is needed. This approach should include the adoption of multiple dimensional measures of poverty, where different measures or indicators of poverty are sequentially added to regression models to assess how much each strengthens or weakens the association.

Second, there is a need to understand complex local realities qualitatively and lived experiences that yield essential differences within and between different SSA country contexts to support theory development. Lastly, more interventions that aim to address both poverty and mental ill health need to be developed and evaluated, especially those that focus on reducing the impact of the poverty-related risk factors that increase the prevalence or severity of MEB disorders among children and adolescents.

Implications for Research and Practice

This chapter attempted to address the question of whether poverty is associated with MEB disorders in SSA. For policymakers, the relatively consistent association between MEB disorders in SSA strengthens the case for the inclusion of children's mental health on the agenda of humanitarian and development agencies. Also, given the multidimensional nature of poverty, interventions that seek to address the burden of MEB disorders in SSA may need to target several indicators of poverty by combining multiple components. More specifically, the findings of this review call for increasing precision in the design, implementation, and evaluation of interventions. For example, strategies for addressing poverty should include psychosocial dimensions in the design, delivery, and evaluation. Also, qualitative evaluation of participants' experiences in these interventions should be included in intervention assessments to capture the unintended consequences of the interventions.

References

Adewuya, A. O., & Ologun, Y. A. (2006). Factors associated with depressive symptoms in Nigerian adolescents. *Journal of Adolescent Health, 39*(1), 105–110.

Ahoulé, D. G., Lalanne, F., Mendret, J., Brosillon, S., & Maïga, A. H. (2015). Arsenic in African waters: A review. *Water, Air, and Soil Pollution, 226*, 302. https://doi.org/10.1007/s11270-015-2558-4

Alem, A., Jacobsson, L., & Hanlon, C. (2008). Community-based mental health care in Africa: Mental health workers' views. *World Psychiatry: Official journal of the World Psychiatric Association (WPA), 7*(1), 54–57. https://doi.org/10.1002/j.2051-5545.2008.tb00153.x

Alkire, S., & Housseini, B. (2014). *Multidimensional poverty in sub-Saharan Africa: Levels and trends (OPHI Working Papers 81)*. Oxford University Press.

Alkire, S., Jindra, C., Robles Aguilar, G., & Vaz, A. (2017). Multidimensional poverty reduction among countries in sub-Saharan Africa. *Forum for Social Economics, 46*(2), 178–191. https://doi.org/10.1080/07360932.2017.1310123

Andrews, G., Skinner, D., & Zuma, K. (2005). Epidemiology of health and vulnerability among children orphaned and made vulnerable by HIV/AIDS in sub-Saharan Africa. Paper presented at the OVC roundtable at the 7th AIDS impact conference, Cape Town, April 2005. *AIDS Care, 18*, 269–276. https://doi.org/10.1080/09540120500471861

Bain, L. E., Awah, P. K., Geraldine, N., Kindong, N. P., Sigal, Y., Bernard, N., & Tanjeko, A. T. (2013). Malnutrition in sub-Saharan Africa: Burden, causes and prospects. *The Pan African Medical Journal, 15*, 120. https://doi.org/10.11604/pamj.2013.15.120.2535

Baird, S., De Hoop, J., & Özler, B. (2013). Income shocks and adolescent mental health. *Journal of Human Resources, 48*(2), 370–403.

Baranne, M. L., & Falissard, B. (2018). Global burden of mental disorders among children aged 5-14 years. *Child and Adolescent Psychiatry and Mental Health, 12*, 19. https://doi.org/10.1186/s13034-018-0225-4

Barbarin, O. A., Richter, L., & DeWet, T. (2001). Exposure to violence, coping resources, and psychological adjustment of South African children. *American Journal of Orthopsychiatry, 71*(1), 16–25.

Barnes, H., Wright, G., Noble, M., & Dawes, A. (2007). *The South African index of multiple deprivations for children: Census 2001*. The Human Sciences Research Council.

Betancourt, T., Scorza, P., Kanyanganzi, F., Fawzi, M. C. S., Sezibera, V., Cyamatare, F., . . . Kayiteshonga, Y. (2014). HIV and child mental health: A case-control study in Rwanda. *Pediatrics, 134*(2), e464–e472.

Betancourt, T. S., Meyers-Ohki, S. E., Stulac, S., Barrera, A. E., Mushashi, C., & Beardslee, W. R. (2012). Global mental health programs for children and families facing adversity: Development of a family strengthening intervention in Rwanda. In J. N. Corbin (Ed.), *Children and families affected by armed conflicts in Africa: Implications and strategies for helping professionals in the United States* (pp. 113–142). National Association of Social Workers Press.

Bhargava, A. (2005). AIDS epidemic and the psychological well-being and school participation of Ethiopian orphans. *Psychology, Health & Medicine, 10*(3), 263–275.

Binagwaho, A., Fawzi, M., Agbonyitor, M., Nsanzimana, S., Karema, C., Remera, E., Mutabazi, V., Shyirambere, C., Cyamatare, P., Nutt, C., Wagner, C., Condo, J., Misago, N., & Kayiteshonga, Y. (2016). Validating the children's depression inventory in the context of Rwanda. *BMC Pediatrics, 16*, 29. https://doi.org/10.1186/s12887-016-0565-2

Bireda, A. D., & Pillay, J. (2017). Daily life with early orphanhood from HIV/AIDS: An exploratory study. *Journal of Psychology in Africa, 27*(6), 557–560.

Boivin, M. J. (2002). Effects of early cerebral malaria on cognitive ability in Senegalese children. *Journal of Developmental & Behavioral Pediatrics, 23*(5), 353–364.

Boris, N. W., Brown, L. A., Thurman, T. R., Rice, J. C., Snider, L. M., Ntaganira, J., & Nyirazinyoye, L. N. (2008). Depressive symptoms in youth heads of household in Rwanda:

Correlates and implications for intervention. *Archives of Pediatrics & Adolescent Medicine, 162* (9), 836–843.

Boutayeb, A. (2010). The impact of infectious diseases on the development of Africa. In V. R. Preedy & R. R. Watson (Eds.), *Handbook of Disease Burdens and Quality of Life Measures.* Springer.

Carter, J. A., Lees, J. A., Gona, J. K., Murira, G., Rimba, K., Neville, B. G., & Newton, C. R. (2006). Severe falciparum malaria and acquired childhood language disorder. *Developmental Medicine and Child Neurology, 48*(1), 51–57.

Carter, J. A., Mung'ala-Odera, V., Neville, B. G., Murira, G., Mturi, N., Musumba, C., & Newton, C. R. (2005). Persistent neurocognitive impairments associated with severe falciparum malaria in Kenyan children. *Journal of Neurology, Neurosurgery, and Psychiatry, 76*(4), 476–481. https://doi.org/10.1136/jnnp.2004.043893

Charlson, F. J., Diminic, S., Lund, C., Degenhardt, L., & Whiteford, H. A. (2014). Mental and substance use disorders in sub-Saharan Africa: Predictions of epidemiological changes and mental health workforce requirements for the next 40 years. *PLoS One, 9*(10), e110208.

Chaudry, A., & Wimer, C. (2016). Poverty is not just an indicator: The relationship between income, poverty, and child well-being. *Academic Pediatrics, 16*(3 Suppl), S23–S29. https://doi.org/10.1016/j.acap.2015.12.010

Closson, K., Dietrich, J. J., Nkala, B., Musuku, A., Cui, Z., Chia, J., ... Kaida, A. (2016). Prevalence, type, and correlates of trauma exposure among adolescent men and women in Soweto, South Africa: Implications for HIV prevention. *BMC Public Health, 16*(1), 1191.

Cluver, L., & Orkin, M. (2009). Cumulative risk and AIDS-orphanhood: Interactions of stigma, bullying, and poverty on child mental health in South Africa. *Social Science & Medicine, 69*(8), 1186–1193.

Cole, S. M., & Tembo, G. (2011). The effect of food insecurity on mental health: Panel evidence from rural Zambia. *Social Science & Medicine, 73*(7), 1071–1079. https://doi.org/10.1016/j.socscimed.2011.07.012

Cortina, M. A., Sodha, A., Fazel, M., & Ramchandani, P. G. (2012). Prevalence of child mental health problems in sub-Saharan Africa: A systematic review. *Archives of Pediatrics & Adolescent Medicine, 166*(3), 276. https://doi.org/10.1001/archpediatrics.2011.592

Daidone, S., Davis, B., Handa, S., & Winters, P. (2019). The household and individual-level productive impacts of cash transfer programs in sub-Saharan Africa. *American Journal of Agricultural Economics, 101*(5), 1401–1431.

Das, J., Do, Q., Friedman, J., McKenzie, D., & Scott, K. (2007). Mental health and poverty in developing countries: Revisiting the relationship. *Social Science & Medicine, 65*(3), 467–480. https://doi.org/10.1016/j.socscimed.2007.02.037

Das-Munshi, J., Lund, C., Matthews, C., Clark, C., Rothon, C., & Stansfield, S. (2016). Mental health inequities in adolescents growing up in post-apartheid South Africa: Cross-sectional survey, SHaW study. *PLoS One, 3*(11), 1–16.

De Milliano, M., & Plavgo, I. (2018). Analyzing multidimensional child poverty in sub-Saharan Africa: Findings using an international comparative approach. *Child Indicators Research, 11*(3), 805–833.

Erskine, H. E., Baxter, A. J., Patton, G., Moffitt, T. E., Patel, V., Whiteford, H. A., & Scott, J. G. (2017). The global coverage of prevalence data for mental disorders in children and adolescents. *Epidemiology and Psychiatric Sciences, 26*(4), 395–402. https://doi.org/10.1017/S2045796015001158

Erskine, H. E., Moffitt, T. E., Copeland, W. E., Costello, E. J., Ferrari, A. J., Patton, G., Degenhardt, L., Vos, T., Whiteford, H. A., & Scott, J. G. (2015). A heavy burden on young minds: The global burden of mental and substance use disorders in children and youth. *Psychological Medicine, 45*(7), 1551–1563. https://doi.org/10.1017/S0033291714002888

Foster, H., & Brooks-Gunn, J. (2015). Children's exposure to community and war violence and mental health in four African countries. *Social Science & Medicine, 146*, 292–299. https://doi.org/10.1016/j.socscimed.2015.10.020

Franke, H. A. (2014). Toxic stress: Effects, prevention and treatment. *Children (Basel, Switzerland), 1*(3), 390–402. https://doi.org/10.3390/children1030390

Gamarel, K. E., Kuo, C., Boyes, M. E., & Cluver, L. D. (2017). The dyadic effects of HIV stigma on the mental health of children and their parents in South Africa. *Journal of HIV/AIDS & Social Services, 16*(4), 351–366. https://doi.org/10.1080/15381501.2017.1320619

Gentz, S. G., Calonge-Romano, I., Martínez-Arias, R., Zeng, C., & Ruiz-Casares, M. (2018). Mental health among adolescents living with HIV in Namibia: The role of poverty, orphanhood, and social support. *AIDS Care, 30*(sup2), 83–91. https://doi.org/10.1080/09540121.2018. 1469727

Gilborn, L., Apicella, L., Brakarsh, J., Dube, L., Jemison, K., Kluckow, M., Smith, T., & Snider, L. (2006). Orphans and vulnerable youth in Bulawayo, Zimbabwe: An exploratory study of psychosocial well-being and psychosocial support. In *Horizons Final Report*. Population Council. Retrieved from https://bettercarenetwork.org/sites/default/files/attachments/Orphans %20and%20Vulnerable%20Youth%20in%20Bulawayo%20Zimbabwe.pdf

Gill, I. S., Revenga, A., & Zeballos, C. (2016). Grow, invest, insure: A game plan to end extreme poverty by 2030 [7892]. Retrieved from World Bank Group: Development economics poverty and Equity Global Practice Group & International Finance Corporation website: http:// documents.worldbank.org/curated/en/924111479240600559/pdf/WPS7892.pdf

Greene, M. E., & Patton, G. (2020). Adolescence and gender equality in health. *The Journal of Adolescent Health, 66*(1S), S1–S2. https://doi.org/10.1016/j.jadohealth.2019.10.012

Gupte, J., te Lintelo, D., & Barnett, I. (2014). Understanding 'urban youth' and the challenges they face in sub-Saharan Africa: Unemployment, food insecurity and violent crime (no. IDS evidence report; 81). IDS.

Hadley, C., & Patil, C. L. (2008). Seasonal changes in household food insecurity and symptoms of anxiety and depression. *American Journal of Physical Anthropology, 135*(2), 225–232. https:// doi.org/10.1002/ajpa.20724

Handa, S., Natali, L., Seidenfeld, D., Tembo, G., Davis, B., & Zambia Cash Transfer Evaluation Study Team. (2018). Can unconditional cash transfers raise long-term living standards? Evidence from Zambia. *Journal of Development Economics, 133*, 42–65.

He, Z., Bishwajit, G., Yaya, S., Cheng, Z., Zou, D., & Zhou, Y. (2018). Prevalence of low birth weight and its association with maternal body weight status in selected countries in Africa: A cross-sectional study. *BMJ Open, 8*(8), e020410. https://doi.org/10.1136/bmjopen-2017-020410

Hjern, A., Weitoft, G. R., & Lindblad, F. (2010). Social adversity predicts ADHD-medication in school children–a national cohort study. *Acta Paediatrica, 99*(6), 920–924.

Huang, K. Y., Abura, G., Theise, R., & Nakigudde, J. (2017). Parental depression and associations with parenting and children's physical and mental health in a sub-Saharan African setting. *Child Psychiatry & Human Development, 48*(4), 517–527.

Ilorah, R. (2009). Ethnic bias, favoritism and development in Africa. *Development Southern Africa, 26*(5), 695–707. https://doi.org/10.1080/03768350903303209

Jack, H., Wagner, R. G., Petersen, I., Thom, R., Newton, C. R., Stein, A., Kahn, K., Tollman, S., & Hofman, K. J. (2014). Closing the mental health treatment gap in South Africa: A review of costs and cost-effectiveness. *Global Health Action, 7*, 23431. https://doi.org/10.3402/gha.v7. 23431

Jebena, M. G., Lindstrom, D., Belachew, T., Hadley, C., Lachat, C., Verstraeten, R., ... Kolsteren, P. (2016). Food insecurity and common mental disorders among Ethiopian youth: Structural equation modeling. *PLoS One, 11*(11), e0165931.

Kamau, J. W., Kuria, W., Mathai, M., Atwoli, L., & Kangethe, R. (2012). Psychiatric morbidity among HIV-infected children and adolescents in a resource-poor Kenyan urban community. *AIDS Care, 24*(7), 836–842.

Kariuki, S. M., Abubakar, A., Murray, E., Stein, A., & Newton, C. R. (2016). Evaluation of psychometric properties and factorial structure of the pre-school child behaviour checklist at the Kenyan Coast. *Child and Adolescent Psychiatry and Mental Health, 10*(1), 1–10.

Kerac, M., Postels, D. G., Mallewa, M., Jalloh, A. A., Voskuijl, W. P., Groce, N., ...& Molyneux, E. (2014, March). The interaction of malnutrition and neurologic disability in Africa. In Seminars in pediatric neurology (Vol. 21, No. 1, pp. 42–49). WB Saunders.

Kessler, R. C. (2012). The costs of depression. *The Psychiatric Clinics of North America, 35*(1), 1–14. https://doi.org/10.1016/j.psc.2011.11.005

Kidman, R., & Heymann, J. (2016). Caregiver supportive policies to improve child outcomes in the wake of the HIV/AIDS epidemic: An analysis of the gap between what is needed and what is available in 25 high prevalence countries. *AIDS Care, 28*(sup2), 142–152. https://doi.org/10. 1080/09540121.2016.1176685

Kidman, R., & Thurman, T. R. (2014). Caregiver burden among adults caring for orphaned children in rural South Africa. *Vulnerable Children and Youth Studies, 9*(3), 234–246. https://doi.org/10. 1080/17450128.2013.871379

Kieling, C., Baker-Henningham, H., Belfer, M., Conti, G., Ertem, I., Omigbodun, O., Conti, G., & Rahman, A. (2011). Child and adolescent mental health worldwide: Evidence for action. *The Lancet, 378*(9801), 1515–1525. https://doi.org/10.1016/S0140-6736(11)60827-1

Kilburn, K., Thirumurthy, H., Halpern, C. T., Pettifor, A., & Handa, S. (2016). Effects of a large-scale unconditional cash transfer program on mental health outcomes of young people in Kenya. *Journal of Adolescent Health, 58*(2), 223–229.

Kim, M. H., Mazenga, A. C., Devandra, A., Ahmed, S., Kazembe, P. N., Yu, X., Nguyen, C., & Sharp, C. (2014). Prevalence of depression and validation of the Beck depression inventory-II and the children's depression inventory-short amongst HIV-positive adolescents in Malawi. *Journal of the International AIDS Society, 17*(1), 18965. https://doi.org/10.7448/IAS.17.1. 18965

Kinyanda, E., Kizza, R., Abbo, C., Ndyanabangi, S., & Levin, J. (2013). Prevalence and risk factors of depression in childhood and adolescence as seen in 4 districts of North-Eastern Uganda. *BMC International Health and Human Rights, 13*(1), 19.

Kinyanda, E., Kizza, R., Levin, J., Ndyanabangi, S., & Abbo, C. (2011). Adolescent suicidality as seen in rural northeastern Uganda: Prevalence and risk factors. *Crisis: The Journal of Crisis Intervention and Suicide Prevention, 32*(1), 43–51. https://doi.org/10.1027/0227-5910/a000059

Kuo, C., & Operario, D. (2010). Caring for AIDS-orphaned children: An exploratory study of challenges faced by carers in KwaZulu-Natal, South Africa. *Vulnerable Children and Youth Studies, 5*(4), 344–352. https://doi.org/10.1080/17450128.2010.516372

Langhaug, L. F., Pascoe, S. J., Mavhu, W., Woelk, G., Sherr, L., Hayes, R. J., & Cowan, F. M. (2010). High prevalence of affective disorders among adolescents living in rural Zimbabwe. *Journal of Community Health, 35*(4), 355–364.

Liddell, C., Kvalsvig, J., Qotyana, P., & Shabalala, A. (1994). Community violence and young South African children's involvement in aggression. *International Journal of Behavioral Development, 17*, 613–628.

Lund, C., De Silva, M., Plagerson, S., Cooper, S., Chisholm, D., Das, J., ...& Patel, V. (2011). Poverty and mental disorders: breaking the cycle in low-income and middle-income countries. *The Lancet, 378*(9801), 1502–1514.

Mabasa, E., Mabapa, N. S., Jooste, P. L., & Mbhenyane, X. G. (2019). Iodine status of pregnant women and children age 6 to 12 years feeding from the same food basket in Mopani district, Limpopo province, South Africa. *South African Journal of Clinical Nutrition, 32*(3), 76–82. https://doi.org/10.1080/16070658.2018.1449370

Maes, K. C., Hadley, C., Tesfaye, F., & Shifferaw, S. (2010). Food insecurity and mental health: Surprising trends among community health volunteers in Addis Ababa, Ethiopia during the 2008 food crisis. *Social Science & Medicine, 70*(9), 1450–1457. https://doi.org/10.1016/j. socscimed.2010.01.018

Magwaza, A. S., Killian, B. J., Petersen, I., & Pillay, Y. (1993). The effects of chronic violence on preschool children living in South African townships. *Child Abuse & Neglect, 17*(6), 795–803.

Makame, V., Ani, C., & Grantham-McGregor, S. (2002). Psychological well-being of orphans in Dar El Salaam, Tanzania. *Acta Paediatrica, 91*(4), 459–465.

Marais, L., Sharp, C., Pappin, M., Lenka, M., Cloete, J., Skinner, D., & Serekoane, J. (2013). Housing conditions and mental health of orphans in South Africa. *Health & Place, 24*, 23–29.

Meinck, F., Cluver, L. D., Orkin, F. M., Kuo, C., Sharma, A. D., Hensels, I. S., & Sherr, L. (2017). Pathways from family disadvantage via abusive parenting and caregiver mental health to adolescent health risks in South Africa. *Journal of Adolescent Health, 60*(1), 57–64.

Miranda, J. J., & Patel, V. (2005). Achieving the millennium development goals: Does mental health play a role? *PLoS Medicine, 2*(10), e291. https://doi.org/10.1371/journal.pmed.0020291

Mpango, R. S., Kinyanda, E., Rukundo, G. Z., Levin, J., Gadow, K. D., & Patel, V. (2017). Prevalence and correlates for ADHD and relation with social and academic functioning among children and adolescents with HIV/AIDS in Uganda. *BMC Psychiatry, 17*(1), 336.

Muktar, M., Roba, K. T., Mengistie, B., & Gebremichael, B. (2018). Iodine deficiency and its associated factors among primary school children in Anchar district, eastern Ethiopia. *Pediatric Health, Medicine and Therapeutics, 9*, 89–95. https://doi.org/10.2147/PHMT.S165933

Nankabirwa, J., Brooker, S. J., Clarke, S. E., Fernando, D., Gitonga, C. W., Schellenberg, D., & Greenwood, B. (2014). Malaria in school-age children in Africa: An increasingly important challenge. *Tropical Medicine & International Health, 19*(11), 1294–1309. https://doi.org/10.1111/tmi.12374

Ng, L. C., Kirk, C. M., Kanyanganzi, F., Fawzi, M. C. S., Sezibera, V., Shema, E., . . . Betancourt, T. S. (2015). Risk and protective factors for suicidal ideation and behavior in Rwandan children. *The British Journal of Psychiatry, 207*(3), 262–268.

Nöstlinger, C., Bartoli, G., Gordillo, V., Roberfroid, D., & Colebunders, R. (2006). Children and adolescents living with HIV positive parents: Emotional and behavioral problems. *Vulnerable Children and Youth Studies, 1*(1), 29–43.

Nyamukapa, C. A., Gregson, S., Wambe, M., Mushore, P., Lopman, B., Mupambireyi, Z., . . . Jukes, M. C. H. (2010). Causes and consequences of psychological distress among orphans in eastern Zimbabwe. *AIDS Care, 22*(8), 988–996.

Olney, D. K., Pollitt, E., Kariger, P. K., Khalfan, S. S., Ali, N. S., Tielsch, J. M., . . . Stoltzfus, R. J. (2007). Young Zanzibari children with iron deficiency, iron deficiency anemia, stunting, or malaria have lower motor activity scores and spend less time in locomotion. *The Journal of Nutrition, 137*(12), 2756–2762.

Pappin, M., Marais, L., Sharp, C., Lenka, M., Cloete, J., Skinner, D., & Serekoane, M. (2015). Socio-economic status and socio-emotional health of orphans in South Africa. *Journal of Community Health, 40*(1), 92–102.

Parcesepe, A. M., Bernard, C., Agler, R., Ross, J., Yotebieng, M., Bass, J., Kwobah, E., Adedimeji, A., Goulet, J., & Althoff, K. N. (2018). Mental health and HIV: Research priorities related to the implementation and scale up of 'treat all' in sub-Saharan Africa. *Journal of Virus Eradication, 4* (Suppl 2), 16–25.

Pascoe, J. M., Wood, D. L., Duffee, J. H., Kuo, A., & Committee on Psychosocial Aspects of Child and Family Health. (2016). Mediators and adverse effects of child poverty in the United States. *Pediatrics, 137*(4), e20160340.

Patel, V., Flisher, A. J., Nikapota, A., & Malhotra, S. (2008). Promoting child and adolescent mental health in low and middle income countries. *Journal of Child Psychology and Psychiatry, 49*(3), 313–334.

Perry-Jenkins, M., Repetti, R. L., & Crouter, A. C. (2000). Work and family in the 1990s. *Journal of Marriage and the Family, 62*, 981–998. https://doi.org/10.1111/j.1741-3737.2000.00981.x

Plagerson, S., Patel, V., Harpham, T., Kielmann, K., & Mathee, A. (2011). Does money matter for mental health? Evidence from the child support grants in Johannesburg, South Africa. *Global Public Health, 6*(7), 760–776.

Richter, L. M., Riesel, R. D., & Barbarin, O. A. (2000). Behavioural problems among preschool children in South Africa: A six-year longitudinal perspective from birth to age five. In N. Singh, J. Leung, & A. Singh (Eds.), *International perspectives on child and adolescent mental health* (pp. 160–182). Elsevier.

Rochat, T. J., Houle, B., Stein, A., Pearson, R. M., & Bland, R. M. (2018). Prevalence and risk factors for child mental disorders in a population-based cohort of HIV-exposed and unexposed African children aged 7–11 years. *European Child & Adolescent Psychiatry, 27*(12), 1607–1620.

Rock, A., Barrington, C., Abdoulayi, S., Tsoka, M., Mvula, P., & Handa, S. (2016). Social networks, social participation, and health among youth living in extreme poverty in rural Malawi. *Social Science & Medicine, 170*, 55–62.

Roelen, K. (2017). Monetary and multidimensional child poverty: A contradiction in terms? *Development and Change, 48*(3), 502–533.

Roos, L. L., Wall-Wieler, E., & Lee, J. B. (2019). Poverty and early childhood outcomes. *Pediatrics, 2019*, e20183426. https://doi.org/10.1542/peds.2018-3426

Russell, A. E., Ford, T., & Russell, G. (2015). Socioeconomic associations with ADHD: findings from a mediation analysis. *PLoS One, 10*(6), e0128248.

Sachs, S. E., & Sachs, J. D. (2007). Mental health in the millennium development goals: Not ignored. *PLoS Medicine, 4*(1), e56. https://doi.org/10.1371/journal.pmed.0040056

Salisbury, K. E., Levin, J., Foster, A., Mpango, R., Patel, V., & Kenneth, D. G. (2020). Clinical correlates and adverse outcomes of ADHD, disruptive behavior disorder and their co-occurrence among children and adolescents with HIV in Uganda. *AIDS Care, 32*, 11. https://doi.org/10.1080/09540121.2020.1742860

Samuels, F., & Stavropoulou, M. (2016). 'Being able to breathe again': The effects of cash transfer programmes on psychosocial wellbeing. *The Journal of Development Studies, 52*(8), 1099–1114.

Silberberg D, Katabira E. Neurological disorders. In: Jamison DT, Feachem RG, Makgoba MW, et al., editors. (2006) Disease and mortality in sub-Saharan Africa. 2nd. : The International Bank for Reconstruction and Development/The World Bank

Slade, M. (2010). Mental illness and well-being: The central importance of positive psychology and recovery approaches. *BMC Health Services Research, 10*(1), 1–14. https://doi.org/10.1186/1472-6963-10-26

Slade, M., & Longden, E. (2015). Empirical evidence about recovery and mental health. *BMC Psychiatry, 15*, 285. https://doi.org/10.1186/s12888-015-0678-4

Ssewamala, F. M., Han, C. K., & Neilands, T. B. (2009). Asset ownership and health and mental health functioning among AIDS-orphaned adolescents: Findings from a randomized clinical trial in rural Uganda. *Social Science and Medicine, 69*, 191–198.

Ssewamala, F. M., Neilands, T. B., Waldfogel, J., & Ismayilova, L. (2012). The impact of a comprehensive microfinance intervention on depression levels of AIDS-orphaned children in Uganda. *Journal of Adolescent Health, 50*(4), 346–352.

Stewart, R. C., Umar, E., Tomenson, B., & Creed, F. (2014). A cross-sectional study of antenatal depression and associated factors in Malawi. *Archives of Women's Mental Health, 17*(2), 145–154. https://doi.org/10.1007/s00737-013-0387-2

Thurman, T. R., Snider, L. A., Boris, N. W., Kalisa, E., Nyirazinyoye, L., & Brown, L. (2008). Barriers to the community support of orphans and vulnerable youth in Rwanda. *Social Science & Medicine, 66*(7), 1557–1567.

Townsend, P. (1979). *Poverty in the United Kingdom: A survey of household resources and standards of living*. University of California Press.

Townsend, P. (1987). Deprivation. *Journal of Social Policy, 16*(02), 125. https://doi.org/10.1017/s0047279400020341

Toye, M., & Downing, R. (2006). *Social inclusion and community economic development*. Retrieved from Canadian CED Network website https://www.ccednet-rdec.ca/files/ccednet/PCCDLN_Final_Report.pdf

Toye, M., & Infanti, J. (2004). *Social inclusion and community economic development: A literature review*. The Canadian CED Network.

Trautmann, S., Rehm, J., & Wittchen, H. U. (2016). The economic costs of mental disorders: Do our societies react appropriately to the burden of mental disorders? *EMBO Reports, 17*(9), 1245–1249. https://doi.org/10.15252/embr.201642951

UNDP. (2018). *The new global MPI 2018.* Retrieved from http://hdr.undp.org/en/2018-MPI

UNICEF. (1989). Convention on the rights of the child.

Ventevogel, P. (2015). The effects of war: Local views and priorities concerning psychosocial and mental health problems as a result of collective violence in Burundi. *Intervention: Journal of Mental Health and Psychosocial Support in Conflict Affected Areas, 13*(3), 216–234. https://doi.org/10.1097/WTF.0000000000000100

Walker, S. P., Wachs, T. D., Gardner, J. M., et al. (2007). Child development: Risk factors for adverse outcomes in developing countries. *Lancet, 369*(9556), 145–157. https://doi.org/10.1016/S0140-6736(07)60076-2

Whiteford, H. A., Degenhardt, L., Rehm, J., Baxter, A. J., Ferrari, A. J., Erskine, H. E., Charlson, F. J., Norman, R. E., Flaxman, A. D., Johns, N., Burstein, R., Murray, C. J. L., & Vos, T. (2013). Global burden of disease attributable to mental and substance use disorders: Findings from the global burden of disease study 2010. *The Lancet, 382*(9904), 1575–1586. https://doi.org/10.1016/S0140-6736(13)61611-6

WHO. (2015). *Lead exposure in African children.* Retrieved from https://apps.who.int/iris/bitstream/handle/10665/200168/9780869707876.pdf;jsessionid=C948CC46CC2DF02FBB05C4CB9CA7175C?sequence=1

WHO. (2016). *Global health estimates 2016: Disease burden by cause, age, sex, by country and by region, 2000-2016.* World Health Organization.

WHO. (2018). *Mental health atlas 2017.* World Health Organization. https://apps.who.int/iris/handle/10665/272735. License: CC BY-NC-SA 3.0 IGO

Wood, K., Chase, E., & Aggleton, P. (2006). 'Telling the truth is the best thing': Teenage orphans' experiences of parental AIDS-related illness and bereavement in Zimbabwe. *Social Science & Medicine, 63*(7), 1923–1933. https://doi.org/10.1016/j.socscimed.2006.04.027

Wright, M. O. D., Masten, A. S., & Narayan, A. J. (2013). Resilience processes in development: Four waves of research on positive adaptation in the context of adversity. In *Handbook of resilience in children* (pp. 15–37). Springer.

Yoder, H. N., Tol, W. A., Reis, R., & de Jong, J. T. (2016). Child mental health in Sierra Leone: A survey and exploratory qualitative study. *International Journal of Mental Health Systems, 10*, 48. https://doi.org/10.1186/s13033-016-0080-8

Yoshikawa, H., Aber, J. L., & Beardslee, W. R. (2012). The effects of poverty on the mental, emotional, and behavioral health of children and youth: Implications for prevention. *American Psychologist, 67*(4), 272–284. https://doi.org/10.1037/a0028015

Improving Child and Adolescent Mental Health in Africa: A Review of the Economic Evidence

Yesim Tozan and Ariadna Capasso

Introduction

Childhood mental disorders are a growing public health concern in low- and middle-income countries (LMICs). A major driving factor is the increasing proportion of children and adolescents[1] among the overall LMIC population, owing to greatly improved childhood survival and slow decline in fertility (United Nations, 2017a). Today, children and adolescents make up about one-third (2.3 billion) of the world's population. While just over one in three persons (36%) is aged under 20 years in LMICs, this age group represents more than half (54%) of the population in Africa (United Nations, 2017b). Economic and social adversity, coupled with high prevalence of diseases that lead to psychopathology, is another important factor contributing to poor mental health outcomes in children and adolescents worldwide, particularly in Africa (Owen et al., 2016). Staggeringly, up to 20% of the world's youth is estimated to suffer from a mental disorder during childhood (Belfer, 2008; Kieling et al., 2011; World Health Organization, 2001).

Significant disparities exist in the availability of mental health services globally. The latest data from the WHO's Mental Health Atlas survey indicated that less than half of African countries had at least two functioning mental health promotion and prevention programs, compared to over 70% globally (World Health Organization, 2018). There are also wide treatment gaps for people with mental disorders across countries. For instance, while 132 and 320 per 100,000 patients are treated for depression in upper middle-income and high-income countries, respectively, only 19 and 34 per 100,000 patients receive treatment for this prevalent disorder in

---

[1] The WHO defines an adolescent as any person between ages 10 and 19 years.

Y. Tozan (✉) · A. Capasso
School of Global Public Health, New York University, New York, NY, USA
e-mail: tozan@nyu.edu

© Springer Nature Switzerland AG 2022
F. M. Ssewamala et al. (eds.), *Child Behavioral Health in Sub-Saharan Africa*,
https://doi.org/10.1007/978-3-030-83707-5_3

low-income and lower middle-income countries (World Health Organization, 2018). The mental health treatment gaps for children are anticipated to be much larger in African countries because very few countries have the ability to dedicate resources towards mental health programs and facilities to meet the specific needs of this age group (World Health Organization, 2018). For instance, in post-conflict Sierra Leone, the treatment gap for children with mental disorders is found to be nearly universal (98.8%) (Yoder et al., 2016). The evidence further shows that most mental disorders in adults emerge during adolescence unless detected and treated early (Carr et al., 2013; Kessler et al., 2007). This backdrop suggests that the burden of mental disorders in LMICs will increase in the coming decades, with major implications for overburdened health systems, particularly in Africa where infectious diseases are still highly prevalent.

The purpose of this chapter is threefold. First, we review the extent, nature, and risk factors of childhood and adolescent mental disorders in LMICs, with a focus on African countries, and discuss the economic consequences for the individual, family, and society as a whole. Second, we report on the state of the economic evidence base on mental health programs and interventions for children and adolescents in low-resource settings, as recommended by the WHO's Comprehensive Mental Health Action Plan 2013–2020. Last, we discuss the most immediate economic considerations relevant to introduction, integration, and scale-up of evidence-based programs and interventions to improve child and adolescent mental health and well-being in such settings.

Extent, Nature, and Risk Factors of Childhood and Adolescent Mental Disorders

Childhood and adolescent mental disorders fall broadly into three categories: neurodevelopmental, behavioral, and emotional (World Health Organization, 2001). A recent review showed that prevalence rates of mental disorders among children and adolescents varied greatly in LMICs, ranging from 8% to 27% for anxiety, nil to 28% for depression, and 0.2% to 87% for post-traumatic stress disorder (PTSD) in armed conflict settings (Yatham et al., 2017). In Africa, behavioral and emotional disorders such as anxiety, depression, conduct disorder, and PTSD are the most frequently reported disorders in children and adolescents (Cortina et al., 2012; Global Burden of Disease Pediatrics et al., 2016). However, there is a dearth of nationally representative and comparable data on mental disorders in African countries, particularly in children and adolescents (Baxter et al., 2013). This is mainly because large-scale mental health surveys require proportionately large research teams and resources. There is also limited availability of mental health services and providers, as well as inadequate monitoring and surveillance of mental disorders, particularly at the primary care level (Jenkins, 2019; Lyons-Ruth et al., 2017). These limitations lead to underdiagnosis and underreporting of mental disorders in African countries (Kieling & Rohde, 2012). Lastly, research points to a strong social stigma for people with mental illness that precludes recognizing and seeking care for mental disorders in LMICs, including African countries (Mascayano et al., 2015; Semrau et al., 2015).

As a result, prevalence estimates for mental disorders are mainly based on data from single-country studies of variable quality and methods, rendering synthesis and comparison of their findings difficult. Nevertheless, a recent meta-analysis pooled data from ten studies across six African countries and estimated that 14% of children aged 0–16 years suffered from some form of psychopathology (Cortina et al., 2012). Individual studies present data for selected mental disorders across different settings. A study in Kenya found a prevalence rate of 13% for anxiety disorders in children aged 1–6 years (Kariuki et al., 2017). A study in adolescents aged 10–12 years reported a prevalence rate of 14% for anxiety and depression disorders and 24% for PTSD in South Africa (Kawakami et al., 2012). Another study in adolescents aged 13–18 years in Nigeria found a prevalence rate of 15% for anxiety disorders, which also showed a remarkable gender difference with 20% in females versus 11% in males (Adewuya et al. 2007). Girls aged 3–19 years were found to be affected more by anxiety disorders also in Uganda with a prevalence rate of about 30% compared to boys at about 23%, with an overall prevalence of about 27% (Abbo et al., 2013). A study among girls aged 12–19 years in Sudan reported a prevalence rate of 39% for depression disorders, including both moderate and severe forms (Shaaban and Baashar, 2003). In Rwanda, 53% of the youth who identified themselves as head of household screened positive for depression (Boris et al., 2008). Although limited, the existing evidence indicates that the burden of mental health problems in children and adolescents is considerable in African countries.

Across the globe, numerous studies have identified chronic adversity, toxic social environment, and exposure to trauma during childhood as major risk factors for psychological problems in children and adolescents (Jonas et al., 2011; Kessler et al., 2010; Patalay & Fitzsimons, 2016). In Africa, the elevated prevalence of mental disorders among youth has also been attributed to risk factors such as living with chronic disease with neuropsychiatric comorbidities such as HIV (Mellins & Malee, 2013; Small et al., 2014; Vreeman et al., 2017) and malaria (Jenkins et al., 2017), being an orphan (Ssewamala et al., 2012), and experiencing deprivation and conflict-related violence and trauma (de Jong et al., 2015; Lund et al., 2010). These findings signify the increased risk of mental disorders among youth living in areas affected by social and economic deprivation and pose a particular concern for African children and adolescents given the high rates of deprivation and social tension experienced in the region.

Economic Consequences of Childhood and Adolescent Mental Disorders

Mental disorders in children and adolescents exert a considerable economic burden on families, but there is limited research in this area in LMICs, and further evidence is needed (Scott et al., 2015). According to the 2017 WHO's Mental Health Atlas Survey, in 43% of African countries, patients pay mostly or entirely out of pocket for mental health services and treatment (World Health Organization, 2018). The economic burden on families also results from other types of out-of-pocket expenditures while seeking care such as transportation, as well as from loss of income to provide and arrange care for a child with mental health needs (World Health Organization, 2008; Zergaw et al., 2008). Several studies have shown that caring for a person with mental illness affects a caregiver's life in various ways, including their quality of life and social and economic status (Ae-Ngibise et al., 2015; Thompson & Doll, 1982). Family members are usually the primary caregivers of persons with mental illness in LMICs (Rathod et al., 2017). Family caregivers not only endure physical strain and emotional stress of caregiving, but they also are usually required to provide financial support to the patient. A recent review found that the caregiver's income level and employment status and the patient's mental illness severity and duration negatively affected the economic burden experienced by caregivers in sub-Saharan Africa (Ae-Ngibise et al., 2015). A study on out-of-pocket costs incurred by caregivers of adult schizophrenic patients in Ghana showed that the total average cost per patient was staggeringly high at US$273 per month, with medications (50%) and transportation (27%) as the key cost drivers (Opoku-Boateng et al., 2017).

Mental disorders during childhood are linked to school absenteeism, reduced academic performance, and early termination of education, all of which are shown to limit employment prospects later in life and result in lower salaries when employed (Chorozoglou et al., 2015; Fergusson et al., 2005; Griswold et al., 2018; Kawakami et al., 2012; Lee et al., 2009; McCrone et al., 2005; Ngui et al., 2010; Scott et al., 2001). To that end, at the individual level, severe mental illness was estimated to be associated with a 33% reduction in median earnings in LMICs, with no significant difference between men and women (Levinson et al., 2010). A study in South Africa showed that severe depression and anxiety disorders in adults were associated with a significant reduction in individual earnings over the past 12 months, resulting in a mean annual income loss of US$4798 per person, totaling to US$3.6 billion per year (Lund et al., 2010). Another study reported a massive loss of productive human capital due to severe mental illness at the societal level through a significant reduction in population-level earnings equivalent to 0.3% of all earnings in LMICs (Levinson et al., 2010). Untreated childhood mental disorders have also been linked to chronic disease in adulthood (e.g., diabetes, heart attack), resulting in decreased quality of life and increased healthcare spending later in life (Deschenes et al., 2018; Monnat & Chandler, 2015).

Overall, the global lost economic output as a result of common mental disorders, including depression and anxiety, was estimated at US$1.15 trillion in the absence of scaled-up treatment (Chisholm & Saxena, 2012). A large body of evidence shows that the onset of many mental and developmental disorders can be prevented with early-life interventions (World Health Organization, 2001). Evidence-based mental health promotion and preventive interventions have been shown to prevent illness and reduce severity of symptoms (Barry et al., 2013). Studies in high-income countries (HICs) have shown a positive return on investment with early-life interventions to address mental disorders during childhood (McDaid, 2018; Scott et al., 2001). Hence, early investments in mental health care may serve to improve health, education, and social and economic outcomes and curb associated future costs.

Historical Perspective on Economic Evaluation of Mental Health Programs and Interventions

Economic evaluation literature dates back to the 1960s and 1970s (Hutton, 2012). The World Bank conducted cost-benefit analysis for a majority of its development projects implemented in LMICs in the 1970s and 1980s and defined it as "any quantitative analysis performed to establish whether the present value of benefits of a given project exceeds the present value of costs" (Independent Evaluation Group, 2010); however, only a few of these analyses were for projects in the health sector. A big push to use economic evaluation for decision-making in health care came from HICs in the 1990s, particularly in the context of drug reimbursements with the creation of the National Institute for Clinical Excellence (NICE) in England and Wales (Hutton, 2012). In the United States, the Panel on Cost-Effectiveness in Health and Medicine was convened around the same time and provided recommendations on cost-effectiveness analysis in health and medicine (Russell et al., 1996). Today, cost-effectiveness and cost-benefit analyses are considered as best practices in decision-making and are widely used policy-making tools to guide allocation of resources to different interventions and programs in the context of increasing budget constraints (Russell, 2015). In an era of increasing demand for evidence-based healthcare spending, evidence on intervention effectiveness alone is insufficient for policy-making. Information on the economic costs and consequences of interventions is equally important for decision-making.

One of the most rigorous cost-benefit analyses in mental health was on psychiatric services in HICs and dates back to 1977 (Glass & Goldberg, 1977). Cost-benefit analyses in the United States suggested that high-quality preschool interventions for mental health had strong returns on investment. For example, by age 21 years, it was estimated that every $1 invested in prenatal interventions returned $3.01; every $1 invested in infancy interventions returned $4.42; and every $1 invested in preschool interventions returned $7.16 (Reynolds et al., 2002). The Foresight report on mental capital and well-being made the economic case for the UK Government to invest on early prevention, detection, and treatment of mental disorders (The Government Office for Science, 2008).

In LMICs, economic evaluation studies in general, and cost-effectiveness analysis in particular, began to appear in the public health literature in the mid-1980s, particularly in the context of interventions to control infectious diseases in Africa, such as eradication of onchocerciasis in West Africa (Evans & Murray, 1987; Prost & Prescott, 1984; Rosenfield et al., 1984), treatment of malaria (Evans et al., 1997; Sudre et al., 1992), and vaccination campaigns (Monath & Nasidi, 1993; Naficy et al., 1998). However, the push for economic evaluations of mental health interventions in LMICs is a more recent development.

Economic evaluations of mental health programs and interventions are often based on retrospective secondary analysis of data from experimental or quasi-experimental studies (Gureje et al., 2007; Siskind et al., 2008). Some studies undertook model-based analysis of data from systematic and non-systematic reviews to project longer term costs and benefits of mental health interventions (Chisholm & Saxena, 2012). In recent years, a growing number of economic studies have used effectiveness and cost data collected prospectively alongside clinical trials of mental health interventions (Ssewamala et al., 2018; Tozan et al., 2019; Zechmeister et al., 2008). While the evidence on the disease and economic burden of mental illness is growing, much less is known about the cost-effectiveness of mental health interventions and programs, as discussed later in the chapter.

The Global Platform for Mental Health

As early as 1940s, world leaders recognized mental health as an integral part of health and well-being (World Health Organization, 1946), as evidenced by the establishment of WHO's Mental Health Division and the World Federation of Mental Health in 1948 (Brody, 2004). The Alma-Ata post-conference report further reaffirmed the importance of mental health as one of the essential elements of primary health care (Ivbijaro et al., 2008; World Health Organization, 1978). Despite these early commitments, funding for mental health lagged behind need. Recognizing the profound global disparities in mental health and the growing burden of mental disorders, WHO member states endorsed the Mental Health Global Action Programme in 2002, followed by the Mental Health Gap Action Programme (mhGAP) in 2008 (World Health Organization, 2008) and the Comprehensive Mental Health Action Plan 2013–2020 later in 2013 (World Health Organization, 2013). These high-level intergovernmental initiatives offered policy recommendations on the delivery of mental health services in low-resource settings based on systematic appraisal of the existing evidence (Jacob, 2017; Kieling et al., 2011), with mhGAP specifically prioritizing childhood mental health disorders (World Health Organization, 2008). In 2015, the Sustainable Development Goals (SDGs) recognized mental health promotion as a priority for global development and called for the adoption of policies and programs to promote mental health and increase access to treatment for mental disorders (Jenkins, 2019). Subsequently, the Lancet Commission on Mental Health was formed to assess the progress towards the SDG targets in this area (Patel et al., 2018).

Economic Considerations Around Mental Health Interventions for Children and Adolescents

The WHO's Mental Health Action Plan 2013–2020 identifies several objectives to guide delivery and scale-up of mental health services and interventions (World Health Organization, 2013). One such objective is the development, implementation, and evaluation of evidence-based mental health interventions, including early and preventive interventions to address mental health disorders in childhood and adolescence (World Health Organization, 2013). Another objective is community-based delivery of mental health interventions with linkages to primary care and in collaboration with informal mental healthcare providers such as teachers and families. During childhood, the Mental Health Action Plan recommends community-based psychosocial and other non-pharmacological interventions, avoiding medicalization and institutionalization. For countries to adopt these intervention approaches and achieve universal access to mental health care, interventions must be not only cost effective, but also affordable and sustainable within the constraints of national healthcare budgets.

Effectiveness and Cost-Effectiveness

Below we review the promising intervention approaches most relevant to children and adolescents living in low-resource settings, and the evidence base on their cost-effectiveness.

Interventions by Nonspecialist Providers

Given the limited availability of mental health professionals, interventions to improve mental health in LMICs are often delivered by paraprofessionals, a strategy known as task-shifting (Javadi et al., 2017). Specifically, interventions delivered by lay counselors and community health workers have been found effective in reducing depressive symptoms in different adult groups, such as recent mothers and persons living with HIV (Javadi et al., 2017). However, the effectiveness of task-shifting in mental health interventions for children and youth is less certain. A review found that only half of mental health promotion interventions for children delivered by community health workers had a significant impact on mental health outcomes (Mutamba 2013). Among children who experienced trauma, trauma-informed cognitive behavioral therapy (CBT) offered by lay counselors relieved trauma- and stress-related symptoms and improved functional impairment in the short term although the effectiveness of the intervention declined over time (Dorsey et al., 2020; Murray et al., 2015). An intervention for HIV-infected mothers and their children in South Africa delivered by community health workers improved children's externalizing behaviors and parent-child communication, but failed to have an effect on their internalizing behaviors and socialization (Eloff et al., 2014). Overall, interventions delivered by lay counselors have been shown to improve overall well-being, relieve trauma symptoms, and strengthen life skills, but have failed to prevent the onset of depression and anxiety among youth (Bell et al., 2008; Puffer et al., 2016; Purgato et al., 2018).

A review focusing on LMICs found that task-shifting interventions improved health system efficiency and lowered healthcare costs, particularly for tuberculosis and HIV/AIDS, at both primary care and community levels (Seidman & Atun, 2017). The review identified only one intervention for mental health. This intervention used a collaborative team approach that included lay healthcare workers to treat anxiety and depressive disorders among adults in primary care settings in India. The cost-effectiveness analysis of the intervention showed that it was less costly and more effective than the physician-only model (Buttorff et al., 2012).

Targeted task-shifting interventions for children and adolescents who are at risk or screened positive for mental disorders are a promising strategy in low-resource settings. However, more research is needed to identify the target populations (age, gender, context, trauma exposure) that will best benefit from these interventions and the optimal settings and approaches to deliver them. Investing in training, supervision, and support of paraprofessionals and quality assurance is potentially a critical factor for the effectiveness of task-shifting interventions (Britto et al., 2015). Future studies should focus on their costs and cost-effectiveness across different settings.

Family-Based Interventions

Most children are intrinsically dependent on adult caregivers for many aspects of their lives, including accessing care. Furthermore, family functioning and caregiver characteristics (e.g., caregiver's physical and mental health, child-caregiver bond, and discipline style) affect children's mental health. Unsurprisingly, many mental health interventions for children aim to modify family relationships and strengthen parenting skills, thus fostering a supportive family environment that can buffer high stress and unstable contexts (Puffer et al., 2016).

Family-based interventions largely fall into two categories: those that are parent focused and seek to build parenting skills specifically focusing on behavior monitoring, effective discipline, nutrition, and health, and those that are family focused and seek to improve the family's overall functioning by strengthening, for example, interpersonal communications, conflict resolution, or family economy and financial management skills (Pedersen et al., 2019). In the context of LMICs, family-based programs have also incorporated psychosocial stimulation (e.g., for undernourished infants) and social protection (e.g., conditional cash transfers and family economic empowerment) to address environmental deprivation (Britto et al., 2015; Pedersen et al., 2019).

Parenting interventions have resulted in improved mental well-being and conduct disorder symptoms in childhood and appeared to prevent the onset of mental health disorders later on (Nystrand et al., 2019; Sandler et al., 2015). A caveat is that a large body of evidence for these interventions comes from HICs, and most studies do not include a mid- or long-term assessment of outcomes (Furlong et al., 2012). While family-based interventions in LMICs are promising, few studies have found significant effects on children's internalizing behaviors (Pedersen et al., 2019). For example, an intervention to improve parenting skills among migrant and displaced Burmese populations in Thailand had no effect on children's internalizing disorders, but improved externalizing behaviors and attention problems compared to control children (Annan et al., 2017). A family-based intervention led by psychologists to improve mental health among children in post-conflict Rwanda reduced depression and anxiety post-intervention and at 6-month follow-up based on caregiver reports, but not according to children self-reports (Betancourt et al., 2014). An analysis of CHAMP+, a program to strengthen family relationships among HIV-infected adolescents, found significant improvement in teen's emotional well-being across three sites (Argentina, South Africa, and the United States); however, anxiety and depression outcomes were not improved (Small et al., 2014). An intensive psychoeducation, nutrition, and early childhood program, Extending the Jamaican Early Childhood Development Intervention, is ongoing for over two decades; it has been shown to reduce adulthood onset of anxiety and depression (Grantham-McGregor & Smith, 2016).

There is limited evidence on the cost-effectiveness of family-based interventions (Furlong et al., 2012). Studies from HICs showed that parent-focused interventions to prevent the onset of anxiety disorders (Mihalopoulos et al., 2015b) and address conduct disorders (Nystrand et al., 2019) are cost effective. Less health economics evidence is available from LMICs. A parenting skill and psychoeducational program for teen mothers in Chile delivered through home visits resulted in improved mental health of mothers. The program cost $2.70 more per month per adolescent than treatment as usual and improved mental health at a cost of US$13.50 over the program period (Aracena et al., 2009). The WHO/UNICEF Parenting for Lifelong Health, a parenting skill-building program to prevent maltreatment of adolescents, found the program to be cost effective; the cost per incident of abuse averted was US $1837, with an estimated lifetime savings of US$2724 (Redfern et al., 2019).

There is strong evidence that parenting programs can be transported effectively to low-resource settings (Gardner et al., 2016). An economic consideration is that most programs have been found to have a dose-response relationship with outcomes: more intensive programs, as measured by duration, frequency, and intensity, are more effective, particularly in early-childhood interventions (Britto et al., 2015).

Therefore, a larger investment may be needed over a more prolonged time in order to attain larger and more sustainable effects. More research to assess the longer term outcomes of interventions and the cost implications of a societal perspective is needed. Programs such as early childhood development intervention in Jamaica are an example of effective programming; however feasibility in low-resource settings needs to be assessed, given competing health priorities and meager public budgets.

School-Based Interventions

A systematic review of health promotion interventions among young people found that most school-based programs had a beneficial effect on emotional and behavioral well-being, self-esteem, and coping skills (Barry et al., 2013). Most of the interventions sought to improve overall well-being and were delivered in high-risk settings, such as conflict-affected and high-HIV/AIDS-prevalence regions while only one intervention aimed specifically to reduce depression. Of the 14 interventions, two resulted in reduced depression, two in reduced anxiety, and two in reduced PTSD, but with limited evidence on their long-term effects (Barry et al., 2013). Another systematic review revealed mixed effects of school-based programs in reducing anxiety, depression, and PTSD among young people in LMICs (Yatham et al., 2017). The review found that program effectiveness varied by sex and age (Yatham et al., 2017). In Mauritius, a school-based program to prevent depression among adolescents decreased depressive symptoms and increased self-esteem and coping skills post-intervention, but improvement in depression symptoms was not maintained at follow-up (Rivet-Duval et al., 2011). In Chile, a similar program did not significantly reduce depression (Araya et al., 2013). Several interventions have focused on reducing depression and anxiety among AIDS-orphaned adolescents in Uganda. A peer-support group intervention significantly reduced depression and anxiety symptoms in the intervention group (Kumakech et al., 2009). Two school-based economic empowerment interventions for AIDS orphans in Uganda, Suubi and Bridges, decreased depression and hopelessness 2 years post-intervention (Ssewamala et al., 2012, 2018).

Despite these promising results, cost-effectiveness studies of school-based interventions are limited both in HICs and LMICs (J. K. Anderson et al., 2019; Mihalopoulos et al., 2011). A three-arm family economic empowerment trial in Uganda, Bridges, cost on average US$418–426 over 2 years. It cost US$212 and US$237 to achieve a 0.2 standard deviation change in depression compared to usual care, and US$263 to US$337 for hopelessness (Ssewamala et al., 2018). At 4-year follow-up, participants in the more intense arm maintained a statistically significant lower level of hopelessness compared to those in the control group, but there were no significant differences in depression scores. The cost of achieving a 0.2 standard deviation reduction in hopelessness score was lower at US$224 (Tozan et al., 2020).

More rigorous research is needed to evaluate the feasibility and cost of school-based screening, prevention, and treatment of mental disorders in LMICs. Evidence suggests that universal programs may be more cost effective in high-risk settings. In other settings, it may be best to improve screening and referrals to increase detection of mental disorders and tailor treatment to children at risk. Furthermore, programs may be more effective in improving the overall well-being, for instance, by enhancing motivation and coping skills, but may not be as effective in preventing the development of depression or anxiety disorders in the long term. However, these temporary mental health improvements may have other long-term societal benefits by reducing school dropout rates and risky behaviors such as hazardous substance use and condomless sex (Goesling et al., 2014; Jewkes et al., 2008; Sarnquist et al., 2017).

Psychosocial Interventions

Psychosocial interventions can reduce the severity of childhood mental health disorders. Such interventions, including psychoeducation, skill training, and CBT, have been used in the prevention and treatment of internalizing disorders among children in LMICs (Barry et al., 2013; Yatham et al., 2017). There is robust evidence from HICs supporting the effectiveness of CBT in the temporary remission of anxiety and depressive symptoms in children and adolescents, albeit with limited longer term effects (Compton et al., 2004; Das et al., 2016; James et al., 2015; Klein et al., 2007; Schwartz et al., 2019). In LMICs, reviews of interventions to treat anxiety, depression, and PTSD among children identified promising interventions, but the evidence was overall of low quality, showing mixed effects on outcomes (Purgato et al., 2018; Yatham et al., 2017). For example, in Zambia, a CBT intervention reduced trauma symptomatology but not in internalizing disorders (Murray et al., 2013a; Murray et al., 2013b). Classroom-based interventions with a CBT component effectively addressed PTSD in children (Yatham et al., 2017). In a proof-of-concept study, a group-delivered CBT intervention for youth was found effective in treating anxiety disorders in Brazil and should be further investigated through clinical trials in other LMICs (de Souza et al., 2013).

CBT interventions have found to be equally effective when administered in group versus individual format in various settings (e.g., schools, communities, clinics) (James et al., 2015; Schwartz et al., 2019). Given the dearth of mental healthcare providers, the administration of CBT by lay providers in group settings may be the most feasible option in low-resource settings. However, a growing body of research has found that digital platforms are another effective way of delivering CBT for the treatment of anxiety and depression in youth (Ebert et al., 2015). Evidence is mainly from HICs, but digital platforms could be a promising mode of administration of CBT given the ubiquity of mobile technology in LMICs and the acceptability and feasibility of mHealth interventions for other health concerns, particularly among young people (Iribarren, Cato, Falzon, & Stone, 2017).

There is limited cost-effectiveness evidence for CBT interventions in children and adolescents in LMICs (Scott et al., 2015). Even in HICs, there is mixed evidence on the cost-effectiveness of CBT interventions for the treatment of anxiety disorders (Ophuis et al., 2017; Scott et al., 2015), and only a limited number of studies have focused specifically on children (Kieling et al., 2011). In HICs, internet-delivered CBT for adults has the strongest evidence of cost-effectiveness (Ophuis et al., 2017). A cost analysis of CBT interventions to treat anxiety disorders estimated a net gain of €9500 (US$10,600 in 2019) per person in HICs (Schwartz et al., 2019; Washington State Institute for Public Policy 2018). A clinical trial in Australia found trauma-informed care using CBT to be highly cost effective in reducing anxiety symptoms among both children and adults (Mihalopoulos et al., 2015a). However, a school-based CBT intervention in England was not cost effective in reducing symptoms of depression (R. Anderson et al., 2014). Group therapy based on CBT principles delivered to war-affected youth in Sierra Leone was not found to be cost effective (McBain et al., 2016), and neither was a school-wide program using CBT for depression in Chile (Araya et al., 2013). A promising focus of cost-effectiveness research in LMICs may be internet- and mobile-based delivery of CBT interventions for prevention of internalizing disorders among children and adolescents.

Affordability

In addition to evidence on cost-effectiveness, country decision makers need to assess the affordability of introducing and scaling up mental health interventions alongside other priority health interventions, particularly in low-resource settings (Lund et al., 2013; Chisholm & Saxena, 2012). This would necessitate an understanding of context-specific needs and resource gaps to deliver interventions (e.g., trained personnel), as well as feasible and acceptable strategies to address the identified gaps (e.g., task-shifting) (Murray et al., 2013a; Thornicroft & Tansella 2009; Kakuma et al., 2011; Mendenhall et al., 2014).

In African countries, the government's mental health expenditure was estimated at US$0.1 per capita, compared to US$2.5 globally (World Health Organization, 2018). A study in South Africa estimated the annual cost of human resources required to scale up child and adolescent mental health services at US$5.99 per child for minimum coverage and US$21.50 per child for full coverage (Lund et al., 2010). In this analysis, the underlying assumption was that it would be possible to obtain trained personnel in the required numbers to deliver services, which was a stark contrast with the then-current realities in the country besides the cost implications.

Another study showed that, starting from a low level of service coverage, the cost of scaled-up provision of a package of evidence-based mental health services by nonspecialist providers would range between US$0.20 and US$0.56 per capita in Ethiopia, Uganda, Nepal, and India (Chisholm & Saxena, 2012). Underlying these estimates are a number of cost drivers in different country contexts, such as local drug prices, type of worker that will deliver services, type of facility (hospital vs. primary health center), and treatment setting (inpatient vs. outpatient care). Due to human resource constraints, task-shifting—delivery of interventions by non-specialist providers—in community platforms may be an effective and efficient strategy to facilitate the introduction of mental health interventions in low-resource settings (Healy et al., 2018).

Levin and Chisholm calculated the cost of scaling up evidence-based school-based programs to improve mental health, with costs ranging from US$0.03 per child in Ethiopia and India to US$0.11 in Mexico, and US$0.24 in Mauritius (Levin & Chisholm, 2016). The authors concluded that school-based delivery of mental health interventions was the most affordable in low-resource settings (Levin & Chisholm, 2016). School-based programs have also the potential to be sustainable as they have been shown to increase community and parental acceptance and buy-in (Kohrt et al., 2018).

The existing evidence suggests that reaching universal mental health coverage for children and adolescents would require investments in early childhood and preventive interventions and family-focused programs. It would also require less emphasis on psychopharmaceuticals, and more investment in treatment through group CBT interventions delivered at schools or in community settings for older children and adolescents and via home visits for young children and caregivers. In addition, considering poverty's multilayered effect on mental health, interventions targeting children and adolescents should include family economic empowerment and financial skill-building components, and consider basic nutritional and social security needs to address the underlying social determinants of poor mental health. Decision makers should prioritize and tailor interventions to disadvantaged families and children (Kieling et al., 2011). Outreach should include educational components to address and counter stigma and discrimination experienced by people with mental and psychosocial disabilities in many settings across the globe (Drew et al., 2011).

As previously discussed, current public spending on mental health in LMICs is insufficient to fund a package of cost-effective interventions. Clearly, a comprehensive response to the growing burden of mental disorders will require resources to bridge these resource gaps. Between 2007 and 2013, less than 1% of international health aid went into mental health (Gilbert et al., 2015). While national governments should play a major role in the financing of mental health care given the potential returns on investment, donors and international development agencies should help to redress the gaps in LMICs. The emergence of a strong global movement on mental health over the past decade may greatly help to direct dedicated sources of funding to break the cycle of neglect that affects mental health programs and interventions in LMICs today.

Sustainability

A key strategy for addressing inequalities in mental health is to integrate mental health care into primary care settings, as also recommended by mhGAP (Ngui et al., 2010). To that end, the importance of robust primary healthcare systems for successful integration and sustainability of mental health services is apparent (Jacob, 2017). However, there are several health system challenges in LMICs, including the weak state of healthcare systems, lack of human and financial resources, and concentration of health services in urban areas (Ngui et al., 2010). These broader challenges are further compounded by a number of barriers to the delivery of mental health services within primary care, including lack of mental health knowledge among primary care staff, lack of access to mental health drugs, high workload among primary care staff, and lack of space in health facilities for confidential consultation of patients (Gwaikolo et al., 2017; Jenkins et al., 2010; Petersen & Lund, 2011).

An appraisal of the state of mental health care and the costs and cost-effectiveness of mental health interventions in South Africa concluded that integrating mental health care with primary care or community services without the use of specialized providers would be the most effective and cost-efficient strategy to increase access to mental health services, including for those at high risk for mental health disorders such as persons living with HIV and with chronic conditions (Jack et al., 2014). All low-income countries were found to have far fewer mental health professionals than required to deliver a core package of mental health interventions for priority mental disorders (Bruckner et al., 2011). In that vein, a study conducted in five LMICs (i.e., Ethiopia, India, Nepal, South Africa, and Uganda) participating in the PRogramme for Improving Mental health carE (PRIME) highlighted the potential for applying existing models of care for HIV, tuberculosis, and other noncommunicable diseases to mental health care through established mechanisms for monitoring adherence to treatment and dropout from care, as well as outreach (Hanlon et al., 2014; Jenkins et al., 2010). The extensive network of community health workers and volunteers in most LMICs was identified as an opportunity to expand mental health care and reduce negative attitudes and stigma associated with mental disorders (Hanlon et al., 2014; Jenkins et al., 2010).

There is increasing evidence for effectiveness of mental health interventions delivered by nonspecialist providers in community settings in LMICs. For instance, a recent review of family-based mental health interventions delivered by nonspecialists targeting youth mental health (Healy et al., 2018) found ten interventions in LMICs, seven from SSA. Similar to Barry's findings (Barry et al., 2013), all of the interventions were conducted in areas with known risk factors for mental health disorders such as areas with high HIV prevalence or affected by conflict. The interventions were predominantly administered to groups, rather than individuals, and in community settings, such as schools, churches, and other common community spaces. Providers included teachers, community members, and lay counselors, including NGO workers.

All interventions had a didactic component targeting HIV risk factors, family-focused skill building, and positive parent-child communication and support, while none of the interventions were directly incorporated into primary care services. The review noted widespread acceptance of program material and delivery by nonspecialist providers, potentially increasing the effectiveness of interventions. Similarly, a recent meta-review focusing on community-based mental health interventions in LMICs identified the following as motivating factors: greater accessibility and acceptability compared to health facilities, greater effectiveness through ongoing contact and use of local providers trusted by communities, family involvement, and economic benefits (Kohrt et al., 2018). There was, however, great variation in the extent to which community-based components were integrated with primary care services. In most cases, child and adolescent interventions appeared to be delivered in groups and in parallel to existing services, typically outpatient clinics.

Use of nonspecialist providers has consistently proved to be feasible, acceptable, and effective and a valuable component of approaches to scaling up mental health programs. A clear next step is to better understand how to increase sustainability, for instance, through establishing and evaluating models of training and supervision of nonspecialist providers to further inform scalability and integration into existing healthcare infrastructure (Murray et al., 2011).

Developing an Economic Evidence Base for Mental Health Programs and Interventions

The true burden of mental health disorders among children and the concomitant treatment gaps in LMICs have not been well established in the literature (Sankoh et al., 2018). However, existing research suggests that there are significant gaps, and that the gaps will increase unless appropriate policy measures are taken. Mental health disorders are costly to individuals, families, and society. Major investments in human resource training and deployment as well as scale-up of community-based outreach programs and interventions are needed.

The limited evidence on the prevalence of mental health disorders among children and adolescents and on the effectiveness and cost-effectiveness of mental health interventions is a major challenge for evidence-based policy-making in this area. The paucity of quality evidence in LMICs is largely reflective of the limited capacity to design and undertake research that addresses these questions (Razzouk et al., 2010), which calls for strengthened collaborations among researchers, government agencies, and nongovernmental organizations.

At present, cost-effectiveness research primarily examines specific interventions, rather than package of interventions. Future cost-effectiveness studies will need to examine a broader range of integrated interventions. National cost-effectiveness estimates may differ greatly from global or regional estimates, and could be important for affecting changes in funding priorities at the country level. For instance, regional cost-effectiveness estimates do not fully account for inefficiencies in fragile health systems, such as high absenteeism and unfilled posts (Jack et al., 2014). Furthermore, there is a need to enumerate the wider social and economic benefits of improving mental health, such as gains in productivity and employment and reductions in costs in other parts of the economy, such as social care expenditures (e.g., child protection and social work services), for a more comprehensive assessment of the returns on investment. While cost-effectiveness evidence can inform decisions on resource allocation, information on economic benefits provides the basis for advocacy for mental health services. Nonetheless, an intervention has to be both cost effective and affordable in order to be of relevance to health policy makers.

There is a growing recognition of the synergies that exist between mental health and other noncommunicable diseases (Stein et al., 2019), and mental health in maternal and child health (Surkan et al., 2011). These linkages provide an opportunity to leverage funding from a range of donors, international development agencies, and governments to support the scale-up of mental health services with the caveat that if these platforms do not function well or are underfunded, mental health programs and interventions will also be ineffective (Patel & Saxena, 2019).

Building political commitment and will is key to the implementation of more integrated models of mental health care and expanding access to mental health services through different delivery platforms. Economic evidence may serve as a basis in making a persuasive argument and guiding policy makers to make informed choices about the importance of investment in mental health care and incorporating mental health services in national health insurance schemes.

References

Abbo, C., Kinyanda, E., Kizza, R. B., Levin, J., Ndyanabangi, S., & Stein, D. J. (2013). Prevalence, comorbidity and predictors of anxiety disorders in children and adolescents in rural north-eastern Uganda. *Child and Adolescent Psychiatry and Mental Health, 7*(1), 21.

Adewuya, A. O., Ola, B. A., & Adewumi, T. A. (2007). The 12-month prevalence of DSM-IV anxiety disorders among Nigerian secondary school adolescents aged 13–18 years. *Journal of Adolescence, 30*(6), 1071–1076.

Ae-Ngibise, K. A., Doku, V. C., Asante, K. P., & Owusu-Agyei, S. (2015). The experience of caregivers of people living with serious mental disorders: A study from rural Ghana. *Global Health Action, 8*, 26957.

Anderson, J. K., Ford, T., Soneson, E., Coon, J. T., Humphrey, A., Rogers, M., . . . Howarth, E. (2019). A systematic review of effectiveness and cost-effectiveness of school-based identification of children and young people at risk of, or currently experiencing mental health difficulties. *Psychological Medicine, 49*(1), 9–19. https://doi.org/10.1017/S0033291718002490

Anderson, R., Ukoumunne, O. C., Sayal, K., Phillips, R., Taylor, J. A., Spears, M., . . . Stallard, P. (2014). Cost-effectiveness of classroom-based cognitive behaviour therapy in reducing symptoms of depression in adolescents: A trial-based analysis. *Journal of Child Psychology and Psychiatry, 55*(12), 1390–1397.

Annan, J., Sim, A., Puffer, E. S., Salhi, C., & Betancourt, T. S. (2017). Improving mental health outcomes of Burmese migrant and displaced children in Thailand: A community-based randomized controlled trial of a parenting and family skills intervention. *Prevention Science, 18*(7), 793–803. https://doi.org/10.1007/s11121-016-0728-2

Aracena, M., Krause, M., Perez, C., Mendez, M. J., Salvatierra, L., Soto, M., . . . Altimir, C. (2009). A cost-effectiveness evaluation of a home visit program for adolescent mothers. *Journal of Health Psychology, 14*(7), 878–887. https://doi.org/10.1177/1359105309340988

Araya, R., Fritsch, R., Spears, M., Rojas, G., Martinez, V., Barroilhet, S., . . . Montgomery, A. A. (2013). School intervention to improve mental health of students in Santiago, Chile: A randomized clinical trial. *JAMA Pediatrics, 167*(11), 1004–1010. https://doi.org/10.1001/jamapediatrics.2013.2361

Barry, M. M., Clarke, A. M., Jenkins, R., & Patel, V. (2013). A systematic review of the effectiveness of mental health promotion interventions for young people in low and middle income countries. *BMC Public Health, 13*, 835.

Baxter, A. J., Patton, G., Scott, K. M., Degenhardt, L., & Whiteford, H. A. (2013). Global epidemiology of mental disorders: What are we missing? *PLoS One, 8*(6), e65514. https://doi.org/10.1371/journal.pone.0065514

Belfer, M. L. (2008). Child and adolescent mental disorders: The magnitude of the problem across the globe. *Journal of Child Psychology and Psychiatry, 49*(3), 226–236. https://doi.org/10.1111/j.1469-7610.2007.01855.x

Bell, C. C., Bhana, A., Petersen, I., McKay, M. M., Gibbons, R., Bannon, W., & Amatya, A. (2008). Building protective factors to offset sexually risky behaviors among Black youths. *Journal of the National Medical Association, 100*(8), 936–944.

Betancourt, T. S., Ng, L. C., Kirk, C. M., Munyanah, M., Mushashi, C., Ingabire, C., . . . Sezibera, V. (2014). Family-based prevention of mental health problems in children affected by HIV and AIDS: An open trial. *AIDS, 28*(Suppl 3), S359–S368. https://doi.org/10.1097/QAD.0000000000000336

Boris, N. W., Brown, L. A., Thurman, T. R., Rice, J. C., Snider, L. M., Ntaganira, J., & Nyirazinyoye, L. N. (2008). Depressive symptoms in youth heads of household in Rwanda. *Archives of Pediatrics & Adolescent Medicine, 162*(9), 836–843. https://doi.org/10.1001/archpedi.162.9.836

Britto, P. R., Ponguta, L. A., Reyes, C., & Karnati, R. (2015). *A systematic review of parenting programmes for young children.* Retrieved from https://www.unicef.org/earlychildhood/files/P_Shanker_final__Systematic_Review_of_Parenting_ECD_Dec_15_copy.pdf

Brody, E. B. (2004). The World Federation for Mental Health: Its origins and contemporary relevance to WHO and WPA policies. *World Psychiatry, 3*(1), 54.

Bruckner, T. A., Scheffler, R. M., Shen, G., Yoon, J., Chisholm, D., Morris, J., . . . Saxena, S. (2011). The mental health workforce gap in low- and middle-income countries: A needs-based approach. *Bulletin of the World Health Organization, 89*(3), 184–194. https://doi.org/10.2471/BLT.10.082784

Buttorff, C., Hock, R. S., Weiss, H. A., Naik, S., Araya, R., Kirkwood, B. R., . . . Patel, V. (2012). Economic evaluation of a task-shifting intervention for common mental disorders in India. *Bulletin of the World Health Organization, 90*(11), 813–821. https://doi.org/10.2471/BLT.12.104133

Carr, C., Martins, C., Stingel, A., Lemgruber, V., & Juruena, M. (2013). The role of early life stress in adult psychiatric disorders: A systematic review according to childhood trauma subtypes. *The Journal of Nervous and Mental Disease, 201*, 1007–1020. https://doi.org/10.1097/NMD.0000000000000049

Chisholm, D., & Saxena, S. (2012). Cost effectiveness of strategies to combat neuropsychiatric conditions in sub-Saharan Africa and South East Asia: Mathematical modelling study. *BMJ, 344*, e609. https://doi.org/10.1136/bmj.e609

Chorozoglou, M., Smith, E., Koerting, J., Thompson, M. J., Sayal, K., & Sonuga-Barke, E. J. (2015). Preschool hyperactivity is associated with long-term economic burden: Evidence from a longitudinal health economic analysis of costs incurred across childhood, adolescence and young adulthood. *Journal of Child Psychology and Psychiatry, 56*(9), 966–975. https://doi. org/10.1111/jcpp.12437

Compton, S. N., March, J. S., Brent, D., Albano, A. M. T., Weersing, R., & Curry, J. (2004). Cognitive-behavioral psychotherapy for anxiety and depressive disorders in children and adolescents: An evidence-based medicine review. *Journal of the American Academy of Child and Adolescent Psychiatry, 43*(8), 930–959. https://doi.org/10.1097/01.chi.0000127589. 57468.bf

Cortina, M. A., Sodha, A., Fazel, M., & Ramchandani, P. G. (2012). Prevalence of child mental health problems in sub-Saharan Africa: A systematic review. *Archives of Pediatrics & Adolescent Medicine, 166*(3), 276–281.

Das, J. K., Salam, R. A., Lassi, Z. S., Khan, M. N., Mahmood, W., Patel, V., & Bhutta, Z. A. (2016). Interventions for adolescent mental health: An overview of systematic reviews. *The Journal of Adolescent Health, 59*(4S), S49–S60. https://doi.org/10.1016/j.jadohealth.2016.06.020

de Jong, J. T., Berckmoes, L. H., Kohrt, B. A., Song, S. J., Tol, W. A., & Reis, R. (2015). A public health approach to address the mental health burden of youth in situations of political violence and humanitarian emergencies. *Current Psychiatry Reports, 17*(7), 60. https://doi.org/10.1007/ s11920-015-0590-0

de Souza, M. A., Salum, G. A., Jarros, R. B., Isolan, L., Davis, R., Knijnik, D., . . . Heldt, E. (2013). Cognitive-behavioral group therapy for youths with anxiety disorders in the community: Effectiveness in low and middle income countries. *Behavioural and Cognitive Psychotherapy, 41*(3), 255–264. https://doi.org/10.1017/S1352465813000015

Deschenes, S. S., Graham, E., Kivimaki, M., & Schmitz, N. (2018). Adverse childhood experiences and the risk of diabetes: Examining the roles of depressive symptoms and cardiometabolic dysregulations in the Whitehall II cohort study. *Diabetes Care, 41*(10), 2120–2126. https://doi. org/10.2337/dc18-0932

Dorsey, S., Lucid, L., Martin, P., King, K. M., O'Donnell, K., Murray, L. K., . . . Whetten, K. (2020). Effectiveness of task-shifted trauma-focused cognitive behavioral therapy for children who experienced parental death and posttraumatic stress in Kenya and Tanzania: A randomized clinical trial. *JAMA Psychiatry, 77*, 464.

Drew, N., Funk, M., Tang, S., Lamichhane, J., Chávez, E., Katontoka, S., . . . Saraceno, B. (2011). Human rights violations of people with mental and psychosocial disabilities: An unresolved global crisis. *The Lancet, 378*(9803), 1664–1675. https://doi.org/10.1016/S0140-6736(11) 61458-X

Ebert, D. D., Zarski, A. C., Christensen, H., Stikkelbroek, Y., Cuijpers, P., Berking, M., & Riper, H. (2015). Internet and computer-based cognitive behavioral therapy for anxiety and depression in youth: A meta-analysis of randomized controlled outcome trials. *PLoS One, 10*(3), e0119895. https://doi.org/10.1371/journal.pone.0119895

Eloff, I., Finestone, M., Makin, J. D., Boeving-Allen, A., Visser, M., Ebersohn, L., . . . Forsyth, B. W. (2014). A randomized clinical trial of an intervention to promote resilience in young children of HIV-positive mothers in South Africa. *AIDS, 28*(3), 347–357. https://doi.org/10. 1097/QAD.0000000000000335

Evans, D. B., Azene, G., & Kirigia, J. (1997). Should governments subsidize the use of insecticide-impregnated mosquito nets in Africa? Implications of a cost-effectiveness analysis. *Health Policy and Planning, 12*(2), 107–114.

Evans, T. G., & Murray, C. J. (1987). A critical re-examination of the economics of blindness prevention under the onchocerciasis control programme. *Social Science & Medicine, 25*(3), 241–249.

Fergusson, D. M., Horwood, L. J., & Ridder, E. M. (2005). Show me the child at seven: The consequences of conduct problems in childhood for psychosocial functioning in adulthood. *Journal of Child Psychology and Psychiatry, 46*(8), 837–849. https://doi.org/10.1111/j.1469-7610.2004.00387.x

Furlong, M., McGilloway, S., Bywater, T., Hutchings, J., Smith, S. M., & Donnelly, M. (2012). Behavioural and cognitive-behavioural group-based parenting programmes for early-onset conduct problems in children aged 3 to 12 years. *Cochrane Database of Systematic Reviews, 2*, 008225. https://doi.org/10.1002/14651858.CD008225.pub2

Gardner, F., Montgomery, P., & Knerr, W. (2016). Transporting evidence-based parenting programs for child problem behavior (age 3-10) between countries: Systematic review and meta-analysis. *Journal of Clinical Child and Adolescent Psychology, 45*(6), 749–762. https://doi.org/10.1080/15374416.2015.1015134

Gilbert, B. J., Patel, V., Farmer, P. E., & Lu, C. (2015). Assessing development assistance for mental health in developing countries: 2007-2013. *PLoS Medicine, 12*(6), e1001834. https://doi.org/10.1371/journal.pmed.1001834

Glass, N. J., & Goldberg, D. (1977). Cost-benefit analysis and the evaluation of psychiatric services. *Psychological Medicine, 7*(4), 701–707.

Global Burden of Disease Pediatrics Committee, Kyu, H. H., Pinho, C., Wagner, J. A., Brown, J. C., Bertozzi-Villa, A., & Vos, T. (2016). Global and national burden of diseases and injuries among children and adolescents between 1990 and 2013: Findings from the global burden of disease 2013 study. *JAMA Pediatrics, 170*(3), 267–287. https://doi.org/10.1001/jamapediatrics.2015.4276

Goesling, B., Colman, S., Trenholm, C., Terzian, M., & Moore, K. (2014). Programs to reduce teen pregnancy, sexually transmitted infections, and associated sexual risk behaviors: A systematic review. *The Journal of Adolescent Health, 54*(5), 499–507. https://doi.org/10.1016/j.jadohealth.2013.12.004

Grantham-McGregor, S., & Smith, J. A. (2016). Extending the Jamaican early childhood development intervention. *Journal of Applied Research on Children: Informing Policy for Children at Risk, 7*, 2.

Griswold, M. G., Fullman, N., Hawley, C., Arian, N., Zimsen, S. R. M., Tymeson, H. D., . . . Gakidou, E. (2018). Alcohol use and burden for 195 countries and territories, 1990–2016: A systematic analysis for the global burden of disease study 2016. *The Lancet, 392*(10152), 1015–1035. https://doi.org/10.1016/s0140-6736(18)31310-2

Gureje, O., Chisholm, D., Kola, L., Lasebikan, V., & Saxena, S. (2007). Cost-effectiveness of an essential mental health intervention package in Nigeria. *World Psychiatry, 6*(1), 42–48.

Gwaikolo, W. S., Kohrt, B. A., & Cooper, J. L. (2017). Health system preparedness for integration of mental health services in rural Liberia. *BMC Health Services Research, 17*(1), 508–508. https://doi.org/10.1186/s12913-017-2447-1

Hanlon, C., Luitel, N. P., Kathree, T., Murhar, V., Shrivasta, S., Medhin, G., . . . Prince, M. (2014). Challenges and opportunities for implementing integrated mental health care: A district level situation analysis from five low- and middle-income countries. *PLoS One, 9*(2), e88437.

Healy, E. A., Kaiser, B. N., & Puffer, E. S. (2018). Family-based youth mental health interventions delivered by nonspecialist providers in low- and middle-income countries: A systematic review. *Families, Systems & Health, 36*(2), 182–197. https://doi.org/10.1037/fsh0000334

Hutton, J. (2012). 'Health economics' and the evolution of economic evaluation of health technologies. *Health Economics, 21*(1), 13–18. https://doi.org/10.1002/hec.1818

Independent Evaluation Group. (2010). *Cost-benefit analysis in world bank projects.* Retrieved from https://openknowledge.worldbank.org/handle/10986/2561

Iribarren, S. J., Cato, K., Falzon, L., & Stone, P. W. (2017). What is the economic evidence for mHealth? A systematic review of economic evaluations of mHealth solutions. *PLoS One, 12*(2), e0170581. https://doi.org/10.1371/journal.pone.0170581

Ivbijaro, G., Kolkiewicz, L., Lionis, C., Svab, I., Cohen, A., & Sartorius, N. (2008). Primary care mental health and Alma-Ata: From evidence to action. *Mental Health in Family Medicine, 5*(2), 67–69.

Jack, H., Wagner, R. G., Petersen, I., Thom, R., Newton, C. R., Stein, A., & Hofman, K. J. (2014). Closing the mental health treatment gap in South Africa: A review of costs and cost-effectiveness. *Global Health Action, 7*, 1. https://doi.org/10.3402/gha.v7.23431

Jacob, K. S. (2017). Mental health services in low-income and middle-income countries. *Lancet Psychiatry, 4*, 87–88. https://doi.org/10.1016/S2215-0366(16)30423-0

James, A. C., James, G., Cowdrey, F. A., Soler, A., & Choke, A. (2015). Cognitive behavioural therapy for anxiety disorders in children and adolescents. *Cochrane Database of Systematic Reviews, 2015*, CD004690. https://doi.org/10.1002/14651858.CD004690.pub4

Javadi, D., Feldhaus, I., Mancuso, A., & Ghaffar, A. (2017). Applying systems thinking to task shifting for mental health using lay providers: A review of the evidence. *Global Mental Health, 4*, e14. https://doi.org/10.1017/gmh.2017.15

Jenkins, R. (2019). Global mental health and sustainable development 2018. *British Journal of Psychiatry, 16*(2), 34–37. https://doi.org/10.1192/bji.2019.5

Jenkins, R., Kiima, D., Okonji, M., Njenga, F., Kingora, J., & Lock, S. (2010). Integration of mental health into primary care and community health working in Kenya: Context, rationale, coverage and sustainability. *Mental Health in Family Medicine, 7*(1), 37–47.

Jenkins, R., Othieno, C., Ongeri, L., Ongecha, M., Sifuna, P., Omollo, R., & Ogutu, B. (2017). Malaria and mental disorder: A population study in an area endemic for malaria in Kenya. *World Psychiatry, 16*(3), 324–325. https://doi.org/10.1002/wps.20473

Jewkes, R., Nduna, M., Levin, J., Jama, N., Dunkle, K., Puren, A., & Duvvury, N. (2008). Impact of stepping stones on incidence of HIV and HSV-2 and sexual behaviour in rural South Africa: Cluster randomised controlled trial. *BMJ, 337*, a507.

Jonas, S., Bebbington, P., McManus, S., Meltzer, H., Jenkins, R., Kuipers, E., … Brugha, T. (2011). Sexual abuse and psychiatric disorder in England: Results from the 2007 adult psychiatric morbidity survey. *Psychological Medicine, 41*(4), 709–719. https://doi.org/10.1017/s003329171000111x

Kakuma, R., Minas, H., van Ginneken, N. et al. (2011). Human resources for mental health care: current situation and strategies for action. *Lancet, 378*(9803), 1654–1663.

Kariuki, S. M., Abubakar, A., Kombe, M. et al. (2017). Burden, risk factors, and comorbidities of behavioural and emotional problems in Kenyan children: a population-based study. *The Lancet Psychiatry, 4*(2), 136–145.

Kawakami, N., Abdulghani, E. A., Alonso, J., Bromet, E. J., Bruffaerts, R., Caldas-de-Almeida, J. M., … Kessler, R. C. (2012). Early-life mental disorders and adult household income in the world mental health surveys. *Biological Psychiatry, 72*(3), 228–237. https://doi.org/10.1016/j.biopsych.2012.03.009

Kessler, R. C., Amminger, P., Aguilar-Gaxiola, S., Alonso, J., Lee, S., & Ustun, T. B. (2007). Age of onset of mental disorders: A review of recent literature. *Current Opinion in Psychiatry, 20*(4), 359–364.

Kessler, R. C., McLaughlin, K. A., Green, J. G., Gruber, M. J., Sampson, N. A., Zaslavsky, A. M., … Williams, D. R. (2010). Childhood adversities and adult psychopathology in the WHO world mental health surveys. *The British Journal of Psychiatry: the Journal of Mental Science, 197*(5), 378–385. https://doi.org/10.1192/bjp.bp.110.080499

Kieling, C., Baker-Henningham, H., Belfer, M. L., Conti, G., Ertem, I., Omigbodun, O., … Rahman, A. (2011). Child and adolescent mental health worldwide: Evidence for action. *Lancet, 378*, 1515–1525. https://doi.org/10.1016/S0140-6736(11)60827-1

Kieling, C., & Rohde, L. A. (2012). Going global: Epidemiology of child and adolescent psychopathology. *Journal of the American Academy of Child and Adolescent Psychiatry, 51*(12), 1236–1237. https://doi.org/10.1016/j.jaac.2012.09.011

Klein, J. B., Jacobs, R. H., & Reinecke, M. A. (2007). Cognitive-behavioral therapy for adolescent depression: A meta-analytic investigation of changes in effect-size estimates. *Journal of the American Academy of Child and Adolescent Psychiatry, 46*(11), 1403–1413. https://doi.org/10.1097/chi.0b013e3180592aaa

Kohrt, B. A., Asher, L., Bhardwaj, A., Fazel, M., Jordans, M. J. D., Mutamba, B. B., … Patel, V. (2018). The role of communities in mental health care in low- and middle-income countries: A meta-review of components and competencies. *International Journal of Environmental Research and Public Health, 15*, 6. https://doi.org/10.3390/ijerph15061279

Kumakech, E., Cantor-Graae, E., Maling, S., & Bajunirwe, F. (2009). Peer-group support intervention improves the psychosocial well-being of AIDS orphans: Cluster randomized trial. *Social Science & Medicine, 68*, 1038–1043. https://doi.org/10.1016/j.socscimed.20

Lee, S., Tsang, A., Breslau, J., Aguilar-Gaxiola, S., Angermeyer, M., Borges, G., . . . Kessler, R. C. (2009). Mental disorders and termination of education in high-income and low- and middle-income countries: Epidemiological study. *The British Journal of Psychiatry, 194*(5), 411–417.

Levin, C., & Chisholm, D. (2016). Cost-effectiveness and affordability of interventions, policies, and platforms for the prevention and treatment of mental, neurological, and substance use disorders. In V. Patel, D. Chisholm, T. Dua, R. Laxminarayan, & M. E. Medina-Mora (Eds.), *Mental, neurological, and substance use disorders: Disease control priorities.* International Bank for Reconstruction and Development/The World Bank.

Levinson, D., Lakoma, M. D., Petukhova, M., Schoenbaum, M., Zaslavsky, A. M., Angermeyer, M., & Kessler, R. C. (2010). Associations of serious mental illness with earnings: Results from the WHO world mental health surveys. *The British Journal of Psychiatry, 197*(2), 114–121. https://doi.org/10.1192/bjp.bp.109.073635

Lund, C., Breen, A., Flisher, A. J., Kakuma, R., Corrigall, J., Joska, J. A., . . . Patel, V. (2010). Poverty and common mental disorders in low and middle income countries: A systematic review. *Social Science & Medicine, 71*(3), 517–528. https://doi.org/10.1016/j.socscimed.2010.04.027

Lund, C., Myer, L., Stein, D. J., Williams, D. R., & Flisher, A. J. (2013). Mental illness and lost income among adult South Africans. *Social Psychiatry and Psychiatric Epidemiology, 48*, 845–851.

Lyons-Ruth, K., Todd Manly, J., Von Klitzing, K., Tamminen, T., Emde, R., Fitzgerald, H., . . . Watanabe, H. (2017). The worldwide burden of infant mental and emotional disorder: Report of the Task Force of the World Association for Infant Mental Health. *Infant Mental Health Journal, 38*(6), 695–705. https://doi.org/10.1002/imhj.21674

Mascayano, F., Armijo, J. E., & Yang, L. H. (2015). Addressing stigma relating to mental illness in low- and middle-income countries. *Frontiers in Psychiatry, 6*, 38–38. https://doi.org/10.3389/fpsyt.2015.00038

McBain, R. K., Salhi, C., Hann, K., Salomon, J. A., Kim, J. J., & Betancourt, T. S. (2016). Costs and cost-effectiveness of a mental health intervention for war-affected young persons: Decision analysis based on a randomized controlled trial. *Health Policy and Planning, 31*(4), 415–424. https://doi.org/10.1093/heapol/czv078

McCrone, P., Knapp, M., & Fombonne, E. (2005). The Maudsley long-term follow-up of child and adolescent depression. Predicting costs in adulthood. *European Child & Adolescent Psychiatry, 14*(7), 407–413. https://doi.org/10.1007/s00787-005-0491-6

McDaid, D. (2018). *Using economic evidence to help make the case for investing in health promotion and disease prevention.* WHO.

Mellins, C. A., & Malee, K. M. (2013). Understanding the mental health of youth living with perinatal HIV infection: Lessons learned and current challenges. *Journal of the International AIDS Society, 16*, 18593. https://doi.org/10.7448/IAS.16.1.18593

Mendenhall, E., De Silva, M. J., Hanlon, C. et al. (2014). Acceptability and feasibility of using non-specialist health workers to deliver mental health care: stakeholder perceptions from the PRIME district sites in Ethiopia, India, Nepal, South Africa, and Uganda. *Social Science & Medicine 118*, 33–42.

Mihalopoulos, C., Magnus, A., Lal, A., Dell, L., Forbes, D., & Phelps, A. (2015a). Is implementation of the 2013 Australian treatment guidelines for posttraumatic stress disorder cost-effective compared to current practice? A cost-utility analysis using QALYs and DALYs. *The Australian and New Zealand Journal of Psychiatry, 49*(4), 360–376. https://doi.org/10.1177/0004867414553948

Mihalopoulos, C., Vos, T., Pirkis, J., & Carter, R. (2011). The economic analysis of prevention in mental health programs. *Annual Review of Clinical Psychology, 7*, 169–201. https://doi.org/10.1146/annurev-clinpsy-032210-104601

Mihalopoulos, C., Vos, T., Rapee, R. M., Pirkis, J., Chatterton, M. L., Lee, Y. C., & Carter, R. (2015b). The population cost-effectiveness of a parenting intervention designed to prevent anxiety disorders in children. *Journal of Child Psychology and Psychiatry, 56*(9), 1026–1033. https://doi.org/10.1111/jcpp.12438

Monath, T. P., & Nasidi, A. (1993). Should yellow fever vaccine be included in the expanded program of immunization in Africa? A cost-effectiveness analysis for Nigeria. *The American Journal of Tropical Medicine and Hygiene, 48*(2), 274–299.

Monnat, S. M., & Chandler, R. F. (2015). Long term physical health consequences of adverse childhood experiences. *The Sociological Quarterly, 56*(4), 723–752. https://doi.org/10.1111/tsq.12107

Murray, L. K., Dorsey, S., Bolton, P., Jordans, M. J., Rahman, A., Bass, J., & Verdeli, H. (2011). Building capacity in mental health interventions in low resource countries: An apprenticeship model for training local providers. *International Journal of Mental Health Systems, 5*(1), 30.

Murray, L. K., Dorsey, S., Skavenski, S., Kasoma, M., Imasiku, M., Bolton, P., . . . Cohen, J. A. (2013a). Identification, modification, and implementation of an evidence-based psychotherapy for children in a low-income country: The use of TF-CBT in Zambia. *International Journal of Mental Health Systems, 7*(1), 24. https://doi.org/10.1186/1752-4458-7-24

Murray, L. K., Familiar, I., Skavenski, S., Jere, E., Cohen, J., Imasiku, M., . . . Bolton, P. (2013b). An evaluation of trauma focused cognitive behavioral therapy for children in Zambia. *Child Abuse & Neglect, 37*(12), 1175–1185. https://doi.org/10.1016/j.chiabu.2013.04.017

Murray, L. K., Skavenski, S., Kane, J. C., Mayeya, J., Dorsey, S., Cohen, J. A., . . . Bolton, P. A. (2015). Effectiveness of trauma-focused cognitive behavioral therapy among trauma-affected children in Lusaka, Zambia: A randomized clinical TrialTrauma-focused cognitive behavioral therapy trauma-focused cognitive behavioral therapy. *JAMA Pediatrics, 169*(8), 761–769. https://doi.org/10.1001/jamapediatrics.2015.0580

Mutamba, B. B., Ginneken, Nv., Paintain, L. S., Wandiembe, S., & Schellenberg, D. (2013). Roles and effectiveness of lay community health workers in the prevention of mental, neurological and substance use disorders in low and middle income countries: a systematic review. *BMC Health Services Research, 13*, 412.

Naficy, A., Rao, M. R., Paquet, C., Antona, D., Sorkin, A., & Clemens, J. D. (1998). Treatment and vaccination strategies to control cholera in sub-Saharan refugee settings: A cost-effectiveness analysis. *JAMA, 279*(7), 521–525.

Ngui, E. M., Khasakhala, L., Ndetei, D., & Roberts, L. W. (2010). Mental disorders, health inequalities and ethics: A global perspective. *International Review of Psychiatry, 22*(3), 235–244. https://doi.org/10.3109/09540261.2010.485273

Nystrand, C., Feldman, I., Enebrink, P., & Sampaio, F. (2019). Cost-effectiveness analysis of parenting interventions for the prevention of behaviour problems in children. *PLoS One, 14*(12), e0225503. https://doi.org/10.1371/journal.pone.0225503

Ophuis, R. H., Lokkerbol, J., Heemskerk, S. C., van Balkom, A. J., Hiligsmann, M., & Evers, S. M. (2017). Cost-effectiveness of interventions for treating anxiety disorders: A systematic review. *Journal of Affective Disorders, 210*, 1–13. https://doi.org/10.1016/j.jad.2016.12.005

Opoku-Boateng, Y. N., Kretchy, I. A., Aryeetey, G. C., Dwomoh, D., Decker, S., Agyemang, S. A., . . . Nonvignon, J. (2017). Economic cost and quality of life of family caregivers of schizophrenic patients attending psychiatric hospitals in Ghana. *BMC Health Services Research, 17* (Suppl 2), 697. https://doi.org/10.1186/s12913-017-2642-0

Owen, J. P., Baig, B., Abbo, C., & Baheretibeb, Y. (2016). Child and adolescent mental health in sub-Saharan Africa: A perspective from clinicians and researchers. *British Journal of Psychiatry, 13*(2), 45–47.

Patalay, P., & Fitzsimons, E. (2016). Correlates of mental illness and wellbeing in children: Are they the same? Results from the UK millennium cohort study. *Journal of the American Academy of Child and Adolescent Psychiatry, 55*(9), 771–783. https://doi.org/10.1016/j.jaac.2016.05.019

Patel, V., & Saxena, S. (2019). Achieving universal health coverage for mental disorders. *BMJ, 366*, l4516. https://doi.org/10.1136/bmj.l4516

Patel, V., Saxena, S., Lund, C., Thornicroft, G., Baingana, F., Bolton, P., . . . UnÜtzer, J. (2018). The Lancet Commission on global mental health and sustainable development. *The Lancet, 392* (10157), 1553–1598. https://doi.org/10.1016/s0140-6736(18)31612-x

Pedersen, G. A., Smallegange, E., Coetzee, A., Hartog, K., Turner, J., Jordans, M. J. D., & Brown, F. L. (2019). A systematic review of the evidence for family and parenting interventions in low- and middle-income countries: Child and youth mental health outcomes. *Journal of Child and Family Studies, 28*(8), 2036–2055. https://doi.org/10.1007/s10826-019-01399-4

Petersen, I., & Lund, C. (2011). Mental health service delivery in South Africa from 2000 to 2010: One step forward, one step back. *South African Medical Journal, 101*(10), 751–757.

Prost, A., & Prescott, N. (1984). Cost-effectiveness of blindness prevention by the onchocerciasis control programme in upper volta. *Bulletin of the World Health Organization, 62*(5), 795–802.

Puffer, E. S., Green, E. P., Sikkema, K. J., Broverman, S. A., Ogwang-Odhiambo, R. A., & Pian, J. (2016). A church-based intervention for families to promote mental health and prevent HIV among adolescents in rural Kenya: Results of a randomized trial. *Journal of Consulting and Clinical Psychology, 84*(6), 511–525. https://doi.org/10.1037/ccp0000076

Purgato, M., Gastaldon, C., Papola, D., van Ommeren, M., Barbui, C., & Tol, W. A. (2018). Psychological therapies for the treatment of mental disorders in low- and middle-income countries affected by humanitarian crises. *Cochrane Database of Systematic Reviews, 7*, CD011849. https://doi.org/10.1002/14651858.CD011849.pub2

Rathod, S., Pinninti, N., Irfan, M., Gorczynski, P., Rathod, P., Gega, L., & Naeem, F. (2017). Mental health service provision in low-and middle-income countries. *Health Services Insights, 10*, 1–7.

Razzouk, D., Sharan, P., Gallo, C., Gureje, O., Lamberte, E. E., de Jesus Mari, J., et al. (2010). Scarcity and inequity of mental health research resources in low- and middle-income countries: A global survey. *Health Policy, 94*(3), 211–220. https://doi.org/10.1016/j.healthpol.2009.09.009

Redfern, A., Cluver, L. D., Casale, M., & Steinert, J. I. (2019). Cost and cost-effectiveness of a parenting programme to prevent violence against adolescents in South Africa. *BMJ Global Health, 4*(3), e001147. https://doi.org/10.1136/bmjgh-2018-001147

Reynolds, A. J., Temple, J. A., Robertson, D. L., & Mann, E. A. (2002). Age 21 cost-benefit analysis of the title I Chicago child-parent centers. *Educational Evaluation and Policy Analysis, 24*(4), 267–303. https://doi.org/10.3102/01623737024004267

Rivet-Duval, E., Heriot, S., & Hunt, C. (2011). Preventing adolescent depression in Mauritius: A universal school-based program. *Child and Adolescent Mental Health, 16*(2), 86–91. https://doi.org/10.1111/j.1475-3588.2010.00584.x

Rosenfield, P. L., Golladay, F., & Davidson, R. K. (1984). The economics of parasitic diseases: Research priorities. *Social Science & Medicine, 19*(10), 1117–1126.

Russell, L. B. (2015). *The science of making better decisions about health: Cost-effectiveness and cost-benefit analysis.* Retrieved from http://www.ahrq.gov/professionals/education/curriculum-tools/population-health/russell.html

Russell, L. B., Gold, M. R., Siegel, J. E., Daniels, N., & Weinstein, M. C. (1996). The role of cost-effectiveness analysis in health and medicine: Panel on cost-effectiveness in health and medicine. *JAMA, 276*(14), 1172–1177.

Sandler, I., Ingram, A., Wolchik, S., Tein, J. Y., & Winslow, E. (2015). Long-term effects of parenting-focused preventive interventions to promote resilience of children and adolescents. *Child Development Perspectives, 9*(3), 164–171. https://doi.org/10.1111/cdep.12126

Sankoh, O., Sevalie, S., & Weston, M. (2018). Mental health in Africa. *The Lancet Global Health, 6* (9), e954–e955. https://doi.org/10.1016/s2214-109x(18)30303-6

Sarnquist, C., Sinclair, J., Omondi Mboya, B., Langat, N., Paiva, L., Halpern-Felsher, B., . . . Baiocchi, M. T. (2017). Evidence that classroom-based behavioral interventions reduce pregnancy-related school dropout among Nairobi adolescents. *Health Education & Behavior, 44*(2), 297–303. https://doi.org/10.1177/1090198116657777

Schwartz, C., Barican, J. L., Yung, D., Zheng, Y., & Waddell, C. (2019). Six decades of preventing and treating childhood anxiety disorders: A systematic review and meta-analysis to inform policy and practice. *Evidence-Based Mental Health, 22*(3), 103–110. https://doi.org/10.1136/ebmental-2019-300096

Scott, J. G., Mihalopoulos, C., Erskine, H. E., Roberts, J., & Rahman, A. (2015). Childhood mental and developmental disorders. In V. Patel, D. Chisholm, T. Dua, R. Laxminarayan, & M. E. Medina-Mora (Eds.), *Mental, neurological, and substance use disorders* (3rd ed.). World Bank.

Scott, S., Knapp, M., Henderson, J., & Maughan, B. (2001). Financial cost of social exclusion: Follow up study of antisocial children into adulthood. *BMJ, 323*(7306), 191.

Seidman, G., & Atun, R. (2017). Does task shifting yield cost savings and improve efficiency for health systems? A systematic review of evidence from low-income and middle-income countries. *Human Resources for Health, 15*(1), 29. https://doi.org/10.1186/s12960-017-0200-9

Semrau, M., Evans-Lacko, S., Koschorke, M., Ashenafi, L., & Thornicroft, G. (2015). Stigma and discrimination related to mental illness in low- and middle-income countries. *Epidemiology and Psychiatric Sciences, 24*(5), 382–394. https://doi.org/10.1017/s2045796015000359

Shaaban, K. M. A., & Baashar, T. A. (2003). A community study of depression in adolescent girls: Prevalence and its relation to age. *Medical Principles and Practice, 12*(4), 256–259.

Siskind, D., Baingana, F., & Kim, J. (2008). Cost-effectiveness of group psychotherapy for depression in Uganda. *The Journal of Mental Health Policy and Economics, 11*(3), 127–133.

Small, L., Mercado, M., Gopalan, P., Pardo, G., Ann Mellins, C., & McKay, M. M. (2014). Enhancing the emotional wellbeing of perinatally HIV infected youth across global contexts. *Global Social Welfare, 1*(1), 25–35. https://doi.org/10.1007/s40609-014-0009-6

Ssewamala, F. M., Neilands, T. B., Waldfogel, J., & Ismayilova, L. (2012). The impact of a comprehensive microfinance intervention on depression levels of AIDS-orphaned children in Uganda. *The Journal of Adolescent Health, 50*(4), 346–352.

Ssewamala, F. M., Wang, J. S., Neilands, T. B., Bermudez, L. G., Garfinkel, I., Waldfogel, J., . . . Kirkbride, G. (2018). Cost-effectiveness of a savings-led economic empowerment intervention for AIDS-affected adolescents in Uganda: Implications for scale-up in low-resource communities. *The Journal of Adolescent Health, 62*(1S), S29–S36. https://doi.org/10.1016/j.jadohealth.2017.09.026

Stein, D. J., Benjet, C., Gureje, O., Lund, C., Scott, K. M., Poznyak, V., & van Ommeren, M. (2019). Integrating mental health with other non-communicable diseases. *BMJ, 364*, l295. https://doi.org/10.1136/bmj.l295

Sudre, P., Breman, J. G., McFarland, D., & Koplan, J. P. (1992). Treatment of chloroquine-resistant malaria in African children: A cost-effectiveness analysis. *International Journal of Epidemiology, 21*(1), 146–154.

Surkan, P. J., Kennedy, C. E., Hurley, K. M., & Black, M. M. (2011). Maternal depression and early childhood growth in developing countries: Systematic review and meta-analysis. *Bulletin of the World Health Organization, 89*(8), 608–615. https://doi.org/10.2471/BLT.11.088187

The Government Office for Science. (2008). *Foresight mental capital and wellbeing project: Final project report.* Retrieved from https://assets.publishing.service.gov.uk/government/uploads/system/uploads/attachment_data/file/292450/mental-capital-wellbeing-report.pdf

Thompson, E. H., & Doll, W. (1982). The burden of families coping with the mentally III: An invisible crisis. *Family Relations, 31*(3), 379–388. https://doi.org/10.2307/584170

Thornicroft, G., & Tansella, M. (2009). *Better mental health care.* Cambridge, UK: Cambridge University Press.

Tozan, Y., Sun, S., Capasso, A., Shu-Huah Wang, J., Neilands, T. B., Bahar, O. S., . . . Ssewamala, F. M. (2019). Evaluation of a savings-led family-based economic empowerment intervention for AIDS-affected adolescents in Uganda: A four-year follow-up on efficacy and cost-effectiveness. *PLoS One, 14*(12), e0226809–e0226809. https://doi.org/10.1371/journal.pone.0226809

Tozan, Y., Sun, S., Capasso, A., Shu-Huah Wang, J., Neilands, T. B., Bahar, O. S., . . . Ssewamala, F. M. (2020). Evaluation of a savings-led family-based economic empowerment intervention for

AIDS-affected adolescents in Uganda: A four-year follow-up on efficacy and cost-effectiveness. *PLoS One, 14*(12), e0226809. https://doi.org/10.1371/journal.pone.0226809

United Nations. (2017a). *Changing population age structures and sustainable development: A concise report*. Retrieved from https://www.un.org/en/development/desa/population/publica tions/pdf/trends/ConciseReport2017/English.pdf

United Nations. (2017b). *World population prospects 2017*. Retrieved from https://population.un. org/wpp/DataQuery/

Vreeman, R. C., McCoy, B. M., & Lee, S. (2017). Mental health challenges among adolescents living with HIV. *Journal of the International AIDS Society, 20*(Suppl 3), 21497. https://doi.org/ 10.7448/IAS.20.4.21497

Washington State Institute for Public Policy (WSIPP). (2018). Benefit-cost results. https://www. wsipp.wa.gov/BenefitCostx. Accessed February 13, 2020.

World Health Organization. (1946). Preamble to the Constitution of the World Health Organization. Paper presented at the International Health Conference, New York, NY.

World Health Organization. (1978). Declaration of Alma-Ata. Paper presented at the International Conference on Primary Health Care, Alma-Ata, USSR.

World Health Organization. (2001). *The World health report: 2001: Mental health: new under-standing, new hope*. Retrieved from http://www.who.int/iris/handle/10665/42390

World Health Organization. (2008). mhGAP: Mental Health Gap Action Programme: scaling up care for mental, neurological and substance use disorders.

World Health Organization. (2013). *Mental health action plan 2013–2020*. Retrieved from https:// www.who.int/publications/i/item/9789241506021

World Health Organization. (2018). *Mental health atlas 2017*. Retrieved from https://apps.who.int/ iris/bitstream/handle/10665/272735/9789241514019-eng.pdf?ua=1

Yatham, S., Sivathasan, S., Yoon, R., da Silva, T. L., & Ravindran, A. V. (2017). Depression, anxiety, and post-traumatic stress disorder among youth in low and middle income countries: A review of prevalence and treatment interventions. *Asian Journal of Psychiatry, 38*, 78. https:// doi.org/10.1016/j.ajp.2017.10.029

Yoder, H. N. C., Tol, W. A., Reis, R., & de Jong, J. T. V. M. (2016). Child mental health in Sierra Leone: A survey and exploratory qualitative study. *International Journal of Mental Health Systems, 10*, 48–48. https://doi.org/10.1186/s13033-016-0080-8

Zechmeister, I., Kilian, R., & McDaid, D. (2008). Is it worth investing in mental health promotion and prevention of mental illness? A systematic review of the evidence from economic evalua-tions. *BMC Public Health, 8*, 20. https://doi.org/10.1186/1471-2458-8-20

Zergaw, A., Hailemariam, D., Alem, A., & Kebede, D. (2008). A longitudinal comparative analysis of economic and family caregiver burden due to bipolar disorder. *The African Journal of Psychiatry, 11*, 191–198.

Child Maltreatment and Mental Health in Sub-Saharan Africa

Besa Bauta and Keng-Yen Huang

Introduction

Child maltreatment continues to be a salient issue and global health burden in low- and middle-income countries (LMICs) given existing challenges with security due to regional conflicts, access to economic opportunities, and resources such as health, education, and social services. Despite recognition that child maltreatment is a critical public health issue in developing countries, and despite efforts made by the WHO and child violence and maltreatment scholars to implement a set of recommended strategies to end violence against children (e.g., implementation and enforcement of laws, shifting norms and values, creating safe environments, parent and caregiver support, income and economic strengthening, providing response and support services, and enhancing education and life skills), progress has been slow. Challenges remain in implementing recommended strategies effectively due to inadequacy of in-country policies, lack of reactive child welfare systems, and lack of systematic research in LMICs. It remains unclear how international guidelines have been applied in LMICs, what research progress has been made in different regions of LMICs, how child maltreatment impacts child physical and mental health, what interventions can mitigate negative effects, and what is the impact for applying different intervention strategies. To address these research and practice knowledge gaps, it is critical to examine existing research and practice around child violence and

B. Bauta (✉)
Silver School of Social Work, New York University, New York, NY, USA
e-mail: Besa.Bauta@nyu.edu

K.-Y. Huang
Department of Population Health, School of Medicine, NYU Langone Health, New York, NY, USA

© Springer Nature Switzerland AG 2022   67
F. M. Ssewamala et al. (eds.), *Child Behavioral Health in Sub-Saharan Africa*,
https://doi.org/10.1007/978-3-030-83707-5_4

maltreatment in LMICs. In this chapter, we provide a summary of the recent publications in basic science, practice, and policy research related to child maltreatment in African settings. First, we present the prevalence and epidemiological research on maltreatment and child health (including physical and mental health). Then, we outline the global agenda for child maltreatment prevention and control, resources, systems, policies in Africa, and challenges in integrating violence prevention services and child mental health care in African settings. Lastly, we outline frameworks and strategies to address child violence, abuse, neglect, and mental health needs in LMIC settings, and offer suggestions and recommendations for future studies.

Child Maltreatment

Typology and Definitions of Child Maltreatment

Child maltreatment, also commonly referred to as child abuse and neglect, can include physical, sexual, and emotional mistreatment. Child maltreatment is an umbrella term that also includes negligent treatment of children, such as lack of appropriate medical care, access to educational opportunities, and exploitation (e.g., trafficking, sexual exploitation, labor) that can result in actual or potential harm to the child's health and well-being (WHO, 2017a, 2017b; Leeb et al., 2008; CDC, 2010, 2014, 2016a). Among the five subtypes of child maltreatment, the most commonly studied in LMICs focuses on physical abuse. This is due to the visibility of this type of abuse, existing physical abuse prevalence studies, and widespread use of disciplinary practices in LMICs, such as corporal punishment. Other types of maltreatment, such as sexual abuse and child neglect, are more difficult to assess and are often confounded by social factors. Sexual abuse is confounded by taboos around sexuality and sexual health while child neglect is confounded by poverty, local labor conditions, and family's socioeconomic status (WHO, 2006, 2016a, 2017a; Conger et al., 2010). Furthermore, children in LMICs are often engaged in activities that would be considered child maltreatment such as child labor, or not attending school in order to support their families with caregiving or other needs (WHO, 2006).

Based on the World Health Organization's (WHO) child maltreatment framework (2005, 2006), and Centers for Disease Control and Prevention (CDC) technical package for policy, norm, and programmatic activities to prevent child abuse and neglect (Fortson et al., 2016), the definitions of maltreatment include four domains:

- Physical abuse includes hitting, kicking, shaking, burning, or other forces against a child.
- Sexual abuse involves coercing a child to engage in sexual activities (e.g., fondling, penetration, and sexual exploitation).

- Emotional abuse refers to behaviors that harm a child's emotional well-being (e.g., name-calling, threatening with physical force, rejection, shaming, and withholding affection).
- Neglect refers to the failure of a caregiver to meet a child's needs including food, shelter, clothing, access to education, recreational activities, and medical care.

Finkelhor and Korbin (1988) expanded the child maltreatment definition through the inclusion of the following dimensions: child meeting societal/cultural definitions of a minor; goal of the action and/or intention was perpetrated by an individual with an intention to cause harm; the act of violence was censured by the culture; and the action met definition of maltreatment as per international standards (such as WHO protocols around Child Maltreatment) (Pierce & Bozalek, 2004). Finkelhor and Korbin (1988) emphasized that child maltreatment dimensions are crucial in understanding and placing maltreatment and child violence within a local context and within social frameworks. They took into consideration who can be defined a minor, and if the act of violence is largely accepted within that culture or social milieu. This definition places an emphasis on how child maltreatment fits within the larger social context.

In their assessment of physical punishment in several countries, Lansford et al. (2010) report that across their study sample including China, Colombia, Italy, Jordan, Kenya, the Philippines, Sweden, Thailand, and the United States, 54% of girls and 58% of boys had experienced mild physical punishment, and 13% of girls and 14% of boys had experienced severe punishment by their parents or other caregivers in their household in the last month. This data reveals that the use of punishment as a discipline practice is commonly utilized by parents and caregivers globally. In Kenya ($n = 100$), 82% of girls and 97% of boys reported being subjected to mild corporal punishment, and 61% of girls and 62% of boys reported experiencing severe physical punishment from their parents or other caregivers. Mild physical punishment included spanking, hitting, or slapping with a bare hand; hitting or slapping on the hand, arm, or leg; and shaking or hitting with an object. Severe physical punishment included hitting or slapping the child on the face, head, or ears, and beating the child repeatedly with an implement to cause pain or discomfort (Lansford et al., 2010). For example, in Uganda, children identified physical punishment both in their home and school setting as one of their major concerns, and 90% reported having experienced some form of physical punishment at home, and 79% at school (GIECPC, 2017; The Republic of Uganda, 2006, 2016). The frequent use of this type of discipline (i.e., both mild and severe physical punishment) within Uganda and other sub-Saharan African countries reflects a normative form of this type of discipline practice and often is the default method for disciplining children in the region. In the case of sub-Saharan African countries, parental discipline practices often include harsh discipline and physical punishment, and these behaviors are not censured by the culture (Lansford et al., 2010; Republic of Uganda, 2006, 2016; GIECPC, 2017).

Risk, Protective Factors, and Impact of Child Maltreatment on Physical and Mental Health

Risk factors for child maltreatment include individual predisposition, family, community, and societal risks. The risks for physical and sexual abuse have been well documented; recent research on the impact of neglect and emotional abuse paints an even more complex profile about the interrelated nature between negative childhood experiences and adult health and mental health (CWIG, 2019; NSCDC, 2020). The consequences of this take years to present in full clinical profiles due to the complex nature of neglect and emotional abuse (Rosen et al., 2018; NSCDC, 2020). Risks for physical abuse include poverty, unemployment, parental exposure to child maltreatment as a child, parental mental health, substance abuse, and interpersonal violence (WHO, 2006; Conger et al., 2010). The risks for sexual abuse include being female, living in a family without biological parents, poor or deteriorating relationship between parents, presence of a stepfather, strength of the relationship between the parent and child, younger maternal age, and parental death (MacMillan & Wathen, 2014; Norman et al., 2012).

The impacts of experiencing child violence, including neglect, include higher prevalence of depression, anxiety, and learning and developmental disabilities as children (CWIG, 2019). Children who have experienced prolonged neglect and toxic stress exhibit altered brain chemistry and inability to regulate psychological and mental health states (NSCDC, 2020). Furthermore, stress increases allostatic load that affects a child's response to threatening situations and their ability to manage external and internal stressors. Dysregulated stress response leads to long-lasting changes in the immune system (ability to manage infections), neuroendocrine system (ability to modulate and maintain hormonal balance), heart and cardiovascular systems (ability to regulate glucose and oxygen production), and metabolic systems (ability to manage energy production, storage, and use) (NSCDC, 2020; McEwen & Akil, 2020). Adults who have experienced child maltreatment have long-term negative physical health consequences including higher predisposition to conditions such as diabetes and high blood pressure which can lead to an increased chance for a heart attack, back problems, chronic fatigue, and persistent headaches, including functional limitations (CWIG, 2019). Child maltreatment has a direct link with increased prevalence of cancer, chronic obstructive pulmonary disease (COPD), lung disease, and many other physical ailments.

Additional consequences of maltreatment include lifelong psychological and behavioral impacts. Survivors of child abuse and neglect have difficulty modulating emotions, communicating, learning, and making decisions due to diminished executive functioning and changes in hippocampus (learning and memory) and orbitofrontal cortex (decision-making) (CWIG, 2019; NSCDC, 2020; McEwen & Akil, 2020). There are also societal influences such as higher abuse of alcohol, narcotic, and illicit substances by adults who were maltreated as children, and increased utilization of emergency treatment and health services (CWIG, 2019). Child abuse and neglect is one of the few conditions with multisystemic influence, from individual to family, community, and national level. Its influence crosscuts many areas of functioning and it is one of the few issues which can be addressed effectively with preventive interventions.

The negative consequences of abuse and neglect are many; however children, adolescents, and even adults that have experienced maltreatment can recover and ameliorate some of the negative effects with promising interventions. Research on brain plasticity shows that with early intervention many of the negative effects of abuse and neglect can be reversed (CWIG, 2015, 2019; NSCDC, 2020). Children who have experienced maltreatment were able to recover neural connections and direct therapeutic intervention was able to stymie some of the negative socio-emotional-developmental effects (Shonkoff & Phillips, 2000). Because child mal-treatment is so common, not everyone that experiences abuse and neglect develops negative socio-emotional and physical effects. There are many genetic, biological, temperamental, and other factors which are protective such as the ability to form nurturing attachments, social connections, and a sense of purpose and agency that can buffer the effect of maltreatment (CWIG, 2019; NSCDC, 2020). Preventive measures include offering concrete supports for parents struggling financially, teaching new parents about child development and positive parenting practices, and helping children build and repair existing social connections.

Poverty and Neglect

There is also a growing body of research that correlates poverty, violence, mental health, and child neglect (Kimbro & Denney, 2015; Drake & Jonson-Reid, 2014). Child neglect occurs when parents are not able to provide for the educational, medical, and psycho-emotional needs of children as predefined by social obligations (Drake & Jonson-Reid, 2014). Neglect occurs at all levels of the socioeconomic gradient; however due to limited financial means poor parents often struggle to meet their children's basic needs (such as food and shelter) with additional obligations such as healthcare and education (Drake & Jonson-Reid, 2014). In regions with limited access to public goods it becomes difficult for even middle-class families to meet all child obligations. For parents experiencing marginal or absolute poverty, meeting those child obligations often seems insurmountable. Absolute poverty or extreme poverty is defined as an individual's or family's inability to access and/or secure necessities (e.g., food, water, sanitation, housing, clothing), whereas relative poverty is defined as an individual and/or family not meeting a set living standard defined by the society that they are part of (Madden, 2000; Wilkinson, 1997). Children in sub-Saharan Africa (SSA) are disproportionally more likely to experi-ence both relative and abject poverty and parents often struggle with maintaining basic needs which creates greater levels of stress (Flisher et al., 2007; Kimbro & Denney, 2015). Patel and his colleagues (Patel, Flisher, Nikapota, & Malhotra, 2008,

Patel, Kieling, Maulik, & Divan, 2013) argue that poverty is strongly associated with mental health outcomes, and that both relative and absolute poverty poses a risk for mental disorders.

Poverty is nuanced, and neither of these definitions truly capture the actual rate of deprivation that families feel, or their experiences of meeting societal standards. The World Bank in its guidelines for measuring poverty notes that the choice of a poverty line to assess relative poverty is arbitrary, and that poverty lines need to resonate with social norms/customs regarding what represents a minimum in that culture (World Bank, 2016). For absolute poverty, the World Bank includes two other constructs: the food-energy intake method (i.e., if income is sufficient to meet food energy requirement) and the cost-basic needs method (i.e., allowance of goods and foods typically utilized and consumed by the poor at local prices). Relative and absolute poverty measures can be combined, and this method considers inequality relative to the position of households to meet basic living standards (World Bank, 2016). Wilkinson (1997) expands on the poverty definition (e.g., relative and absolute poverty) and argues that besides material factors, social influences also affect poverty rates, which in turn creates additional social and health inequalities.

Wilkinson further argues that the widening socioeconomic differences account for the current widening in the social-health gradient and limiting of access to both goods and services. Services can include access to health care, and goods can include housing, food, and other household items that lead to both safety and security, and lack of access to these resources can be considered child neglect (Wilkinson, 1997). Kimbro and Denney (2015), in their assessment of a family's transition into food insecurity and child behavioral outcomes, found that there were consistent negative impacts on children's overall health based on parental reports, and limited self-control and interpersonal skills, as well as increased externalizing behaviors based on teacher's reports. The data came from the Great Recession of 2007–2009, where many US household incomes fell below 300% of the federal poverty level. Their findings underscore the importance of food security not only on child development but also on reducing individual- and family-level stress which often leads to child abuse and neglect. Thinking about how neglect is applied in an SSA context is critical since the region suffers from periodic food insecurity. Because the relative definition of neglect assumes parent's or caregiver's inability to meet the basic needs of a child, it is important to disentangle poverty from true neglect and assess for bias when reporting children of poor families (Drake & Jonson-Reid, 2014).

Prevalence/Patterns of Child Maltreatment in Sub-Saharan Africa

Child maltreatment is a significant public health issue that affects the lives of 3.3 million children annually in the United States and significantly more globally (Zimmerman & Mercy, 2010; Leeb et al., 2008; CDC, 2014; Children's Bureau,

2011). Maltreatment includes acts of commission such as physical, sexual, and emotional abuse, or acts of omission such as educational, exploitation, or medical neglect. Most children experience neglect (78%) and/or physical abuse (18%), with significantly fewer cases being reported for sexual (9%) and psychological abuse (8%) globally (Leeb et al., 2008; CDC, 2010, 2014, 2016a; WHO, 2005, 2006, 2017a, 2017b). Overall abuse and neglect in children are grossly underreported, with a greater propensity for underreporting for cases of sexual and emotional abuse. This is due to the sensitive nature of the abuse, as well as the difficulty with identification of psychological abuse and lack of definitional clarity on the child maltreatment categories, especially neglect (National Academy of Sciences, 1993).

The impact of child maltreatment is greater than other types of adverse or negative exposure such as children experiencing the separation or the divorce of a parent, parental death, being treated or judged unfairly due to race or ethnicity, parents serving time in jail, or children witnessing domestic violence (Child Trends, 2019; CWIG, 2019). The Northwest Foster Care Alumni Study in the United States found that children in foster care (already exposed to child abuse and neglect) exhibit post-traumatic stress disorder (PTSD) at twice the rates of combat veterans and are more likely to experience repeat child maltreatment or multiple traumas/polytrauma (Pecora et al., 2005, 2010; Nilsson et al., 2015). Polytrauma is defined as an individual experiencing multiple negative life events and/or injuries that are either limiting or lasting and have a cumulative effect on health and mental health (Nilsson et al., 2015). Olema et al. (2014) concluded that even in the context of war, the impact of child maltreatment surpassed the damage caused by exposure to war trauma. Their study simultaneously assessed the effect of psychological damage caused by both exposure to war and child maltreatment in war-affected Northern Uganda. Both parents and children were severely affected by war and child mal-treatment and those two trauma types were independently associated with psycho-logical disorders. The most important finding was that only child maltreatment accounted for PTSD symptoms and negative mental health in the parents, which has ramifications for caregiving, intergenerational transmission of trauma, and child maltreatment. Child maltreatment was more damaging than exposure to war vio-lence, partly due to the nature of child abuse and neglect which is interpersonal compared to war violence which is often external, and the violence can be rational-ized differently by the victim.

The seminal study on child maltreatment also known as the Adverse Childhood Experiences (ACE), a CDC-Kaiser study, collected health and mental health data from adult patients receiving general health services in Southern California (Felitti et al., 1998; CWIG, 2019). The study collected data from 17,000 patients who completed surveys regarding their childhood experiences and current health and mental health status. One of the key findings was the high prevalence of child maltreatment in this sample (CWIG, 2019). The prevalence rate for abuse in the United States was approximately 19.87 per 100,000 (population), for neglect it was 12.5, and for household dysfunction the average prevalence rate was approximately 17.4 per 100,000 across the five distinct categories (e.g., abuse, mental illness, incarceration, separation, and divorce among parents and caregivers) (Leeb et al.,

2008; CDC, 2014, 2016a, 2016b; Felitti et al., 1998). A key finding was that abused and neglected children experience higher rates of both emotional and behavioral challenges because of maltreatment and trauma that has lifelong consequences (Sheldon et al., 2011). Additionally, as per CDC (2014) data, children under the age of 4 living in stressful family environments, high-risk communities, and low social capital have greater rates of poverty and are more likely to experience elevated risk for abuse and neglect and these experiences are common among all populations (Conger et al., 2002a, 2010).

In low- and middle-income countries (LMICs), child abuse and neglect research is still in preliminary stages. Most studies have focused on developing surveillance (or data collection) systems for monitoring maltreatment trends and prevalence rates, as well as measuring related risks (Leeb et al., 2008; WHO, 2005, 2006, 2016b; UNICEF, 2017). For example, the United Nations International Children's Emergency Fund (UNICEF) (, 2014) initiated the Multiple Indicator Cluster Survey (MICS) project in 1995 to carry out international household surveys to assess the situation that children and women live in. Although the focus of MICS is to assess the impacts of Millennium Development Goals (MDGs) on children and women, child abuse- and protection-related indicators were included in the survey. Key indicators included *child survival* (under-5 mortality, neonatal mortality), *child health* (pneumonia, diarrhea, malaria, immunization), *child nutrition* (malnutrition, low birthweight, infant and young child feeding), *maternal health, water and sanitation, education, early childhood development, child disability, child protection* (birth registration, child labor, child marriage, violence against children), and *HIV/ AIDS*. More than 100 LMICs have data that can be used to assess rates of child maltreatment and determine if countries are meeting their MDGs and Sustainable Development Goals (SDGs) and World Health Organization (WHO) targets (UNICEF, 2014).

MICS has provided useful data resources to understand child maltreatment/ protection prevalence (e.g., violence against children, child labor, and child marriage) in LMICs. Data is available for Eastern and Southern Africa and West and Central Africa. Data from a total of 363 surveys between 2010 and 2017 covered domains such as disparities by household wealth, under-5 mortality rates, child health, child mortality, nutrition, maternal health, early childhood, education, HIV/AIDS, child protection, sanitation, and water access (UNICEF, 2016, 2017). UNICEF has designated seven specific domains for child protection including requiring countries to provide data on (1) child protection, (2) protection systems, (3) violence against children, (4) justice for children, (5) birth registrations, (6) child protection and emergencies, and (7) strengthening families and communities, and other general child protection measures that fall outside of these predetermined categories (UNICEF, 2017). The challenge for countries themselves as well as UNICEF is the availability of data and countries' internal systems and capacity to collect and respond to child maltreatment and implement child protection measures. Examining child protection and response systems globally, at least 73% of countries have achieved that target; however SSA countries less than 40% have achieved this target by having fully functioning and responsive child protection systems, which means that at least 732 million children or half of the global population of youth aged 6–17 years are not protected from physical punishment at school and at home, and a big percentage of those children live in SSS and other developing countries and regions (UNICEF, 2017).

Child Maltreatment Research in SSA

Mechanisms of Child Maltreatment on Child Health and Development: An Integrated Theoretical Framework

There are several theoretical approaches that are applicable to child abuse and neglect research both in high-income countries (HICs) and LMICs. They include the social ecological model, social determinants of health, adverse childhood experiences, and family stress model. These theories focus on the socio-ecological context of the child and the caregiving environment, with a special emphasis on the health and mental health of the caregiver, including the level of stress or duress that the family experiences during the child's formative developmental years. The dominant paradigm in understanding causal pathways in child maltreatment is Bronfenbrenner's (1979) social-ecological theory. The social-ecological theory (Bronfenbrenner, 1979, 1986, 1994) acknowledges the myriad of factors from the individual level of the child to the child's microsystem (e.g., family including siblings and peers) to the exosystem (e.g., extended family, neighborhood, school), and the larger microsystem (e.g., dominant culture, sociopolitical and economic conditions, as well as existing laws and services), that can be interrupted and lead to abuse and neglect. The model (Fig. 1) accounts for the interrelated nature of child maltreatment, including the relationship between individual-, family-, and community-level factors that can lead to and perpetuate child maltreatment cross-generationally (Myers, 2011; Cicchetti & Rizley, 1981).

Other conceptual frameworks for assessing the impact of child maltreatment at a multifactorial level are the social determinants of health (SDG) (Fig. 2) and adverse childhood experiences (ACEs) (Fig. 3). SDGs take into consideration both socio-environmental factors and intermediary determinants of health, including material circumstances (e.g., living conditions, food availability) and behavioral, biological, and psychosocial factors (Solar & Irwin, 2010). The focus of SDGs includes ensuring stable and responsive relationships for children, safe and secure environments, nutrition, and health-promoting behaviors (e.g., perinatal health, physical, oral, socio-emotional, mental, and behavioral health); these constructs map directly onto the ACE framework by Felitti and Anda (Felitti et al., 1998; National Academy of Sciences, 2016b).

The adverse childhood experiences are composed of five distinct stages (Fig. 3). The first stage includes exposure to adverse childhood events such as abuse and neglect. These early experiences affect a child's socio-emotional and cognitive

Fig. 1 Social-ecological theory (SET) (Gonzales, 2020). Adapted by permission from Springer Nature: Theories and Models in Systems Thinking by M. Gonzales. In: Systems Thinking for Supporting Students with Special Needs and Disabilities. Copyright 2020

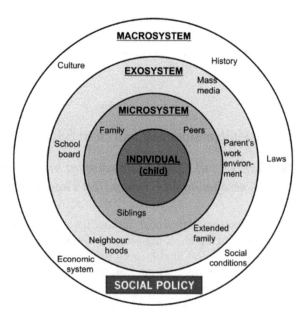

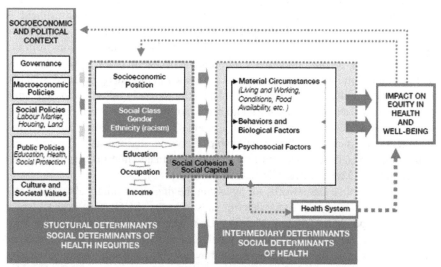

Fig. 2 World Health Organization (WHO) conceptual framework for Social Determinants of Health (SDH) (Solar & Irwin, 2010). Reproduced from A conceptual framework for action on the social determinants of health. Social Determinants of Health Discussion Paper 2 (Policy and Practice), O. Solar & A. Irwin, Page No. 6, Copyright 2010. Used with permission

development, which is the second adverse stage in the ACE model. Cumulative child adverse events and socio-emotional-cognitive delays lead to the third stage in late childhood and early adolescence. This stage includes the adoption of health risk behaviors such as smoking, drinking, and experimentation with gateway drugs. The

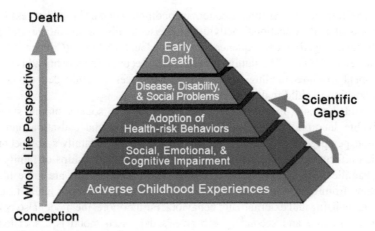

Fig. 3 Adverse childhood experiences (ACEs) (Felitti et al., 1998). Reprinted from American Journal of Preventive Medicine, 14(4), Vincent J. Felitti, et al., Relationship of Childhood Abuse and Household Dysfunction to Many of the Leading Causes of Death in Adults. The Adverse Childhood Experiences (ACE) Study, pp. 245–258, Copyright 1998, with permission from Elsevier

SOURCE: Conger, McLoyd, Wallace, et al., 2002.

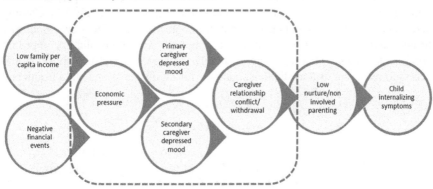

Fig. 4 Family stress model (FSM) (Conger, McLoyd, Wallace et al., 2002a). Copyright © 2002 by American Psychological Association. Reproduced with permission

model is progressive regarding adoption of risky behaviors which lead to the final stages of disease, disability in stage four, and eventually early death in stage five. The second quadrant of the SDGs/intermediary determinants overlaps with ACE stages two to four, including social-emotional-cognitive impairment, health risk behaviors, disease, disability, and social problems.

The last model assesses how stress is an enabling factor in child maltreatment. The family stress model (FSM) (Fig. 4) highlights how economic problems can lead to disrupted familial relationships, including marital instability, which in turn can lead to child maltreatment due to elevated stress levels within the family system (Conger et al., 2010). It also considers economic pressure and how social position influences families across time. Economic conditions such as limited access to jobs/ occupational and educational activities increase family disadvantage and stress, which have negative consequences for adults and children (Conger, McLoyd, Wallace et al., 2002a). The family stress model of economic hardship adds a critical component to understanding the economic influences on child development and predisposition to child maltreatment.

This interactionist model of the relationship between socioeconomic status and family life incorporates assumptions from both the social causation and social selection perspectives (citation), and underscores how a family's socioeconomic position affects the life course development and interrelationships of family members. Families that experience greater negative financial events are more likely to withdraw from caregiving activities, and their children are more likely to exhibit both internalizing and externalizing behaviors. Furthermore, the model also confirms that both primary and secondary caregiver's depressed mood is associated with adverse child events (Conger, McLoyd, Wallace et al., 2002a). Their findings suggest that a supportive and stable caregiver relationship protects children from possible adverse consequences of economic hardship. Conger, McLoyd, Wallace et al. (2002a) highlight a child's caregiving environment (i.e., low or noninvolved parenting) and later presentation of mental health issues.

Transactional child maltreatment model (TCMM) (Fig. 5) is proposed as a unifying model to understand the causal links between family/caregiver functioning and child outcomes (including physical, psychological, and socio-developmental health), and the effect that society and community have on enabling or impeding child maltreatment. TCMM integrates family's socioeconomic status/position and access to resources as a mediational pathway for family stress and child health and

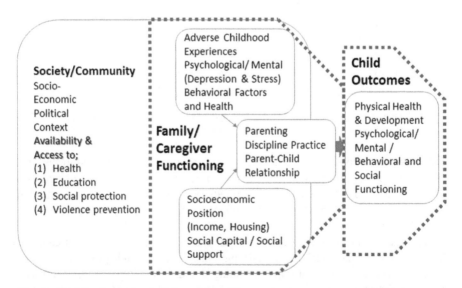

Fig. 5 Conceptual model of child maltreatment experience, parenting, and child outcomes: transactional child maltreatment model (TCMM)

mental health outcomes. The TCMM model incorporates individual experiences of abuse and neglect including their influence on parenting and caregiving relationship. The model also takes into account access to resources and how that impacts issues related to neglect including having access to basic needs as well as health, education, and other social services.

For example, the lack of housing, social capital, and social support can lead to increased stress, which may impact the quality of caregiving and supervision. The social-ecological/systems theory (SET) guides the overall model and the nested components relate to the bidirectional transactions between each system (i.e., society/community, family/caregiver, and child). This model combines Bronfenbrenner's social-ecological framework as an overarching concept but focuses on active pathways that can lead to child maltreatment. These are often the transactional components between the family and community (e.g., family residing in higher crime areas and lower resource settings), or between the family/caregiver and the child (e.g., the family experiencing greater stress due to lack of resources is more likely to resort to negative discipline practices). The transactional model focuses on the intermediary constructs between systems and highlights how those intermediate pathways facilitate or mitigate child abuse and neglect within families and communities. For example, families can experience greater stress due to financial constraints; however because of availability of community resources those stressful patterns are mitigated, whereas in other cases the level of caregiver stress and negative or less supportive environments can facilitate child maltreatment because of the duplicity of those negative factors. The transactional aspect between systems is enabling or limiting factors for maltreatment in addition to the existing perspectives that trauma, stress, and resources serve as active agents in child maltreatment.

Intergenerational Transmission of Child Maltreatment and Impacts on Physical and Mental Health

Intergenerational transmission of child maltreatment is when parents who were victims of childhood maltreatment abuse or neglect their own children (Valentino et al., 2012; Schelbe & Geiger, 2017; Cicchetti et al., 2016). Parents who were maltreated as children are more likely to maltreat their own offspring, and more often suffer from depression and personality disorders (Thornberry & Henry, 2013). Understanding patterns of maltreatment within families helps stop the intergenerational maltreatment (Thornberry & Henry, 2013; Schelbe & Geiger, 2017). One of the theories that focus on the etiology of intergenerational transmission of maltreatment is the social-learning theory (Cicchetti et al., 2016; Wareham et al., 2009), which includes learned patterns of behavior and reinforcement. The second proposed framework argues for a genetic predisposition towards aggression and aggressive behavior (Tomison, 1996), where aggressiveness is assumed to be an

80 B. Bauta and K.-Y. Huang

individual characteristic such as temperament and the predisposition towards aggressive behavior is inherited cross-generationally. The third framework includes a combination of environmental factors, such as genetic changes due to epigenetic effects (i.e., environment changing genotype/phenotype due to stress or adversity) (Mehta et al., 2013; McGowan et al., 2009; Yang et al., 2013; CWIG, 2019).

Mehta and colleagues in their study of epigenetic effects of childhood maltreatment found that there were changes in DNA methylation for the maltreated group and its effects were two times greater compared to the control group. This might reflect true genetic differences in the pathophysiology of PTSD, and level of exposure to trauma during childhood. Epigenetic markers associated with gene expression changes were up to 12-fold higher in PTSD patients with a history of childhood abuse. This suggests that although all patients with PTSD may show similar symptoms, abused children who subsequently develop PTSD may experience a systematically and biologically different form of the disorder compared to those without childhood abuse. These results suggest that differences in trauma exposure and pathophysiological processes in stress-related disorders associated with child maltreatment have a complex clinical presentation in cases of PTSD and other mental health conditions in adults who were exposed to maltreatment as children (Mehta et al., 2013). Yang et al.'s (2013) study suggests that epigenetic mechanisms may be associated with increased risk for health problems later in life among maltreated children. Cicchetti et al. (2016) found that maltreated children exhibited changes in gene expression which conferred significant risk for both physiological and psychological systems. Altered gene expression leads to nonreactive immune systems, higher rates of cancer, and cardiovascular disease, including increased mental health conditions such as depression, anxiety, and bipolar disorder. These enduring vulnerability factors and altered gene expression confer future risk to subsequent generations of children whose parents had experienced child maltreatment (CWIG, 2019; Cicchetti et al., 2016).

Cross-generational patterns of child maltreatment are also influenced by caregivers' own childhood experience, as well as their current socioeconomic status, educational attainment, gender, race, age, marital status, and community factors. Parents who are depressed, lack social bonds, and are socially isolated tend to respond to young children more aggressively due to stress (Shonkoff & Phillips, 2000). Intergenerational patterns of child abuse and neglect (i.e., CAN/CM) are far more complex and nuanced than originally understood, and exposure to child maltreatment does not always lead to negative health effects or IGM (CWIG, 2016; Children's Bureau, 2011) if there are protective factors in place. Intergenerational transmission of maltreatment is affected by many factors and requires a multifactorial approach in understanding it true etiology and consequences (Tomison, 1996). Individual resilience and presence of other caring and supportive relationships in childhood mitigate some of maltreatment's negative effects and having representations of caring and nurturing relationships provides a template for modeling pro-social behavior (Wareham et al., 2009; Cicchetti et al., 2016). This in turn can lead to improved (and/or buffered) reaction to stressful environments and improved parenting practices, or the willingness to seek support (Cicchetti et al., 2016; Bandura & Walters, 1971).

Global Agenda for Child Maltreatment Prevention and Control

The World Health Organization's (2016a) INSPIRE Report provides a road map for addressing child maltreatment and violence against children. It proposes seven strategies for ending violence against children, which include (1) implementation and enforcement of laws, (2) adjusting norms and values (e.g., around corporal punishment), (3) creating safe environments for children, (4) parent and caregiver support, (5) income and economic strengthening for at-risk families, (6) response and support services, and (7) education and life skills. The report reiterates the importance of reinforcing protections guaranteed under the UN Convention on the Rights of the Child (CRC), which requires states to provide legislative, administrative, social, and educational measures to protect children from all types of violence (WHO, 2016b; De Bruin, 2010; Baker et al., 2016; UNICEF, 2015).

The second international measure to ensure that LMICs support child maltreatment protection policies includes achieving key targets of the 2030 guideline for addressing maltreatment in LMICs as outlined in the Sustainable Development Goals (SDGs). The SDGs include several key targets for child maltreatment by 2030, which include Target 16.2 that stipulates an end to "abuse, exploitation, trafficking, and all forms of violence against and torture of children" and Target 5.2, which requires that "all forms of violence against all women and girls in the public and private spheres, including trafficking and sexual and other types of exploitation," are eliminated; Target 16.1 requires significant reductions in "all forms of violence and death rates everywhere" (WHO, 2016b).

WHO recommends that preventive and interventive (P&I) strategies for child maltreatment must include reduction of risk factors and building child protection mechanisms at the individual, family, community, and societal levels. The WHO guide to preventing child maltreatment includes targeting interventions at each level of the child's ecology in a developmentally appropriate way (Butchart et al., 2006; Zielinski & Brandshaw, 2006). Specifically, interventions and services need to consider the following five domains: (1) health interventions (e.g., medical and mental health interventions, such as trauma therapy), (2) social interventions (e.g., child protection services, foster care placements, respite care), (3) educational interventions (e.g., specialized education plans for children with learning and other difficulties, and specialized training plans), (4) legal interventions (e.g., child protection, prosecution for perpetrators, claim damages), and (5) financial assistance (e.g., housing, food, transportation, educational expenses) (Butchart et al., 2006; Hardcastle et al., 2015). The guide recommends that all maltreatment and preventive interventions should consider local and community contexts and culture in the design and implementation of interventions (WHO, 2006; Lau, 2006; Castro et al., 2010).

Child Maltreatment Resources, Systems, and Policies in SSA Countries

The state of child maltreatment laws, policies, and interventions in SSA varies greatly by country and regionally within countries. Countries need to crosswalk international conventions and design policies and procedures that address the core components of child protection. Interpretation of international mandates, lack of uniformity in the implementation of conventions, and issues around transportability of maltreatment interventions to SSA create challenges in designing uniform child protection systems. The lack of resources and other competing priorities around health usually impinge on the implementation of child violence prevention measures at the local and regional levels. Child maltreatment interventions need adaptations that are sensitive to the unique needs of children and families living in LMIC/SSA contexts. Child maltreatment and violence prevention interventions most often are developed within HICs and transported to LMICs. Some of these interventions lack specificity and relativity to local contexts. These interventions tend to be resource heavy and not easily adapted to low-resource settings, or environments with fledgling child protection systems and policies. A greater focus on assessing LMIC resources for child protection including system-sustaining practices is an integral component when designing or transporting evidence-based or evidence-informed interventions.

Child Maltreatment Prevention and Intervention Programs (Evidence in SSA)

Families and children living in LMICs often reside in communities that lack adequate health or educational resources (Laird, 2016). These system-level issues often lead to child neglect, a child maltreatment domain associated with poverty, lack of resources, and inequity (UNICEF, 2017). The most influential factor in the reduction of child maltreatment, specifically child neglect, is instituting policies that provide economic opportunities and reduce economic disparities (UNICEF, 2014, 2017). Addressing poverty and gender-based issues ensures that young children are protected in all caregiving environments. Reduction of environmental risks such as unsafe living conditions, availability of water and sanitation systems, and limiting exposure to environmental toxins would reduce unintended accidents and injuries in young children. For abuse and neglect prevention to be effective, individuals and caregivers need appropriate information on child developmental milestones and long-term effects of exposure to risk factors, including violence, and child abuse and neglect (CWIG, 2019; NSCDC, 2020). The local community needs to have access to preventive healthcare services (e.g., prenatal/postnatal services, low-cost baby well-care, access to vaccinations, and dental services) (IOM, 2014). Most importantly individuals and families at risk need access to quality and effective care services such as home visiting services, and training in effective and positive parenting practices (NSCDC, 2020; CWIG, 2019; Butchart et al., 2006). Programs need to respond to caregivers' needs by developing and deploying practical strategies on how to support core life skills, developing positive and responsive relationships, and reducing parental stress. Additionally, countries need to institute safety-net policies and basic needs programs that address issues with income, and ensure that families have affordable housing, access to proper nutrition, education, and medical services (NSCDC, 2020). Reduction of systemic and economic inequities would have the greatest impact on reduction of neglect and maltreatment rates.

Emerging Frameworks and Strategies (for Addressing Service, Evidence-Based Intervention, Implementation, and Research Gaps)

To mitigate or reduce child maltreatment, interventions need to influence multiple spheres of a child's life, including home, school, and community. Interventions for child abuse and neglect fall under three broad categories: (1) awareness campaigns, (2) prevention, and (3) intervention strategies (e.g., evidence-based/evidence-informed programs). Knerr et al.'s (2013) systematic review of parenting interventions in LMICs that targeted abusive and harsh parenting, improved parent/child relationship, and enhanced positive parenting identified only 12 studies that reported favorable results. They noted that most research on parenting interventions is conducted in HICs, and very few in LMICs. Furthermore, there was great variability in both the implementation of evidence-based/informed interventions and outcomes among the interventions that were transported to LMICs/SSA. In the review, they identified only two studies that were effective in improving parental knowledge and parent/child interaction in LMICs. They further argued that parents and children living in LMIC contexts can benefit from interventions where the fidelity of the model was maintained even after modification to local context. Some of the challenges in implementing evidence-based interventions in LMICs include the costs associated with implementation, including training and educational resources, having qualified health professionals to administer the intervention, and technological challenges such as maternal and parenting interventions requiring video feedback for supervision of practice (Cluver et al., 2016b; Ward et al., 2020). There is an urgent need for interventions that can be adapted to low-resource contexts and meet the challenges that exist in LMICs (Ward et al., 2020).

Intervention approaches that have been transported to LMICs/SSA include individual-level interventions focused on enhancing problem-solving skills and psychoeducation about children, child-parenting interventions focusing on enhancing parent/child relationship and interactions, and group-parenting interventions focused on psychoeducation and problem-solving using social-learning theory

(Cluver et al., 2016a). School-based interventions such as the Good School Toolkit developed by Raising Voices in Uganda include both psychoeducation and awareness components with the aim of reducing physical violence in school settings (Devries et al., 2015). Furthermore, this intervention approach included behavior change techniques for students, teachers, and school administrators, as well as awareness measures built in for the parents and community. Devries et al. (2015) used the transtheoretical model as a key driver of the behavior change strategy. The model specified behavior change techniques for staff, students, and administration and included setting goals at the school and individual level, developing action plans with deliverables, facilitating reflection on violence, providing alternative forms of nonviolent discipline, and encouraging empathy. Their intervention influenced both the individual and school levels. There was a substantial change among caregivers in attitudes and behaviors related to using physical punishment as a discipline method (reduction from 53% to 11%), and an overall reduction in physical violence in school. The intervention also improved students' feeling of safety, which in turn had a direct effect on both mental health and educational outcomes as measured by test scores post-intervention. This intervention is unique in that it was designed in Uganda with stakeholder engagement regarding both the intervention and implementation approaches. Lastly, training programs that raise awareness of abuse and neglect in health care, education, or service settings have been shown effective in identifying and referring cases of suspected abuse and neglect in children (National Academies, 2016a; NSCDC, 2020).

Parenting interventions for young children need to take stock of the political and cultural landscapes, and engage various stakeholders in building support, financial resources, and political capital in supporting maltreatment interventions in communities (National Academies, 2016a; Cluver et al., 2016b). Child maltreatment interventions need to be sensitive to the cultural context when designed to provide either universal (i.e., preventive services), selective (i.e., targeted to specific populations or risk groups), or indicated interventions (i.e., where there has been clear substantiation of abuse and neglect) (NSCDC, 2020; Hardcastle et al., 2015; Castro et al., 2010; Lau, 2006).

In sum, the goals of maltreatment interventions include promoting safety, stability, and nurturing relationships, in order to allow children to grow up trauma free and healthy. The effectiveness of child maltreatment interventions depends on collaborative and coordinated approaches across a variety of sectors, such as education, health, and legal systems, both in the identification and treatment of abuse and neglect cases (IOM, 2014; Butchart et al., 2006). Coordination across sectors is inherently dependent on the robustness of country's health and child welfare systems. In resource-poor settings, even with exposure to adversity, most children grow up to be healthy and productive adults. Most families and children are resilient in the face of adversity, and they usually draw from internal strengths and family social resources to mitigate risks in the home or community. Interventions for maltreatment need to leverage those strengths to make lasting change and ensure that those changes achieve outcomes in child health and well-being.

Challenges in Addressing Child Maltreatment Care and Welfare Services in SSA

The lack of data on child maltreatment in SSA relates to the sensitive nature of child maltreatment and the lack of child protection structures that can validate and process abuse and neglect cases. Collection of maltreatment data and research efforts are needed to determine the extent of this issue in SSA and translate existing surveillance data into policy and intervention action. Child maltreatment often occurs at the interpersonal level, with influences from both the micro- and exosystem. Ecological influences on the sequelae of child maltreatment create an added complexity in studying this phenomenon and disentangling effects of the subcomponents of maltreatment (e.g., physical, sexual, emotional, and neglect) (Zielinski & Brandshaw, 2006; Atilola, 2014). Results from studies on child maltreatment in the sub-Saharan Africa need to be reflective of the cultural norms of the region, in terms of both physical abuse and neglect. Laird (2016) in the analysis of nutritional and medical neglect in sub-Saharan Africa suggests that in SSA, conditions of relative/absolute poverty and food insecurity, as well as grossly inadequate public services, affect parents' ability to meet their children's basic needs. Furthermore, the definition of "child neglect" is an ethnocentric concept that requires testing for fit and relevance before being applied to LMIC contexts. The transportability of international conventions such as the Convention on the Rights of the Child (CRC) and its definitions and Western notions of parenting might not be reflective of the reality of caregiving in low- and middle-income countries. Child maltreatment interventions that include multiple components often have difficulty isolating main effects and require greater resources and funding to make them sustainable, which makes it difficult to transport these interventions to LMICs (Gardner et al., 2015; Baker et al., 2016; MacMillan & Wathen, 2014). Measuring outcomes is easier at the individual rather than community or population levels due to various confounders in the environment (National Academy of Sciences, 1993). Only better research evidence in these areas can inform better policy development, prevention plans, and intervention solutions.

LMICs face a variety of barriers that makes the transportability and implementation of evidence-based and evidence-informed interventions a challenge. Programs such as Parenting for Lifelong Health with significant decrease in physical/emotional abuse and neglect among caregivers should be adopted. These low-cost implementation approaches with minimal resource needs can serve as a model for other programs (Cluver et al., 2016b). Key design components should also include implementation by community health or lay workers with minimal equipment requirements (Ward et al., 2020). Interventions with sustainability measures built in should be the ones considered for implementation in LMICs. There are several challenges in implementing and scaling up evidence-based child and parenting interventions in SSA and LMICs; however, limited availability of tested interventions in low-resource settings and interventions that are applicable to SSA context should not be among them. Interventions that can change cultural norms around physical abuse as a normative practice are the ones that have long-lasting effects on reducing child maltreatment and intergenerational effects on individual and community violence (Cluver et al., 2016b; Baker et al., 2016).

Conclusion

Child maltreatment is a serious social and public health issue with lasting consequences for children, youth, families, and communities. Therefore, a thorough understanding of how and why maltreatment occurs is critical in informing prevention efforts, especially in low-resource settings (CWIG, 2016, 2019). Additional studies are needed to identify individual and contextual risk factors that may contribute to maltreatment practices, and elucidate mechanisms of maltreatment impact on family functioning and children's health and development in LMICs. Models that focus on the transactional components between the individual and family, or family and outside systems, are essential in understanding pathways to and prevalence of maltreatment within families and communities. Transactional Child Maltreatment Model (TCMM) is proposed as an intermediary model that assesses the interplay from the individual to family level, including how those mediational pathways either sustain or mitigate child abuse and neglect. Further examination is needed to isolate the enabling pathways in various resource settings (e.g., wealthy compared to resource-poor). Child maltreatment research to date has identified that poverty-associated stressors are key drivers for neglect and parents that experience economic challenges such as poverty have higher levels of stress which impacts their and their children's health and mental health. It is one pathway that is associated with larger socioeconomic factors. Physical and sexual abuse can have different pathways which can include stress, prior history of trauma or sexual abuse, and cultural factors that view physical punishment as an appropriate discipline method for young children or adolescents. Changing cultural norms around physical abuse and use of corporal punishment requires a concerted effort across various sectors (e.g., health, mental health, policy, and practice) to change norms around discipline. It also requires resources and focus by international bodies, countries, and communities on alternative approaches to caregiving practices that focus on reducing stress and building resilience within individuals, families, and communities.

The prevention of child maltreatment has direct returns on health, mental health, and well-being for both children and adults. Reduction of maltreatment includes societal benefits such as having a healthier population, and reduction of health and mental health service utilization among individuals and families. Interventions that provide caregivers with problem-solving skills and insight to address stress and conflict in a relational way without resorting to physical punishment as a discipline method have been shown to reduce child maltreatment and improve child outcomes. At the societal level, legal and human rights reforms, along with national laws and policies that promote social, economic, and individual rights, are principal factors in ensuring legal protection mechanisms for preventing child abuse and neglect. Another crucial component is ensuring that judicial, health, and social systems are functional and have the authority to adjudicate and redress cases of child abuse and neglect. Based on the myriad of negative effects to child maltreatment exposure it is surprising that more attention and resources are not levied against this significant public health issue. Child maltreatment is a public health issue that has cross-generational ramifications; addressing the root causes is key in improving the health and well-being of future generations.

References

Atilola, O. (2014). Where lies the risk? An ecological approach to understanding child mental health risk and vulnerabilities in Sub-Saharan Africa. *Psychiatry Journal, 2014*, 11.

Baker, P. M., Reid, A., & Schall, M. W. (2016). A framework for scaling up health interventions: Lessons from large-scale improvement initiatives in Africa. *Implementation Science, 11*, 12.

Bandura, A., & Walters, R. H. (1971). *Social learning theory* (pp. 1–46). General Learning Press. Retrieved from http://www.esludwig.com/uploads/2/6/1/0/26105457/bandura_sociallearningtheory.pdf

Bronfenbrenner, U. (1979). *The ecology of human development: Experiments by nature and design.* Harvard University Press.

Bronfenbrenner, U. (1986). Ecology of the family as a context for human development: Research perspectives. *Developmental Psychology, 22*(6), 723–742.

Butchart, A., Phinney-Harvey, A., Mian, M., Fürniss, T., & Kahane, T. (2006). Preventing child maltreatment: A guide to taking action and generating evidence. World Health Organization & International Society for Prevention of Child Abuse and Neglect, . Retrieved from http://whqlibdoc.who.int/publications/2006/9241594365_eng.pdf

Castro, F. G., Barrera, M., & Holleran Steiker, L. K. (2010). Issues and challenges in the design of culturally adapted evidence-based interventions. *Annual Review of Clinical Psychology, 6*, 213–239.

Centers for Disease Control and Prevention. (2010). *Promoting safe, stable, and nurturing relationships: A strategic direction for child maltreatment prevention.* Retrieved from https://www.cdc.gov/violenceprevention/pdf/cm_strategic_direction%2D%2Donepager-a.pdf

Centers for Disease Control and Prevention. (2014). *Child maltreatment: Facts at a glance.* Retrieved from https://www.cdc.gov/violenceprevention/pdf/childmaltreatment-facts-at-a-glance.pdf

Centers for Disease Control and Prevention. (2016a). Child abuse and neglect prevention. *Violence Prevention, 2016*, 28. Retrieved from https://www.cdc.gov/violenceprevention/childmaltreatment/

Centers for Disease Control and Prevention. (2016b). *Child maltreatment. Adverse Childhood Experiences (ACE) study.* Violence Prevention, Retrieved 1 April, 2016, from https://www.cdc.gov/violenceprevention/acestudy/

Child Trends. (2019). *Adverse experiences.* Retrieved from https://www.childtrends.org/?indicators=adverse-experiences

Child Welfare Information Gateway (CWIG). (2015). *Understanding the effects of maltreatment on brain development.* U.S. Department of Health and Human Services, Children's Bureau. Retrieved from https://www.childwelfare.gov/pubPDFs/brain_development.pdf

Child Welfare Information Gateway (CWIG). (2016). *Intergenerational patters of child maltreatment: What the evidence shows.* Issue Brief, August 2016. Children's Bureau, Administration for Children Youth and Families, U.S. Department of Health, and Human Services. Retrieved from https://www.childwelfare.gov/pubPDFs/intergenerational.pdf

Child Welfare Information Gateway (CWIG). (2019). *Long-term consequences of child abuse and neglect.* U.S. Department of Health and Human Services, Administration for Children and Families, Children's Bureau. Retrieved April 2019 from https://www.childwelfare.gov/pubPDFs/long_term_consequences.pdf

Children's Bureau. (2011). *Child maltreatment.* U.S. Department of Health & human services. Retrieved from http://www.acf.hhs.gov/sites/default/files/cb/cm11.pdf

Cicchetti, D., Hetzel, S., Rogosch, F. A., Handley, E. D., & Toth, S. L. (2016). An investigation of child maltreatment and epigenetic mechanisms of mental and physical health risk. *Development and Psychopathology, 28,* 1305–1317. https://doi.org/10.1017/S0954579416000869

Cicchetti, D., & Rizley, R. (1981). Developmental perspectives on the etiology, intergenerational transmission, and sequelae of child maltreatment. *New Directions for Child and Adolescent Development, 11,* 31–55.

Cluver, L., Meinck, F., Shenderovich, Y., Ward, C. L., et al. (2016a). A parenting programme to prevent abuse of adolescents in South Africa: Study protocol for a randomized control trial. *Trials, 17,* 328.

Cluver, L., Meinck, F., Yakubovich, A., Doubt, J., et al. (2016b). Reducing child abuse amongst adolescents in low- and middle-income countries: A pre-post-trial in South Africa. *BMC Public Health, 16,* 567.

Conger, R. D., Conger, K. J., & Martin, M. J. (2010). Socioeconomic status, family processes, and individual development. *Journal of Marriage and Family, 72*(3), 685–704.

Conger, R. D., McLoyd, V. C., Wallace, L. E., Sun, Y., Simons, R. L., & Brody, G. H. (2002a). Economic pressure in African American families: A replication and extension of the family stress model. *Developmental Psychology, 38*(2), 179–193.

Conger, R. D., Wallace, L. E., Sun, Y., Simons, R. L., McLoyd, V. C., & Brody, G. H. (2002b). Economic pressure in African American families: A replication and extension of the family stress model. *Developmental Psychology, 38,* 179–193.

De Bruin, I. (2010). *National plan of action for orphans and vulnerable children.* Establishing, reviewing and implementation national plans of action for orphans and vulnerable children in southern and eastern Africa: Lessons learned and challenges. Multi-sectoral workshop on legal and policy frameworks protecting children, Pretoria, South Africa, April 20–21, 2010. Retrieved from http://www.crin.org/en/docs/NPA%20Report%20-%20English.pdf

Devries, K. M., Knight, L., Child, J. C., Mirembe, A., et al. (2015). The good school toolkit for reducing physical violence from school staff to primary school students: A cluster-randomized controlled trial in Uganda. *The Lancet Global Health, 385,* e378–e386.

Drake, B., & Jonson-Reid, M. (2014). Poverty and child maltreatment. In J. Korbin & R. Krugman (Eds.), *Handbook of Child maltreatment. Child maltreatment (contemporary issues in research and policy).* Springer. https://doi.org/10.1007/978-94-007-7208-3_7

Felitti, V. J., Anda, R. F., Nordenberg, D., Williamson, D. F., Spitz, A. M., Edwards, V., Koss, M. P., & Marks, J. S. (1998). Relationship of childhood abuse and household dysfunction to many of the leading causes of death in adults. The adverse childhood experiences (ACE) study. *American Journal of Preventive Medicine, 14*(4), 245–258.

Finkelhor, D., & Korbin, J. (1988). Child abuse as an international issue. *Child Abuse & Neglect, 12,* 3–23.

Flisher, A. J., Lund, C., Funk, M., Banda, M., Bhana, A., Doku, V., Drew, N., et al. (2007). Mental health policy development and implementation in four African countries. *Journal of Helath Psychology, 12*(3), 505–516.

Fortson, B. L., Klevens, J., Merrick, M. T., Gilbert, L. K., & Alexander, S. P. (2016). *Preventing child abuse and neglect: A technical package for policy, norm, and programmatic activities.* National Center for Injury Prevention and Control, Centers for Disease Control and Prevention. Retrieved from https://www.cdc.gov/violenceprevention/pdf/can-prevention-technical-package.pdf

Gardner, F., Montgomery, P., & Knerr, W. (2015). Transporting evidence-based parenting programs for child problem behavior (age 3-10) between countries: Systematic review and meta-analysis. *Journal of Clinical Child and Adolescent Psychiatry, 0,* 1–14.

Global Initiative to End All Corporal Punishment of Children (GIECPC). (2017). *Corporal punishment of children in Uganda, January 2017.* Retrieved from http://www.endcorporalpunishment.org/assets/pdfs/states-reports/Uganda.pdf

Gonzales, M. (2020). Theories and models in systems thinking. In *Systems thinking for supporting students with special needs and disabilities.* Springer. https://doi.org/10.1007/978-981-33-4558-4_1

Hardcastle, K. A., Bellis, M. A., Hughes, K., & Sethi, D. (2015). *Implementing child maltreatment prevention programmes: What the experts say.* World Health Organization. Retrieved from http://www.euro.who.int/__data/assets/pdf_file/0009/289602/Maltreatment_web.pdf?ua=1

Institute of Medicine (IOM). (2014). *Investing in global health systems: Sustaining gains, transforming lives.* The National Academies Press. Retrieved from http://www.nationalacademies.org/hmd/Reports/2014/Investing-in-Global-Health-Systems-Sustaining-Gains-Transforming-Lives.aspx

Kimbro, R. T., & Denney, J. T. (2015). Transitions into food insecurity associated with behavioral problems and worse overall health among children. *Health Affairs, 34*(11), 1949–1955.

Knerr, W., Gardner, F., & Cluver, L. (2013). Improving positive parenting skills and reducing harsh and abusive parenting in low- and middle-income countries: A systematic review. *Prevention Science, 14*(4), 352. https://doi.org/10.1007/s11121-012-0314-1

Laird, S. (2016). Protecting children from nutritional and medical neglect in sub-Saharan Africa: A five-country study. *International Journal of Social Welfare, 25,* 47–57.

Lansford, J. E., Alampay, L. P., Al-Hassan, S., Bacchini, D., Bombi, A. S., et al. (2010). Corporal punishment of children in nine countries as a function of child gender and parent gender. *International Journal Of Pediatrics, 2010,* 1–12.

Lau, A. S. (2006). Making the case for selective and directed cultural adaptations of evidence-based treatments: Examples from parent training. *Clinical Psychology: Science and Practice, 13*(4), 295–310.

Leeb, R. T., Paulozzi, L., Melanson, C., Simon, T., & Arias, I. (2008). *Child maltreatment surveillance: Uniform definitions for public health and recommended data elements, version 1.0.* Centers for Disease Control and Prevention, National Center for Injury Prevention, and Control. Retrieved from https://www.cdc.gov/violenceprevention/pdf/CM_Surveillance-a.pdf

MacMillan, H. L., & Wathen, C. N. (2014). *Research brief: Interventions to prevent Child maltreatment.* PreVAiL, Preventing Violence Across the Lifespan Research Network.

Madden, D. (2000). Relative or absolute poverty lines: A new approach. *Review of Income and Wealth, 46*(2), 181–199.

McEwen, B. S., & Akil, H. (2020). Revisiting the stress concept: Implications for affective disorders. *The Journal of Neuroscience, 40*(1), 12–21.

McGowan, P. O., Sasaki, A., D'alessio, A. C., Dymov, S., Labonté, B., Szyf, M., & Meaney, M. J. (2009). Epigenetic regulation of the glucocorticoid receptor in human brain associates with childhood abuse. *Nature Neuroscience, 12*(3), 342–348.

Mehta, D., Klengel, T., Conneely, K. N., Smith, A. K., Altmann, A., Pace, T. W., Rex-Haffner, M., Loeschner, A., Gonik, M., Mercer, K. B., Bradley, B., Müller-Myhsok, B., Ressler, K. J., & Binder, E. B. (2013). Childhood maltreatment is associated with distinct genomic and epigenetic profiles in posttraumatic stress disorder. *Proceedings for the National Academy of Sciences, 110* (20), 8302–8307.

Myers, J. E. B. (2011). *The APSAC handbook on child maltreatment.* SAGE Publications.

National Academies of Sciences, Engineering, and Medicine (NAS). (1993). *Understanding child abuse and neglect.* Panel on Research on Child Abuse and Neglect, national Research Council, p. 408. Retrieved from https://www.nap.edu/catalog/2117/understanding-child-abuse-and-neglect

National Academies of Sciences, Engineering, and Medicine (NAS). (2016a). *Parenting matters: Supporting parents of children ages 0–8*. The National Academies Press.

National Academies of Sciences, Engineering, and Medicine (NAS). (2016b). *A framework for educating health professionals to address the social determinants of health*. The National Academies Press.

National Scientific Council on the Developing Child (NSCDC). (2020). *Connecting the brain to the rest of the body: Early childhood development and lifelong health are deeply intertwined: Working Paper No. 15*. Retrieved from www.developingchild.harvard.edu

Nilsson, D., Dahlstöm, Ö., Priebe, G., & Svedin, C. G. (2015). Polytraumatization in an adult national sample and its association with psychological distress and self-esteem. *Brain and Behavior: A Cognitive Neuroscience Perspective, 5*(1), 62–74. https://doi.org/10.1002/brb3.298

Norman, R. E., Byambaa, M., De, R., Butchart, A., Scott, J., & Vos, T. (2012). The long-term health consequences of child physical abuse, emotional abuse, and neglect: A systematic review and meta-analysis. *PLoS One, 9*(11), 1–31.

Olema, D. K., Catani, C., Ertl, V., Saile, R., & Neuner, F. (2014). The hidden effects of child maltreatment in a war region: Correlates of psychopathology in two generations living in northern Uganda. *Journal of Traumatic Stress, 27*, 35–41.

Patel, V., Flisher, A. J., Nikapota, A., & Malhotra, S. (2008). Promoting child and adolescent mental health in low- and middle-income countries. *Journal of Child Psychology and Psychiatry, 49*(3), 313–334.

Patel, V., Kieling, C., Maulik, P. K., & Divan, G. (2013). Improving access to care for children with mental disorders: A global perspective. *Archives of Disease in Childhood, 98*(5), 323–327.

Pecora, P. J., Kessler, R. C., Williams, J., O'Brien, K., Downs, A. C., English, D., White, J., Hiripi, E., White, C. R., Wiggins, T., & Holmes, K. E. (2005). *Improving family foster care: Findings from the northwest Foster Care alumni study*. Casey Family Programs. Retrieved from http://www.casey.org/resources/publications/pdf/improvingfamilyfostercare_es.pdf

Pecora, P. J., White, C. R., Murdock, L. A., O'Brien, K., Kessler, R. C., Sampson, N., & Hwang, I. (2010). Rates of mental, emotional, and behavioral disorders among alumni of family foster care in the United States: The Casey National Study. In E. Fernandez & R. Barth (Eds.), *How does foster care work? International evidence on outcomes* (pp. 166–186). Jessica Kingsley.

Pierce, L., & Bozalek, V. (2004). Child abuse in South Africa: An examination of how child abuse and neglect are defined. *Child Abuse & Neglect, 28*, 817–832.

Rosen, A. L., Handley, E. D., Cicchetti, D., & Rogosch, F. C. (2018). The impact of patterns of trauma exposure among low income children with and without histories of child maltreatment. *Child Abuse & Neglect, 80*, 301–311. https://doi.org/10.1016/j.chiabu.2018.04.005

Schelbe, L., & Geiger, J. M. (2017). *Intergenerational transmission of child maltreatment* (pp. 25–86). Springer.

Sheldon, G. H., Berwick, D., & Hyde, P. S. (2011). *Joint letter to state child welfare, Medicaid, and mental health authorities on the use of psychotropic medication for children in foster care*. U.S. Department of Health and Human Services. Retrieved from https://www.childwelfare.gov/systemwide/mentalhealth/effectiveness/jointlettermeds.pdf

Shonkoff, J. P., & Phillips, D. A. (Eds.). (2000). *Committee on integrating the science of early childhood development. From neurons to neighborhoods: The science of early childhood development* (p. 39). National Academies Press. Retrieved from http://site.ebrary.com/lib/columbia/Doc?id=10038720&ppg=60

Solar, O., & Irwin, A. (2010). A conceptual framework for action on the social determinants of health. In *Social determinants of health, discussion paper 2 (policy and practice)*. World Health Organization. Retrieved from http://www.who.int/sdhconference/resources/ConceptualframeworkforactiononSDH_eng.pdf

The Republic of Uganda. (2006). *Creating safer schools: Alternatives to corporal punishment*. A report by the Republic of Uganda, Raising Voices, and UNICEF. Retrieved from https://www.unicef.org/uganda/Alternatives_to_VAC_160812.pdf

The Republic of Uganda. (2016). *Learners' Booklet—Facts and tips on keeping safe in schools!* For primary schools P4-P7. The Republic of Uganda – Ministry of Education, Science, Technology and Sports, and UNICEF Uganda. Retrieved from https://www.unicef.org/uganda/RTRR_Primary_School_booklet_final_5.2016.pdf

Thornberry, T. P., & Henry, K. L. (2013). Intergenerational continuity in maltreatment. *Journal of Abnormal Child Psychology, 41*(4), 555–569. https://doi.org/10.1007/s10802-012-9697-5

Tomison, A. M. (1996). *Intergenerational transmission of maltreatment. Causes of intergenerational transmission of maltreatment.* Australian Institute of Family Studies. Child Family Community Australia (CFCA), NCPC. Retrieved from https://aifs.gov.au/cfca/publications/intergenerational-transmission-maltreatment#cau

United Nations International Children's Emergency Fund (UNICEF). (2015). *Situation analysis of children in Uganda.* Ministry of Gender, Labour and Social Development and UNICEF. Retrieved from http://www.unicef.org/uganda/UNICEF_SitAn_7_2015_(Full_report).pdf

United Nations International Children's Emergency Fund (UNICEF). (2016). *UNICEF data: Monitoring the situation of children and women.* Uganda—Key demographic indicators. Retrieved from https://data.unicef.org/country/uga/

United Nations International Children's Emergency Fund (UNICEF). (2014). *Multiple indicator cluster survey (MICS).* Statistics and monitoring. Retrieved from http://www.unicef.org/statistics/index_24302.html

United Nations International Children's Emergency Fund (UNICEF). (2017). *Annual results report 2017: Child protection.* Retrieved from https://www.unicef.org/media/47761/file/Child_Protection_2017_Annual_Results_Report.pdf

Valentino, K., Nuttall, A. K., Comas, M., Borkowski, J. G., & Akai, C. E. (2012). Intergenerational continuity of child abuse among adolescent mothers: Authoritarian parenting, community violence, and race. *Child Maltreatment, 17*(2), 172–181. https://doi.org/10.1177/1077559511434945

Ward, C. L., Wessels, I. M., Lachman, J. M., Hutchings, J., Cluver, L. D., Kassanjee, R., Nhapi, R., Little, F., & Gardner, F. (2020). Parenting for lifelong health for young children: A randomized controlled trial of a parenting program in South Africa to prevent harsh parenting and child conduct problems. *Journal of Child Psychology and Psychiatry, 61*, 503–512. https://doi.org/10.1111/jcpp.13129

Wareham, J., Boots, D. P., & Chavez, J. M. (2009). A test of social learning and intergenerational transmission among batterers. *Journal of Criminal Justice, 37*(2), 163–173. https://doi.org/10.1016/j.jcrimjus.2009.02.011

Wilkinson, R. G. (1997). Socioeconomic determinants of health. Health inequalities: Relative or absolute material standards? *BMJ, 314*, 591–595.

World Bank. (2016). Choosing and estimating a poverty line. *Poverty analysis, measuring poverty.* Retrieved from http://web.worldbank.org/WBSITE/EXTERNAL/TOPICS/EXTPOVERTY/EXTPA/0,,contentMDK:20242879~menuPK:435055~pagePK:148956~piPK:216618~theSitePK:430367,00.html

World Health Organization. (2005). *Child and adolescent mental health policies and plans.* WHO. Retrieved from http://www.who.int/mental_health/policy/Childado_mh_module.pdf

World Health Organization. (2006). *Preventing child maltreatment: A guide to taking action and generating evidence.* World Health Organization and International Society for Prevention of Child Abuse and Neglect. Retrieved from http://apps.who.int/iris/bitstream/10665/43499/1/9241594365_eng.pdf

World Health Organization. (2016a). *Child maltreatment.* Retrieved from http://www.who.int/mediacentre/factsheets/fs150/en/

World Health Organization. (2016b). *INSPIRE: Seven strategies for ending violence against children.* Retrieved from http://apps.who.int/iris/bitstream/10665/207717/1/9789241565356-eng.pdf?ua=1

World Health Organization. (2017a). *Child maltreatment ("child abuse")*. Retrieved from http://www.who.int/violence_injury_prevention/violence/child/en/

World Health Organization. (2017b). *Violence info. Child maltreatment, studies of child maltreatment prevalence*. Retrieved from http://apps.who.int/violence-info/child-maltreatment/

Yang, B. Z., Zhang, H., Ge, W., Weder, N., Douglas-Palumberi, H., Perepletchikova, F., ... Kaufman, J. (2013). Child abuse and epigenetic mechanisms of disease risk. *American Journal of Preventive Medicine, 44*(2), 101–107.

Zielinski, D. S., & Brandshaw, C. P. (2006). Ecological influences on the sequelae of child maltreatment: A review of the literature. *Child Maltreatment, 11*(1), 49–62.

Zimmerman, F., & Mercy, J. (2010). *A better start: Child maltreatment prevention as a public health priority. Zero to three*. Retrieved from http://www.zerotothree.org/maltreatment/child-abuse-neglect/30-5-zimmerman.pdf

Part II
Current Efforts in Policy, Research, and Practice in Child Behavioral Health: Case Examples

Child Behavioral Health in Ghana: Current Efforts in Policy Research and Practice

Emmanuel Asampong and Abdallah Ibrahim

Introduction

Child behavioral health is the outcome of the interaction that takes place between a child's emotions and behaviours, their ability to function in everyday life, and their concept of self in their environment (Ogundele, 2018). There is a growing recognition in most African countries that investing in child behavioral health is important (Rathod et al., 2017). Investing in child behavioral health would put children on the path to healthy and productive lives as they transition into adulthood. As the future leaders, innovators, and reformers, investments in children's health, including behavioral health, will also enable the society to realize future benefits that will manifest in higher national productivity and economic growth. Thus, it is important that developing countries such as Ghana are interested in the healthy upbringing of children, their well-being, and overall growth, and devote necessary attention and resources to behavioral health from an early age. Unfortunately, despite what we know, efforts to address child behavioral health are neglected in most African countries, including Ghana. In a few places where it is given attention, the investments remain too minimal to make the much-needed impact.

In the box below are two cases of young "Kwofie" and "Ama" who both had behavioral issues while growing up in the city of Accra. Each of them had been enrolled in school, but their attendance to school has always been a subject for concern for their guardians and teachers. Unfortunately, there is no system in place

E. Asampong (✉)
Department of Social and Behavioral Sciences, School of Public Health, University of Ghana, Legon, Ghana
e-mail: easampong@ug.edu.gh

A. Ibrahim
Department of Health Policy, Planning and Management, School of Public Health, University of Ghana, Legon, Ghana

© Springer Nature Switzerland AG 2022
F. M. Ssewamala et al. (eds.), *Child Behavioral Health in Sub-Saharan Africa*,
https://doi.org/10.1007/978-3-030-83707-5_5

to attend to the needs of "Kwofie" and "Ama" as they continue to be consistently absent from school.

"Kwofie" is an 8-year-old boy who lives with his parents in Accra. He is considered a burden to the family as he skips school, sometimes sneaks away from home, and engages in other social vices. Kwofie will follow friends aimlessly in their neighbourhood and sometimes scavenge for scrap metals to sell. As Kwofie grows, society is unlikely to benefit from his potential because of the neglect he faced. Currently, Kwofie's behavioral health that needs to prepare him to be a productive adult is not being addressed. Similarly, "Ama", a 10-year-old girl, lives with an aunty in Accra. She is also considered to have behavioral issues because she strays on her way to school to join her peers to engage in petty selling of sachet water and mentholated toffees on some major streets in Accra. Her aunty leaves home at dawn to engage in her business and therefore is unable to ensure that Ama really attends school. On days she goes to school and is given assignment to do as homework, there is nobody to guide her, so she fails to do the homework. Consequently, she absents herself from school the following day to avoid being punished by her teacher.

These situations are far too common among children in Ghanaian communities and in many of the African countries. Children in Ghana who do not have committed parents or guardians to put them through school and provide for them as growing children deviate from the usual path of grown-up children who are well taken care of. Some boys end up using illicit drugs and engage in other social vices at an early stage in their lives. On the other hand, some of the girls by their physical and social vulnerabilities such as entering puberty at an earlier age drop out of school, and are subjected to child marriage which robs them of the realization of their full human potential. They often get impregnated and others are hit and killed as they run in between moving vehicles in traffic to carry out their petty trading.

Meeting both Kwofie and Ama's behavioral health needs would have prepared them to become focused and dependable adults. However, this would require known and working behavioral health systems. The lack of investment in the behavioral health and well-being of children exposes them to the perils of society and deprives them of a productive future. In this chapter, we focus on some pertinent behavioral health issues among children in Ghana, as well as existing research on how available behavioral health services function in practice.

A Situational Analysis of Children in Ghana

There are varying definitions of who is considered a child across Africa. The 1992 Constitution of the Republic of Ghana stipulates that "a child is any person below the age of 18 years, i.e. the age of majority at which one is entitled to vote in national and local elections". The terminology per the constitution refers to individuals from birth to the age of 17 years. This understanding seems to be consistent with international definition in most global democracies. Perhaps for more clarity and reinforcement of who a child is, Section One of the Children's Act in Ghana also defines a child as a person below the age of 18 years (ACPF, 2012). It is worth mentioning, however, that childhood in Ghana is largely a social construct where one remains a child when he/she is under the authority, control, and care of some persons considered as adults in society.

Ghana's current population is estimated at 30.42 million (UN Population Division, 2019). This estimated figure is an increase over the official 2010 population and housing census figure of 24.2 million, which indicated a large youthful population. A little more than one person in four (26.5%) in Ghana then was a child less than 10 years. More than one-third (37.3%) of them were less than 15 years old, with another 20% between 15 and 24 years of age. In other words, a majority (57%) of Ghana's population is below the age of 24. Even though there has been reported declining fertility in recent years, Ghana's population is still considered to be young (Ghana Statistical Service, 2014).

Investing in the lives and health of children has the potential for some positive change in their lives, especially in the developing world where investment in child behavioral health is limited. The treatment gap estimated for the developing world is about 90% (WHO, 2003). In Ghana, there is more than 90% treatment gap for mental health services and it is likely to be even higher for children (WHO, 2014). Availability of behavioral health services is limited to populations in largely urban areas due to limited funding. Archaic behavioral health laws in the country also emphasize institutionalized system of care with limited emphasis on patient rights, rather than community-based services. Yet, it is critical that countries ensure that measures are put in place to make children transition smoothly into adulthood. Perhaps, it is along this path that an act, entitled the Children's Act, 1998, was enacted in Ghana. This Act is a comprehensive law for children, which consolidated and revised existing law and filled in gaps. Among other things, it sets out the rights of the child and parental duties and provides for the care and protection of children. Indeed, there are several provisions in the act that seek to protect the overall well-being of children in Ghana.

Many of these enactments are usually enforced by state agencies, such as the ministries, municipal, and district assemblies (MMDAs); nongovernmental organizations (NGOs); and civil society organizations (CSOs). In a related development, a Child and Family Welfare Policy document put together by the Ministry of Gender, Children and Social Protection in Ghana with support from UNICEF and other local and international organizations and civil society alluded to the Children's Act, in addition to the UN Convention on the Rights of the Child.

Besides, Article 28 of the 1992 Fourth Republic Constitution of Ghana (Ministry of Gender, Children and Social Protection, 2015) emphasizes a child as one who is still largely dependent on an adult for the necessaries of life. Further, Article 37(2) (b) of the Constitution of Ghana states that the "state shall enact appropriate laws to assure the protection and promotion of all other basic human rights and freedoms, including the rights of the disabled, the aged, children and other vulnerable groups in the development processes" (NPC, 2014). All these are manifestations and commitment of the state and other institutions to ensure that children are provided with the requisite protection that will enable them to realize their developmental milestones smoothly.

Historically, caring for children was not the exclusive responsibility of the biological parents. Indeed, everybody in the household and community exercised some level of control and supervision over children (Dzramedo et al., 2018). It was therefore the responsibility of both parents and community members to socialize children as they go through the developmental stages. For example, one could come home from school at a time when the parents had not returned from work or returned home from farmland. Hence, these children would be catered for by neighbours or other people in the community until the parents returned. It is worth noting that it was common for a child to be disciplined by some family elders in our Ghanaian neighbourhoods for misbehaving and upon the return of the child's parents, they would rather show their appreciation to elders for instilling discipline to the child. However, now, parents are more likely to pick a quarrel with anybody who disciplines their children in their absence. It is also worth mentioning that it was very common for other family members, such as an uncle, to give a young child a present for having passed the then "Common Entrance Examination", which was the primary gauge of a child's readiness for secondary school in Ghana. In fact, children were mostly socialized in closely connected communities and extended family networks with certain entrenched traditions that must be upheld at all costs, especially in rural areas where the extended family played a major role in the socialization processes of children.

The extended family system is observed as a social arrangement where individuals have extensive mutual commitments and responsibilities to their relations outside of the nuclear family itself (Awinongya, 2013). Indeed, in those days when the social support system was so strong and effective, it was not unusual for one to provide care to non-biological children (Boakye-Boaten, 2010). Over the years, there has been some rapid social change that has impacted the social support system. For example, rural-urban migration, which has been increasing exponentially, has dealt a great blow to this otherwise stable traditional structure, thus making some children to be cared for by other people and institutions other than their lineage groups. This has been associated with the potential of exposing such children to all kinds of challenges where they are unhappy, and do not get the love and understanding needed for appropriate nurturing (James & Roby, 2019). Consequently, it is currently not possible to guarantee the effectiveness of the social support system that existed and provide a system of support and well-being to children. In effect, children across parts of Ghana are exposed to various challenges that have potential negative mental health outcomes. Some children for instance are made to engage in activities that are not suitable for them.

Adverse Circumstances Encountered by Children in Ghana

In many parts of the country, it is not unusual for children to be seen hawking at a time when they must be in school. The Ghana Living Standard Survey (GLSS) in 2013 indicated that 23.4% of children aged 5–14 years were engaged in some form of economic activity (Ghana Statistical Service, 2014). Those children were mainly involved in the services industry, mining and quarrying, apprenticeships, and household help. There are usually associated consequences such as diminished commitment to education in terms of school attendance, enrolment, and performance (Odonkor, 2007). Some children are also trafficked from poorer regions of the country to urban centres where they are forced into exploitative labour and other practices such as early marriage and female genital cutting, both of which are detrimental to children's behavioral health (UNODC, 2019). That is not to say that only trafficked children are made to go through these practices. Many other children do, but it is most common in situations where they are not under the care of their biological parents. It must be said that many of these practices are illegal based on existing laws in Ghana, yet some people grossly overlook the law and perpetrate them regardless of the consequences that come with them. In certain instances, it has been argued that those existing laws are not properly enforced.

Early marriage for instance is linked to negative health consequences for children such as poorer maternal and reproductive health, increased risk of HIV and other sexually transmitted infections, intimate partner violence, and maternal mortality (Kidman, 2016). It is, however, common in some parts of the country. Although the legal age for girls to marry is 18 years, nearly 6% of girls between the ages of 12 and 17 years are married (Domfe and Oduro, 2018).

Another cultural practice in Ghana that is generally outlawed, but continues to thrive, is female genital circumcision. A study by Action Aid Ghana (2013) found that half of the girls aged less than 15 years in the Bawku Municipality of the Upper East Region of Ghana had undergone female genital cutting, a dangerous practice that can cause pelvic infection from the use of unsterilized instruments and scar tissue that can cause prolonged and obstructed labour. It cannot be overemphasized that such children also experience psychological challenges just for having been taken through that ordeal, including anxiety disorders, post-traumatic stress disorder (PTSD), depression, and somatic (physical) complaints (e.g., aches and pains) with no organic cause (WHO, 2017).

The Value of Education in Ghana

In recent times, the majority of families in Ghana perceive education as an avenue through which one can become "somebody" in future. Education is therefore regarded as an important tool for individuals and national development. Every effort is therefore made to take children to school (Meyer et al., 2004). In schools, teachers are regarded as important observers and are required to report any child abuse occurring in the household (Welsh Office, 1995). Besides, the expectation is that the school is a safe environment where children suffering from any form of abuse, either in the family or in the community, can be listened to or empowered to report (Mortimer et al. 2012). The reality, however, is rather that many children are afraid of abuse reports such that some tend to absent themselves from school (Jones & Pells, 2016). This usually emanates from the use of corporal punishment in homes and schools mostly through caning where fear is instilled in a child to prompt obedience despite the United Nations Committee on the Rights of the Child having strongly recommended that Ghana should prohibit the use of corporal punishment and remove from teachers' guidelines all references to disciplinary measures using physical force (United Nations, 1997).

A study by Twum-Danso (2010) found that over 70% of children cited school as the place they were most likely to experience physical punishment. Physical punishment has been shown to weaken the bond between children and parents, slow down mental development, reduce school performance, and increase the probability that the child will physically abuse others (Strauss et al., 2014). The consequences of such punishment tend to be disruptive to the self-concept and self-esteem of child victims that ultimately affect their level of confidence (Peterson et al., 2014). Unfortunately, many parents and teachers are not aware of or do not use alternative forms of discipline (UNICEF, 2010; Antonowicz, 2010), even though non-physical forms of child discipline, such as positive reinforcement, have been shown to be more effective than punishing strategies for shaping positive behaviours (Bernier et al., 2012). Every growing child misbehaves from time to time which is normal. Some children, however, may have more serious behavioral challenges. These problems can result from temporary stressors in the child's life or they may be symptoms/manifestations of underlying behaviour disorders, such as oppositional defiant disorder (ODD), conduct disorder (CD), and attention-deficit hyperactivity disorder (ADHD) (Woodard et al., 2019).

For some of the children who are physically abused, studies have shown that they tend to have higher levels of aggression and antisocial behaviour (Cicchetti et al., 2012). A study that looked at school children who were classified as physically harmed found that children with a history of physical harm were more aggressive as compared to those who did not experience any physical harm (Peterson et al., 2014). Evidence from other longitudinal studies indicates continued problems of aggression and anger as well as development of conduct disorders (Jonson-Reid et al., 2012). Children who are maltreated struggle more in their social interactions with peers (Noll et al., 2017). Some physically abused children also experience authoritarian control, anxiety-provoking behaviour, and a lack of parental warmth (Friedman & Billick, 2015). In certain instances, there is an intentional application of force against the child, and the outcome is a high likelihood of harm for the child's health, survival, development, or dignity (World Health Organization and International Society for Prevention of Child Abuse and Neglect, 2006). All these may manifest in the form of withdrawal or avoidance (Ferrara et al., 2016), or fear and anger (Odhayani et al., 2013). For these children, there is the possibility for them to see themselves in a defective manner, thus a defective self-concept that translates into a feeling of insignificance, thus a low self-esteem. This trend of development often makes children lack the confidence that is required to enable them to thrive among their peers. Such circumstances usually tend to affect the academic performance of the children because they remain quiet in class and are unable to ask any question should they not understand lessons taught.

Administrative and Policy Response

Several policy decisions have been taken to address challenges as and when they manifest and to ensure that children get the care they need. As indicated earlier, at the governmental level, there are provisions in the 1992 Republican Constitution of Ghana that provide the protection for children against any harm.

The promulgation and ratification of the UN Convention on the Rights of the Child in the year 1990 provided a standard set of rights globally for all children. This was an opportunity for governments to enact legislation, policies, and structures for setting in motion the mechanisms for these rights to be realized. The convention provided for the protection of children from harm and exploitation. In response, the Government of Ghana became the first country in the world to ratify the treaty—committing to adopt it into national law.

Following the path of the United Nations, member states of the African Union, which, at the time, was the Organization of African Unity, had agreed in 1990 to develop the African Charter on the Rights and Welfare of the Child, otherwise known as the Children's Charter. This Charter set out rights and defined universal principles and norms for the status of children. It was to emphasize the specific issues, cultural values, and experiences impacting the African child. The Children's Charter was adopted on 11 July 1990 and came into effect in 1999.

Generally, there has been several reforms, all aimed at reinforcing the rights of children. Later developments culminated in the passage of "The Children's Act" (Act 560) by the Parliament of Ghana in June 1998. The Act clearly stipulates the mechanisms and structures for its implementation at the national, regional, district, and individual levels. For example, there is the Commission on Human Rights and Administrative Justice, set up by the Constitution of Ghana as part of the support for children's access to legal aid. The commission has offices in all districts to serve as referral points on child rights.

In 2015, the Government of Ghana through the Ministry of Gender, Children and Social Protection in Ghana with support from UNICEF and other local and international organizations and civil society developed the Child and Family Welfare policy. The goal of the policy was to provide guidance to the role of specialized services, especially the expectations on the Department of Social Welfare and Community Development at district level to more closely interact with families and communities and help facilitate solutions when problems arise with emphasis on promoting welfare and restoring the well-being of the child, the family, and the community. It is also supposed to give greater flexibility and discretion to social workers at local level. The Ministry of Gender, Children and Social Protection is supposed to lead and coordinate implementation of the Policy while other key line ministries, departments, and agencies were identified to perform various roles and responsibilities as critical contributors to successfully reform the Child and Family Welfare system (Ministry of Gender and Social Protection, 2015).

Nevertheless, there are still reports of both physical and emotional abuse that leads to traumatic experiences and various behavioral disorders among children in Ghana (Badoe, 2017). This can partly be attributed to the lack of adequate notifications of violations of children's rights made to governmental agencies that are mandated to implement the demands of the child rights law, such as the Department of Social Welfare, the Domestic Violence and Victim Support Unit (DOVVSU) of the Ghana Police Service, and other civil society organizations notably Child Rights International, Ghana.

In instances where adequate notifications are given, the delays in addressing issues become a major hindrance for most people to report cases for proper redress. Perhaps, it is because one cannot see a proper harmonization of the efforts of all these institutions that are interested in child welfare matters. It appears therefore that behavioral challenges that result from child abuses and how such challenges could be addressed are done at individual institutional levels where one can hardly see a befitting redress ultimately.

The Government of Ghana in 2012 embraced the WHO community-based approach to mental healthcare and passed the mental health bill. This bill replaced the earlier 1972 mental health decree which was largely at variance with international best practices. This legislation refocused the way in which mental health services are to be provided, shifting from an institutional model to a community-based approach. It was also to address issues of stigma and discrimination against persons with mental health challenges. This notwithstanding, there is an estimated treatment gap of about 98% in Ghana, meaning that for every 100 people suffering from a behavioral disorder, only about 2 are likely to access treatment (WHO, 2007). It is probably for this reason that efforts are being made to strengthen community services which is required to decentralize management of mental health to the communities and foster early detection and treatment of mental disorders (Yaro et al., 2020).

Child Behavioural Health Research

There has been limited research on child behavioral health in Ghana and the existing research is geographically scattered (Cortina et al., 2012). One major challenge with regard to behavioral health research is the use of several local languages in the country. In many Ghanaian communities, the local population speak several languages with varying degrees of proficiency. Another issue is that the research tools, such as questionnaires devised in high-income countries, are sometimes challenging to adapt to low-resource settings. For example, it is important in both psychiatry research and clinical practice to describe psychopathology across different settings, which may require incorporating the perspectives of parents, teachers, and even children. This can be a difficult activity because there are usually limited resources, as well as different contextual factors underpinning the role of parents, teachers, and children in high-income versus less resourced countries.

It is worth noting that existing research in Ghana has identified mental and other behavioral health challenges that children have experienced (Asare & Danquah, 2016). However, evidence-based interventions that can address them and support families to address these challenges have been limited (UNICEF, 2015).

High-quality research on child mental health in both low- and middle-income countries is necessary to understand the scale of the problem (Kieling et al., 2011). However, there is a global trend of minimal resources allocated to behavioral health activities, especially in Ghana.

Most of the research has been undertaken by few psychiatrists and psychologists occasionally assisted by expatriate researchers or clinicians (Read & Doku, 2012). Much of the research has been small in scale. Available resources for behavioral health research in Ghana have mostly come from the Western world, including major donors such as the United Kingdom Department for International Development and the European Union (Eaton & Ohene, 2016).

Behavioural health generally has been described as a neglected area in Ghana's healthcare system (Read & Doku, 2012). There are also few capacities to provide needed behavioral health services by clinicians, social workers, and trained behavioral health researchers in the field. The result has been limited in the quantity and quality of research and in the clinical intervention services for behavioral health. A plausible explanation for this can be found in a systematic review of mental health research in Ghana between 1995 and 2009 where available literature revealed that 98 articles were published. This suggests an average of about seven articles on mental health per year. The authors reviewed 66 of the articles and found topics covered to include hospital- and community-based prevalence studies, psychosis, depression, substance misuse, self-harm, and help seeking (Read & Doku, 2012). They noted that much of the research was small in scale and thus largely speculative in its conclusions. This obviously is an indication for child behavioral health research to be intensified.

Cultural Attitudes to Mental Health in Ghana

Health-seeking behaviours of many Ghanaians are mostly informed by their perception of the source of their predicament. Different people from diverse cultures hold varied opinions, beliefs, and understanding with respect to the antecedents of mental illness (Nieuwsma et al., 2011). In Ghana, some think that supernatural phenomena such as being possessed by evil spirits and witchcraft are the major causes of mental illness (Crabb et al., 2012). Other people hold the view that mental health challenges are due to individuals' personal failures and often seen as a disgrace to the family. It is for that reason that many families will rather conceal the mental illness of a family member and not seek the appropriate treatment.

There are issues of stigma against families that may have a member suffering from a mental illness (Tawaih et al., 2015). That means that the effects of stigma are extended to the rest of the other family members who may not have any mental illness (van der Sanden et al., 2016). In 2012, there was a large-scale decongestion exercise undertaken at the premier psychiatric hospital (Accra Psychiatric Hospital) in Ghana. The exercise was aimed at reuniting over 600 treated patients with their families. Apparently, the facility was overwhelmed with the number of treated patients, yet they remained in the facility for several years because relatives who sent them there had refused to receive them home. In some instances, the communities from which they came from would not welcome them back. Others had also provided wrong contacts at the time they sent their relatives to the facility. It had therefore become difficult locating those family members. Even among those who were initially accepted in their homes, some of them returned to the hospital to escape from harassment and ridicule that they experienced within their communities. This was highly publicized on the Joy News outlet and other news websites on 13th January 2013.

Similarly, professionals who provide mental healthcare are sometimes ridiculed as having been affected by the very illness they care for. In effect, courtesy stigma, also referred to as "stigma by association", manifests in a public disapproval of these professionals because of their association with a stigmatized condition, an individual, or group. In view of that, most people do not want to specialize in behavioral health, neither do they want their relatives to do any specialization in mental health (Schulze, 2012; Opoku Agyeman & Ninnoni, 2018). This has implications for the number of people who are willing to take up behavioral health practice as a profession (Kapungwa et al., 2010; Jack-Ide et al., 2013). This is a plausible explanation for the few psychiatrists in Ghana. For instance, with over 30 million people in Ghana, it is estimated that there are only 18–25 psychiatrists (Ofori-Atta et al., 2018; Agyapong et al., 2016).

Child Behavioural Health Services in Ghana

Generally, the mental health system in Ghana is inundated with the absence of adequate number of mental health professionals, up-to-date mental health facilities, and highly underfunded mental health services (Roberts et al., 2014). Additionally, there is the challenge of providing quality diagnoses (Atakora & Asampong, 2020). Mental health services in Ghana are available at most levels of care. However, most of the care is provided through three specialized psychiatric hospitals in Ghana. In fact, two of these hospitals are in Accra, the capital city, and the other is located in Ankaful, a suburb of Cape Coast in the Central Region. It must be said that all these facilities are in the southern part of the country. It has therefore been difficult for people with behavioral health needs in the middle and northern sectors of the country to easily access such specialized services located in the south. Among the three hospitals, only one has a children's ward. That means that children who are admitted at the other two hospitals do not get a dedicated ward and are therefore mixed up with adults.

There are few community-based services being provided, but these are private and mainly run by religious organizations or entities. Great efforts are being made to change the model of service provision to one that emphasizes care in the community. In fact, Ghana's 1972 mental health decree had strongly emphasized institutional care to the detriment of providing mental healthcare in primary healthcare settings, contradictory to both national and international policy directives. Furthermore, procedures for involuntary admission in the 1972 law did not sufficiently protect people against unnecessary admission. Indeed, serious mistreatment of people with mental disorders has been widely reported (Juma et al., 2020). Some have been involuntarily incarcerated in institutions for decades without legal recourse or effective treatment opportunities.

In principle and as a matter of policy, mental health services in the public sector of Ghana are free. Therefore, financing of the psychiatric hospitals has mostly been provided by the government and supplemented by internally generated funds and donations. The main challenge has always been the inadequate funds that are provided to mental health facilities and what those funds are used for. In 2011 for instance, an amount of 4,516,163 Ghana Cedis (approximately 903,203 US dollars) was allocated to all three psychiatric hospitals in Ghana (Roberts et al., 2014). That amount summed up to only 1.4% of the total national health budget. The funds allocated were meant to cover overhead costs, including basic medical supplies and maintenance. Other fundings that supplement the government funds usually come from other countries and international partners, notable among them being the Department for International Development (DFID), as well as some NGOs such as BasicNeeds that also receive external funding to enable them to donate some medicines to the facilities, especially when government supplies and funds are insufficient (Shand, 2019). In effect, many people still spend large amounts on transportation and other opportunity costs to access services. Besides, in instances where there is shortage of medicines, some patients have been compelled to purchase their own medicines.

The lack of facilities across the country coupled with certain traditional beliefs makes many people seek assistance from the informal behavioral health services such as traditional and faith-based practitioners whose services vary in terms of quality and level of efficacy (Ofori Atta et al., 2010). These practitioners treat a wide range of illnesses based on the cultural contextualization of ill health (Kpobi & Swartz, 2019). Some of them use herbs while others use spiritual psychicism. There are also those who combine both methods (Addy, 2003). These practitioners therefore operate within communities where they are known to their clients (Kpobi & Swartz, 2019). We must acknowledge that there have been calls for a collaboration between biomedical system and various alternative systems (Akpalu et al., 2010), knowing very well that most people continue to access the services of alternative healers other than only those in the formal sector.

In recognition of the presence of these informal healers, BasicNeeds-Ghana, in collaboration with the Ghana Health Services (GHS) and the Mental Health Authority of Ghana (MHAG), as well as the Christian Health Association of Ghana (CHAG) through a grant from the Department for International Development (DFID) provided training to 400 traditional and 400 spiritual healers (informal healthcare providers) on how to identify mental disorders and collaboration with formal health system (Yaro et al., 2020). It must however be mentioned that these informal places are also reported to be associated with intense stigmatization, discrimination, and inhumane treatment of the people who go there to seek for spiritual and traditional healing (Dako-Gyeke and Asumang, 2013).

With regard to personnel as discussed earlier, there are not many professionals who can render the requisite services to children with behavioral health issues. Report indicates that the doctor-to-patient ratio within the mental health setting of Ghana is 1:1.7 million (Abdul Karim, 2016). Besides, there are 123 mental health outpatient services in Ghana, but there are no services exclusively for children and adolescents, although 14% of all those treated in mental health outpatient units are children and adolescents (Roberts et al., 2014).

Children are usually taken to traditional or faith-based healers because of beliefs that mental and neurological problems have spiritual causes (Akol et al., 2018). As mentioned earlier, these practitioners mostly resort to interventions such as the use of herbal medicines, rituals, and spiritual practices. Some of these practitioners put victims in chains as a means of restraining them. This approach tends to infringe on the human rights of innocent children with behavioral health disorders. Thus, there is considerable stigma among many of these children who face rejection from their communities and in some cases their own families and the public at large. Children at the Accra Psychiatric Hospital Children's ward, for instance, tend to be excited when they see visitors and will always try hugging these visitors. The general observation has been hesitation and sometimes reluctance on the part of some of the visitors to freely respond appreciably to the children. All these reactions stem from the fact that they may have been misinformed about mental illness to the extent that some even think that it is contagious.

Educational Interventions and Raising Awareness?

As a way of addressing the stigma around mental health, there are few programmes designed to educate communities about the nature of mental illness, measures to take as a way of prevention, and where people can access help. This has mostly been through the electronic media (radio and television). An example was Unilever, Ghana Limited, a company engaged in manufacturing of fast-moving consumer goods through Adams JWT Ghana, an advertising and branding communications company, that sponsored a 1-h weekly programme named "Geisha Obaatampa Do" on one of the multimedia outlets (Adom FM), where a drama on an adolescent development and mental health issues aired and allowed listeners to call into the programme with comments and questions. Two resourced persons that included a mental health professional and a social advocate were always present in the studio to speak to all the mental health-related issues. One would have thought that such an educative programme would have been sustained, but that was not the case.

Indeed, addressing stigma is essential to ensuring that persons with behavioral health challenges can lead lives of dignity and gain access to resources they need. Ahuja et al. (2017), for instance, supported the effectiveness of education and contact-based strategies as approaches for reducing mental illness stigma. Unfortunately, the development of anti-stigma programmes is still insufficient in low- and middle-income countries (Mascayano, 2015). Going forward, we need to ensure that sustainable educative programmes in relation to mental health are put in place to reach out to the public.

Conclusion

Ghana as a country has developed several national policies backed by legal instruments, all aimed at ensuring the welfare of children. In the last decade, there has been the establishment of the Ministry of Gender, Children and Social Protection, also an indication that the place of children in the country cannot be overemphasized. Further, to the extent that Ghana has signed on to and ratified several international treaties pertaining to the welfare of children is an ample testimony that children are to be nurtured properly. At best, these are fine writings and agreements that can be found on paper. In practical terms however, the current attention given to children and their behavioral health cannot be said to have reached the desired level. Some children in Ghana continue to experience some of the ills of society coupled with school dropouts who end up on the streets engaging in all kinds of risky behaviours.

Children who have behavioral health challenges do not have the benefit of dedicated places where they can seek help devoid of any stigmatizing tendencies. Besides, there are no contextualized screening tools that have been developed. As a result, one cannot be definite about the diagnosis that is made. Consequently, the need for increased research activities focusing on child behavioral health has become paramount than ever. Results derived from these researches can help shape existing policies and inform the development of newer evidence-based policies that will address existing challenges. Achieving this feat will help Ghana position herself to say that child behavioral health not only is said to be upheld but actually can also be seen to be upheld.

Recommendations

From the foregoing, it is obvious that child behavioral health has been a neglected area for a long time. The time has thus come for the needed attention to be provided. In doing so, the following recommendations are suggested:

1. There is a need for appropriate measurement and screening tools/scales that will take into account context-specific issues. This will require that some qualitative studies that explore context-specific social expectations and standards for behaviour in childhood are undertaken.
2. There is a need to incorporate behavioral health services in all regional and district hospitals by establishing behavioral health units. This will ensure that there is an equitable distribution of accessible behavioral healthcare services across all the regions.
3. There is a need for extensive and continuous research into behavioral health problems, promotion, and prevention. This will require collaboration between academics, various health institutions, and NGOs. Findings can be used as a proven basis to inform policy and practice.

References

Abdul-Karim, M. A. (2016). *Mental health care; Ghana among worst in Africa*, in press, Daily Graphic. Retrieved from http://www.graphic.com.gh/news/health/mental-health-care-ghana-among-worst-in-africa.html

ACPF. (2012). *Child law resources, Volume 2: Reporting status of African States*. Retrieved http://www.africanchildinfo.net/clr/vol2

Action Research on Female Genital Mutilation in the Bawku Municipality, Upper East Region: By BEWDA in collaboration with Actionaid. January, 2013.

Addy, M. E. (2003). *Putting science into the art of healing with herbs*. Ghana Universities Press.

Agyapong, V. I. O., Farren, C., & McAuliffe, E. (2016). Improving Ghana's mental healthcare through task-shifting-psychiatrists and health policy directors' perceptions about government's commitment and the role of community mental health workers. *Globalization and Health, 12*, 57.

Ahuja, K. K., Dhillon, M., Juneja, A., & Sharma, B. (2017). Breaking barriers: An education and contact intervention to reduce mental illness stigma among Indian college students. Psychosocial intervention. *Agostology, 26*, 103–109.

Akol, A., Molan, K. M., Babirye, J. N., & Engebrestsen, I. M. S. (2018). "We are like co-wives": Traditional healers' views on collaborating with the formal child and adolescent mental health system in Uganda. *BMC Health Services Research, 18*, 258.

Akpalu B, Lund C, Doku V, (2010). et al. Scaling up community-based services and improving quality of care in the state psychiatric hospitals: The way forward for Ghana. The African Journal of Psychiatry 13:109–115. https://doi.org/10.4314/ajpsy.v13i2.54356.

Antonowicz, L. (2010). *Too often in silence: A report on school-based violence in west and Central Africa. UNICEF, plan, save the children and action aid.* Retrieved from http://www.unicef.org/cotedivoire/too_often_in_silence_report.pdf.

Asare, M., & Danquah, S. A. (2016). Observation report from clinical practice in Ghana: Children and adolescent depression. *Journal of Child Adolescent Behavior, 4*, 286.

Atakora, M., & Asampong, E. (2020). A study of the diagnostic practices for mental disorders in Ghana. *Journal of Clinical Review & Case Reports, 5*(4), 189.

Awinongya, M. A. (2013). The understanding of family in Ghana as a challenge for a contextual ecclesiology. In *LIT*. Deutsche Nationalbibliothek.

Badoe, E. (2017). A critical review of child abuse and its management in Africa. *African Journal of Emergency Medicine, 7*, 32–33.

Bernier, S., Simpson, C. G., & Rose, C. A. (2012). Positive and negative reinforcement in increasing compliance and decreasing problematic behavior. *National Teacher Education Journal, 2012*, 45–51.

Boakye-Boaten, A. (2010). Changes in the concept of childhood: Implications for children in Ghana. *Journal of International Social Research, 3*(10), 104–115.

Cicchetti, D., Rogosch, F. A., & Thibodeau, E. L. (2012). The effects of child maltreatment on early signs of antisocial behavior: Genetic moderation by tryptophan hydroxylase, serotonin transporter, and monoamine oxidase a genes. *Development and Psychopathology, 24*(3), 907–928.

Cortina, M. A., Sodha, A., Fazel, M., & Ranchandani, P. G. (2012). Prevalence of child mental health problems in sub-Saharan Africa: a systematic review. *Archives of Pediatrics and Adolescent Medicine, 166*(3), 276–281. https://doi.org/10.1001/archpediatrics.2011.592

Crabb, J., Stewart, C. R., Kokota, D., Masson, N., Chabunya, S., & Krishnadas, R. (2012). Attitudes towards mental illness in Malawi: A cross-sectional survey. *Biomedicalcentral Public Health, 12*, 541.

Dako-Gyeke, M., & Asumang, E. S. (2013). Stigmatization and discrimination experiences of persons with mental illness: Insights from a qualitative study in Southern Ghana. *Social Work & Society, 11*(1), 1–14.

Domfe, G., Oduro, A. D. (2018). *Prevalence and trends in child marriage in Ghana.* Centre for Social Policy Studies (CSPS) Technical Publications Series No. 1/18.

Dzramedo, J. E., Amoako, B. M., & Amos, P. M. (2018). The state of the extended family system in Ghana: Perceptions of some families. *Research on Humanities and Social Sciences, 8*, 24.

Eaton, J., & Ohene, S. (2016). *Providing sustainable mental health Care in Ghana: A demonstration project.* National Academies Press.

Ferrara, P., Guadagno, C., Sbordone, A., Amato, M., Spina, G., Perrone, G., Cutrona, C., Basile, M. C., Ianniello, F., Fabrizio, G. C., Pettoello-Mantovani, M., Verrotti, A., Villani, A., & Corsello, G. (2016). Child abuse and neglect and its psycho-physical and social consequences: A review of the literature. *Current Pediatric Reviews, 12*(4), 301–310.

Friedman, E., & Billick, S. B. (2015). Unintentional child neglect: Literature review and observational study. *The Psychiatric Quarterly, 86*(2), 253–259.

Ghana Statistical Service. (2014). Ghana - Ghana Living Standards Survey 6 (With a Labour Force Module) 2012–2013, Round Six. GHA-GSS-GLSS6–2012-v1.0.

Jack-Ide, I. O., Uys, L. R., & Middleton, L. E. (2013). Mental health care policy environment in Rivers state: Experiences of mental health nurses providing mental health care services in neuro-psychiatric hospital, Port Harcourt, Nigeria. *International Journal of Mental Health Systems, 7*, 8.

James, S. L., & Roby, J. L. (2019). Comparing reunified and residential care facility children's wellbeing in Ghana. 'The role of hope'. *Children and Youth Services Review, 96*, 316–325.

Jones, H., Pells, K. (2016). *Undermining learning: Multi-country longitudinal evidence on corporal punishment in schools.* Innocenti Resarch Brief. UNICEF. Retrieved from http://disde.minedu.gob.pe/handle/123456789/4063.

Jonson-Reid, M., Kohl, P. L., & Drake, B. (2012). Child and adult outcomes of chronic child maltreatment. *Pediatrics, 129*(5), 839–845.

Juma, K., Wekesah, F. M., Kabiru, C. W., & Izugbara, C. O. (2020). Burden, drivers, and impacts of poor mental health in young people of west and Central Africa: Implications for research and programming. In M. McLean (Ed.), *West African youth challenges and opportunity pathways. Gender and cultural studies in Africa and the diaspora*. Palgrave Macmillan.

Kapungwe, A., Cooper, S., Mwanza, J., Mwape, L., Sikwese, A., Kakuma, R., Lund, C., & Flisher, A. J. (2010). Mental illness stigma and discrimination in Zambia. *African Journal of Psychiatry, 13*, 192–203.

Kidman, R. (2016). Child marriage and intimate partner violence: A comparative study of 34 countries. *International Journal of Epidemiology, 46*(2), 662–675.

Kieling, C., Baker-Henningham, H., Belfer, M., Conti, G., Ertem, I., Omigbodun, O., Rohde, L. A., Srinath, S., Ulkuer, N., & Rahman, A. (2011). Child and adolescent mental health worldwide: evidence for action. *Lancet 378*, 1515–1525. https://doi.org/10.1016/S0140-6736(11)60827-1

Kpobi, L., & Swartz, L. (2019). Indigenous and faith healing in Ghana: A brief examination of the Formalising process and collaborative efforts with the biomedical health system. *African Journal of Primary Health Care & Family Medicine, 11*(1), 2035.

Mascayano, F., Armijo, J. E., & Yang, L. H. (2015). Addressing stigma relating to mental illness in low- and middle-income countries. *Frontiers in Psychiatry, 6*, 1–4.

Meyer, A., Eilertsen, D. E., Sundet, J. M., Tshifularo, J. G., & Sagvolden, T. (2004). Cross-cultural similarities in ADHD-like behaviour amongst south African primary school children. *South African Journal of Psychiatry, 34*, 123–139.

Ministry of Gender, Children and Social Protection. (2015). *Child and family welfare policy*.

Mortimer, J., North, A., Katz, M., Stead, J. (2012). *You have someone to trust: Outstanding safeguarding practice in primary schools*. Office of the Children's Commissioner. [Online]. Retrieved from http://dera.ioe.ac.uk/15496/1/You_Have_Someone_to_Trust_FINAL_Sept_2012%5B1%5D.pdf

Nieuwsma, J. A., Pepper, C. M., Maack, D. J., & Birgenheir, D. G. (2011). Indigenous perspectives on depression in rural regions of India and the United States. *Transcultural Psychiatry, 48*(5), 539–568.

Noll, J. G., Reader, J. M., & Bensman, H. (2017). Environments recreated: The unique struggles of children born to abused mothers. In D. Teti (Ed.), *Parenting and family processes in child maltreatment and intervention. Child Maltreatment Solutions Network*. Springer.

NPC Policy Brief No. III. (2014). Population ageing in Ghana and its implications.

Odhayani, A. A., Watson, W. J., & Watson, L. (2013). Behavioural consequences of child abuse. *Canadian Family Physician, 59*(8), 831–836.

Odonkor, M. (2007). Addressing child labour through education: A study of alternative/complementary initiatives in quality education delivery and their suitability for cocoa-farming communities. Retrieved from http://citeseerx.ist.psu.edu/viewdoc/download?doi=10.1.1.732.5631&rep=rep1&type=pdf

Ofori-Atta, A., Attafuah, J., Jack, H., et al. (2018). Joining psychiatric care and faith healing in a prayer camp in Ghana: Randomised trial. *British Journal of Psychiatry, 212*(1), 34–41.

Ofori-Atta, A., Read, U., & Lund, C. (2010). A situation analysis of mental health services and legislation in Ghana: Challenges for transformation. *African Journal of Psychiatry, 13*, 99–108.

Ogundele, M. O. (2018). Behavioral and emotional disorders in childhood: A brief overview for paediatricians. *World Journal of Clinical Pediatrics, 7*(1), 9–26.

Opoku Agyeman, S., & Ninnoni, J. P. (2018). The effects of stigma on mental health nurses: A study at ankaful psychiatric hospital. *An International Journal of Nursing and Midwifery, 2*, 1.

Petersen, A. C., Joseph, J., & Feit, M. (2014). *Committee on child maltreatment research, policy, and practice for the next decade: Phase II; Board on Children, Youth, and Families; Committee on Law and Justice; Institute of Medicine; National Research Council*. National Academies Press.

Rathod, S., Pinninti, N., Irfan, M., Gorczynski, P., Rathod, P., Gega, L., & Naeem, F. (2017). Mental health service provision in low- and middle-income countries. *Health Services Insights, 10*, 1178632917694350.

Read, U. M., & Doku, V. C. K. (2012). Mental health research in Ghana: A literature review. *Ghana Medical Journal, 46*, 2.

Roberts, M., Mogan, C., & Asare, J. B. (2014). An overview of Ghana's mental health system: results from an assessment using the World Health Organization's Assessment Instrument for Mental Health Systems (WHO-AIMS). *International Journal of Mental Health Systems, 8*, 16.

Schilze, B. (2012). Stigma and mental health professionals: A review of the evidence on an intricate relationship. *International Review of Psychiatry, 19*(2), 137–155.

Shand, W. (2019). *New Climate Economy (NCE), 2020. The finance landscape in Ghana: Mobilising investment in sustainable urban infrastructure.* Paper for the Coalition for Urban Transitions. London and Washington. Retrieved from http://newclimateeconomy.net/content/cities-working-papers

Strauss, M. A., Douglas, E. M., & Medeiros, R. A. (2014). *The primordial violence: Spanking children, psychological development, violence, and crime.* Routledge.

Tawiah, P. E., Adongo, P. B., & Aikins, M. (2015). Mental health-related stigma and discrimination in Ghana: Experience of patients and their caregivers. *Ghana Medical Journal, 49*(1), 30–36.

Twum-Danso, A. (2010). *Children's perceptions of physical punishment in Ghana.* Nuffield Foundation. Retrieved from http://www.icyrnet.net/UserFiles/File/Children_Perceptions_of_%20Physical_%20Punishment_Ghana.pdf

UNICEF. (2010). *Child disciplinary practices at home: Evidence from a range of low- and middle-income countries.* United Nations Children's Fund.

UNICEF and Global Affairs Canada. (2015). Building a national child protection system in Ghana: From evidence to policy and practice.

United Nations (1997). *Committee on rights of child concludes fifteenth session.* Retrieved from http://www.un.org/press/en/1997/19970606.hr4330.html

UNODC. (2019). Child trafficking in Ghana.

van der Sanden, R. L., Pryor, J. B., Stutterheim, S. E., Kok, G., & Bos, A. E. (2016). Stigma by association and family burden among family members of people with mental illness: The mediating role of coping. *Social Psychiatry and Psychiatric Epidemiology, 51*(9), 1233–1245.

Welsh Office. (1995). *Protecting children from abuse: The role of the education service.* Welsh Office Circular 52/95.

Woodard, T. J., Ume, U., & Davis, R. (2019). An introduction to oppositional defiant disorder and conduct disorder. *US Pharmacology, 44*(11), 29–32.

World Health Organisation. (2003). *Investing in mental health.* Retrieved from www.who.int/mental_health/media/en/investing_mnh.pdf

World Health Organization. (2007). Ghana a very progressive mental health law. In *Mental improvements for nations development.* WHO.

World Health Organization. (2014). *Mental health Ghana situational analysis.* Retrieved from http://www.who.int/mental_health/policy/country/ghana/en/

World Health Organization. (2017). *Sexual and reproductive health: Health risks of female genital mutilation (FGM).* Retrieved from http://www.who.int/reproductivehealth/topics/fgm/health_consequences_fgm/en/

World Health Organization and International Society for Prevention of Child Abuse and Neglect. (2006). The nature and consequences of child maltreatment. In *Preventing child maltreatment: A guide to taking action and generating evidence.* WHO.

Yaro, P. B., Asampong, E., Tabong, P. T. N., Anaba, S. A., Azuure, S. S., Dokurugu, A. Y., & Nantogmah, F. A. (2020). Stakeholders' perspectives about the impact of training and sensitization of traditional and spiritual healers on mental health and illness: A qualitative evaluation in Ghana. *International Journal of Social Psychiatry, 5*, 1–9. https://doi.org/10.1177/0020764020918284

Children and Child Behavioral Health in Nigeria: Current Efforts in Policy, Research, and Practice

Ednah Ndidi Madu and Hadiza Osuji

Introduction

Mental health disorders in adolescence are a significant problem globally. According to the World Health Organization (WHO, 2018), mental health conditions account for 16% of the global burden of disease and injury in people aged 10–19 years. Depression is the leading cause of illness, and suicide the leading cause of death among this young population. The onset of all mental health conditions is around the age of 14 years, and most of the cases are undetected and, therefore, untreated (Kessler et al., 2007). This is due in part to the lack of mental health services for adolescents and youth at risk or with mental health disorders. Many young people with mental health problems encounter difficulties in finding appropriate comprehensive resources, support, care, and treatment to their complex and multilayered needs. Globally, depression and anxiety in particular have increased over time (Reem et al., 2019). The burden from depression alone has been estimated to likely increase to be the single biggest burden of all health conditions by 2030 (WHO, 2012). The consequences of not addressing adolescent mental health conditions extend to adulthood, impairing both physical and mental health, and limiting opportunities to lead fulfilling lives as adults. Promoting psychological well-being and protecting adolescents from adverse experiences and risk factors that may impact their potential to thrive are critical for their well-being during adolescence and for physical and mental health into adulthood.

Although the WHO's push for mental health to be included in the Millennium Development Goals (the Mental Health Gap Action Plan) has raised the profile of

E. N. Madu
College of Nursing and Public Health, Adelphi University, Garden City, NY, USA

H. Osuji (✉)
Silver School of Social Work, New York University, New York, NY, USA
e-mail: hosuji@yahoo.com

© Springer Nature Switzerland AG 2022
F. M. Ssewamala et al. (eds.), *Child Behavioral Health in Sub-Saharan Africa*,
https://doi.org/10.1007/978-3-030-83707-5_6

child mental health universally, many countries especially low- and middle-income countries are still lacking behind in the efforts to improve child and adolescent mental health (CAMH). In sub-Saharan Africa specifically, prevalence rate for childhood mental health problems is as high as 20% (Cortina et al., 2012), yet few economic or human resources are dedicated to the mental health of children and young people. There is a dearth of mental health policy framework uniquely pertaining to children and adolescents. Hence, there is no clear pathway to access treatment, especially inpatient facilities, and, when treatment does occur, the providers are rarely mental health specialists (Owen et al., 2016). Moreover, many regions are confronted with political turmoil, economic upheavals, and other health challenges including Ebola, malaria, tuberculosis, and high infant and maternal mortality (Mwaniki, 2018; Omigbodun, 2008), which largely distract the public's and politicians' attention from CAMH. Further, few studies have estimated prevalence rates, assessed needs, or tested interventions in African countries. Consequently, the magnitude of CAMH problem as a significant burden on public health does not receive the much-deserved recognition by the public or policy makers (Omigbodun, 2008).

In Nigeria for example, a significant number of children have been found to be suffering from mental health problems (Adewuya et al., 2007; Adelekan et al., 1999; Chinawa et al., 2014; Jegede et al., 1990). Nearly 30% of Nigerians out of a population of over 200 million are believed to suffer from mental health disorders (Suleiman, 2016). Nigeria is the country with the largest population in Africa and has been ranked as the seventh most populous country in the world (Mwaniki, 2018). The *World Factbook* projects population of Nigeria to grow from more than 186 million people in 2016 to 392 million in 2050 [Central Intelligence Agency (CIA), 2021]. This will make her the world's fourth most populous country. The sustained high population growth rate is expected to continue in the foreseeable future due to population momentum and high birth rate (CIA, 2021). According to the World Poverty Clock report compiled by Brookings Institution, Nigeria had the largest number of people living in extreme poverty in early 2018 and this number continues to grow (Kharas et al., 2018). Physical, social, and family dysfunction and unfavorable family environment are among the most important negative contributors to children mental health (Cortina et al., 2012). Social conditions such as the recent violent attacks of Boko Haram (an Islamist terrorist movement) in the Northeastern part of Nigeria are killing and injuring thousands of the populace, leading to millions fleeing the conflict zone. The massive social upheaval caused by the Fulani Herdsmen, nomadic or seminomadic Fulani people whose primary occupation is raising livestock, has now turned Fulani militia clashing with farmers (Amnesty, 2018). Cattle trample farmers' fields, farmers kill cattle, and herdsmen seek revenge leading to thousands being killed. These contribute to the threat on the state of CAMH in Nigeria as well as child and adolescent mental illness.

The prevalence of major depressive disorder (MDD) among Nigerian adolescents is comparable to the prevalence found in Western countries and continues to increase (Adewuya et al., 2007). In primary care settings in Ibadan, Nigeria, 20% of children and adolescents were found to have mental health problems (Gureje et al., 1994). A multistage cross-sectional study conducted by Lasebikan et al. (2012) to determine the prevalence of psychiatric morbidity in selected semi-urban primary care centers in Lagos Island, Nigeria, found a high prevalence of psychiatric morbidity consisting of approximately 60% unexplained somatic complaint disorder, 50% depressive disorder, and roughly 11% alcohol-use disorder. Despite the improbable prevalence of mental health problems among children and adolescents in Nigeria, the notion of mental health is often culturally or socially dodged and most of the child and adolescent health initiatives in Nigeria lack a child and adolescent mental health strategy. Thus, CAMH issues have remained obscure to the country's current efforts in policy and practices (Atilola et al., 2014).

CAMH Research

CAMH research has attracted attention globally, though requiring better representation from the African continent, particularly in Nigeria with a population of approximately two million people. An integrative review by Weems and Overstreet (2008) was conducted in New Orleans, United States, after the Hurricane Katrina disaster. Child and adolescent mental health research studies with ecological need-based perspective in the context of the hurricane were reviewed. Empirical data on the effects on youth were utilized with the goal of learning from the horrible disaster for practice and policy improvements. Considering the overwhelming burden of mental health resulting from reduced attention to mental health in most African countries, more CAMH research representations from African countries are needed. However, some countries seem to be rising up to the challenge.

In South Africa, Flisher et al. (2012) acknowledged the key role which reducing the burden of mental disorders in childhood plays in reducing its progression later into adulthood. In their research paper which focused on service needs for children and adolescents, the authors commenced with a discussion of the prevalence of child and adolescent psychiatric disorders. Legal and policy contexts of child and adolescent psychiatric services were described, a framework for child and adolescent mental health service provision was presented, and steps for reducing the extent of unmet service need were considered. Based on the stark realities of unmet need and constitutional rights of children and adolescents to appropriate mental health care, Flisher et al. (2012) concluded their paper by making a call to scale up child and adolescent mental health services in South Africa. In Botswana, a retrospective study by Olashore et al. (2017) sought to determine the pattern of presentation of child psychiatric disorders and the predictors of poor treatment outcome in the national psychiatric hospital in Botswana. In addition to identifying baseline information regarding mental health in children, the study highlighted the need for further research, and to develop more specialized mental healthcare services for improved outcomes in children with mental health disorder in the country.

In West African countries, there is a great need for mental health services as well as research focused on CAMH. For example, the psychosocial impact of war has led to the growing amount of research on children in Sierra Leone (Yoder et al., 2016), and need for mental health services (Shackman & Price, 2013). In a systematic review on school mental health in Nigeria, Atilola and Ola (2016) showed that epidemiological data and needs assessments were significantly limited in epistemological philosophy and cultural contextualization evidenced by a "preponderance of non-representative data, quantitative assessments, and de-contextualized interpretation of results and conclusions." The dearth of research focused on CAMH epidemiology and services in Nigeria plays a role in impeding CAMH policy development as well as implementing evidence-based practices. Consequently, there is a growing concern and an increasing call for the development of a robust base for CAMH research in Nigeria to provide the scientific estimates and strategies to address the CAMH burden. Omigbodun (2008) for example averred that CAMH researchers in sub-Saharan Africa should take up the burden of research geared towards charting a course for developing CAMH policy in the region. Additionally, the research should be developed to tap from local experience and expertise rather than foreign policy which may not contextually fit into the local context and challenges. Consequently, there is an urgent need to generate more culturally nuanced CAMH research data.

Facilities and Structures

Illustrative of the foregoing situation, Atilola et al. (2014) used information from UNICEF's State of the World's Children as proxy data to speculate on the state of child mental health in Nigeria in order to bring the status of CAMH to the attention of policy makers. They found that in addition to the dearth of CAMH research, facilities were limited, and many of the existing mental health hospitals and primary healthcare centers are in dilapidating conditions. A report by the World Health Organization [(WHO), 2008] indicated that many of the existing mental health hospitals are too old to be amenable to repair, and thus, new hospitals may have to be built to replace the old ones. Hawkins' (2014) study findings revealed that in a 74-bed hospital, there were only 6 (8%) beds, with a bed-to-population ratio of 3: 100,000, falling into the category of critical bed shortage (<12 per beds for every 100,000), with many patients lying on the bare floor during the study duration. This finding is resonated by the aversion of some other scholars who found that many mental health hospitals particularly in the tropics placed patients in cells without water facilities, toilets, or beds, so the patients had to urinate and defecate in the wards (Aborisade & Fayemi, 2016; Omaka, 2014; Solomon et al., 2014). Further, overcrowding is another dismal feature as the recommendation of two patients per room is violated (Phalen 2014; Thirunavukarasu, 2011; Thirunavukarasu & Thirunavukarasu, 2010; WHO, 2008). Many hospitals used single-person cells to house several patients which is both dehumanizing and unacceptable (Nwaopara, 2016; Thirunavukarasu, 2011; World Health Organization, 2008).

The Child and Adolescent Mental Health (CAMH) Center of the Federal Neuropsychiatric Hospital located in Oshodi, Lagos State, is currently the largest CAMH center in Nigeria. The center was founded in 1999 and utilizes a multimodal approach to manage CAMH cases. In addition, it provides training programs in the field of child psychiatry. The CAMH center had engaged in widespread campaign and media efforts to alert the public about child mental health issues which yielded responses. However, the goals are yet to be realized.

In 2011, the John D. and Catherine T. MacArthur Foundation approved a grant for building CAMH capacity in Africa. Through this grant, the Centre for Child and Adolescent Mental Health (CCAMH) was established at the University of Ibadan, Nigeria. In addition to Africa, the center has guest faculty from institutions in three other continents including Asia, Europe, and North America. The research activities of the program focus on collecting epidemiological data about the prevalence and nature of CAMH problems in Nigeria from which public policy and services can be developed. In addition, the program aims at developing a cadre of professionals who would be a resource to Nigeria and other parts of sub-Saharan Africa. Finally, the center targets to drive full intersectoral collaboration between all major stakeholders involved in child mental health services in the community to improve CAMH services and outcomes. Yet, the desired goal of the center is far from being established.

Infrastructural Gap and Investment

Profound shortage of human resources and basic infrastructure needed to provide adequate mental health services leads to tragically high and persistent unmet needs (Becker & Kleinman, 2012; Uwakwe & Otakpor, 2014). The expenditure for mental health care is very low with only approximately 1% of the 3% gross domestic product (GDP) that is disbursed for health being allocated to mental health institutions and services (Becker & Kleinman, 2012). The WHO recommends 5% of funds be used for mental health, and in many countries, it is about 15% (WHO, 2014).

The centricity of an unbiased access to mental health care and the protection of rights is expedient in healthcare systems of developed and developing countries (Jacob et al., 2007). Mental health systems are a subsystem of the healthcare system of any country. Therefore, how these services are organized, delivered, and financed is significantly a consequence of how the overall health service systems are run (Olson, 2006). Better and improved service provision is the primary objective of any mental health system, which therefore ensures that organizations, institutions, and resources are geared towards achieving the primary objective in terms of the mental health of the populace.

The WHO conceptualizes optimal actions for improved service provision as "establishing national policies, programs, and legislation on mental health, providing services for mental disorders in primary care, ensuring accessibility to essential psychotropic medication, developing human resources, promoting public education and involving other sectors and promoting and supporting relevant research" (WHO-AIMS, 2006). Despite this, mental health systems in low- and middle-income sub-Saharan African countries, Nigeria inclusive, face challenges in ensuring optimal mental healthcare services (Saraceno et al., 2007). Most low-income countries do not have mental health legislation or policies to direct relevant treatment and programs lack appropriately trained mental health personnel (World Health Organization, 2008). For example, Socrates Mbamalu (2019) reported that the Yaba Psychiatric Hospital which had a budget of 133 million naira ($372,000) only received 13 million naira ($36,000) from the federal government which led to the loss of half of the resident psychiatrists. Consequently, the shortfalls not only affect the quality of services, but also limit access to mental health care. In some countries, coordinated efforts to close mental health gaps are embarked on, particularly after catastrophic events. For example, Ravioli and colleagues (2013) provide an overview of the mental health response to the 2010 Haiti earthquake. The authors discussed the consideration of complexities that relate to the emergency response, mental health and psychosocial response in disasters, long-term planning of systems of care, and development of safe, effective, and culturally appropriate mental health services in the Haitian context. In other countries, however, for example Kenya, mental health policy is lagging. The Kenya Mental Health Act 1989 is reported to be outdated, leading to lack of a comprehensive national mental health law (Ndetei et al., 2017).

With respect to children and adolescents, significant gaps are noted regarding understanding the effectiveness of treatments used for the management of child mental disorders, as well as factors that influence the processes involved. The need to develop a more robust base for CAMH epidemiological and service research has therefore been recommended (Owen et al., 2016). The very low level of expenditure on mental health care is manifested in the decaying infrastructure. Even if services were well organized, many of the cases could not receive the needed adequate orthodox psychiatric care due to the shortage of mental health professionals to cater for the health needs of the nation (Uwakwe & Otakpor, 2014; Ewhrudjakpor, 2010). Most of the mental health professionals that are available are located within the urban and southern parts of Nigeria (Gureje, 2003). Consequently, the psychiatrist-patient ratio in Nigeria is dismal, thus widening the mental health treatment gap.

The Mental Health Services on the Ground

In a systematically gathered information from the five Anglophone West African countries (Gambia, Sierra Leone, Ghana, Nigeria, and Liberia), the state of resources and mental health services/care are in various stages of development, and generally characterized by inadequate human resources and long policy neglect. The region has however made some important contributions to community service development and global mental health research. The reported challenges include manpower development, policy and legislation updates, as well as increased attention to policy and budget (Esan et al., 2014).

The Nigerian Federal Ministry of Health (2013) reported that government services are provided mainly in large tertiary institutions (federal neuropsychiatric hospitals) and University Teaching Hospital psychiatric departments. Some states have psychiatric hospitals and some federal medical centers have a psychiatric department. The geographical focus of all these services is in the urban areas, which makes access to care difficult for the majority of the population who reside in the rural areas. There are less than 150 psychiatrists in the country (around one per one million population) and very few neurologists, with many newly trained specialists leaving the country to work abroad. There are around five psychiatric nurses per 100,000 population and only very few other mental and neurological health professionals like clinical psychologists, social workers, neuro-physiotherapists, and occupational therapists. The systems that support delivery of services are currently weak, with a lack of accessibility to psychotropic drugs and difficulty with the incorporation of mental and neurological health measures in health information systems.

The main cause of inequitable access to mental health facilities is the lack of appropriate legislation in Nigeria. This in turn violates the principles of the primary healthcare system, essentially providing a vertical rather than an integrated service. Information about the level of mental health service provision in Nigeria is limited. It is therefore difficult to identify areas of need, make informed decisions about policy direction, and monitor progress. A consequence of this information gap is the continued neglect of mental health issues, as well as huge unmet service needs for CAMH problems in the community (WHO-AIMS, 2006).

The Mental Health Policy Context in Nigeria

Nigeria's current mental health legislation stems from a lunacy ordinance that was enacted in 1916 (Ogunlesi et al., 2012). The lunacy ordinance was instituted by the British colonizers in Nigeria and assumed the status of a law in 1958. The law sought to address mental health disorders and disabilities and defines mental illness as lunacy which includes persons with unsound mind (Sanni & Adebayo, 2014; Ude, 2015; Westbrook, 2011). Consequently, the definition of mental health on the bases of this act was problematic due to its derogative nature towards people with mental health needs. Thus, the Lunacy Act failed to protect the rights of persons with mental health disorders. In addition, the Act did not meet the WHO's definition and description of mental health and persons with mental health issues. As such, it did not meet the international requirements for a good policy (Ude, 2015). The Nigerian legislation was perceived to be established based on colonial ideology of social control, rather than as institutions where persons with mental health challenges could receive therapeutic treatment and proper care. Subsequently, an attempt to repeal and replace the law with a new mental health bill was proposed by Sen. Ibiapuye

Martyns-Yellowe and Sen. Dalhatu Tafida in 2003 (Ude, 2015). The bill was finally withdrawn from the Senate in 2009 after unsuccessful attempts to pass the legislative process.

The Mental Health Act was reintroduced to the National Assembly by Hon. Samuel Adejare and Hon. Solomon Adeola in 2013. The proposed Mental Health bill redefines mental health disorders, replacing "lunatic" with an updated, internationally focused definition of mental health disorders; removes the discretionary power given to medical practitioners and magistrates to determine who was mentally ill; provides protection for the rights of persons with mental disorders; ensures equal access to treatment and care; discourages stigma and discrimination; and sets standards for psychiatric practice in Nigeria (Sanni & Adebayo, 2014; Ude, 2015). Discouraging discrimination in the perception of persons with mental health issues aligns with the WHO report, which recognized the importance of optimal mental health in the overall well-being of individuals, societies, and countries, recommending urgently needed policies to break down mental health stigma and discrimination and implement effective policies for prevention and treatment (WHO, 2001).

The reintroduction of the Mental Health Act with the updated internationally focused definition of mental health disorders has important policy and practice implications. To achieve the desired target of WHO-recommended practice guidelines, advocacy driven by all stakeholders will most likely reinforce governmental enactment of laws that meet contemporary benchmarks, improve mental healthcare delivery, and provide a better basis for later legislative revisions. In practice, the rights of vulnerable persons in need of mental health services would most likely be protected if discriminatory or derogatory terms are avoided, as the use of such terminologies could further discourage care-seeking attitudes of persons who would otherwise benefit from such care.

Although the current mental health bill has better provisions for persons with mental health challenges as well as for the society, efforts made to represent it as an executive bill endorsed by the Federal Ministry of Health have yet to be materialized.

Conclusion

For too long, CAMH in Nigeria has been largely overlooked. Nigeria is the most populous country in Africa. Yet, it is still lagging behind with regard to mental health personnel and official attention to CAMH services and policy strategy. In addition, the lack of current and representative epidemiological data on the mental health of Nigerian children continues to be a barrier to advocacy for CAMH policy initiatives. The need to improve research infrastructure and capacity in low- and middle-income countries (LMIC) has been severally highlighted (Saxena et al., 2006; Patel et al., 2007). Consequently, most of the problems in relation to CAMH can be addressed through capacity building and training. Research and training partnerships with support from high-income countries are critical to building research capacity in the country. Further, in view of the importance of CAMH to national development, continued search for ways to bring the state of CAMH in Nigeria to the attention of policy makers remains critical. It is pertinent that Nigeria develops and implements both a policy and legal framework for addressing CAMH as well as integrating mental health into primary care facilities to provide person-centered and holistic services. Furthermore, it is necessary to undertake the widespread education of the Nigerian public on the recognition of mental health disorders as a disease particularly among children and adolescents, create networks for societal and family support, and decrease the stigmatization of people suffering from mental health disorders.

References

Aborisade, R. A., & Fayemi, J. A. (2016). A qualitative exploration of the coping strategies of female offenders in Nigerian prisons. *International Journal of Criminology and Sociological Theory, 9*, 1–14.

Adegboyega O., & Ogunwale, O. A. (2012). Mental health legislation in Nigeria: current leanings and future yearnings. *International Psychiatry 9*(3) 62–64. https://doi.org/10.1017/S1749367600003234

Adelekan, M., Ndom, R. J., Ekpo, M., & Oluboka, O. (1999). Epidemiology of childhood behavioural disorders in Ilorin, Nigeria—findings from parental reports. *West African Journal of Medicine, 18*, 39–48.

Adewuya, A. O., Ola, B. A., & Aloba, O. O. (2007). Prevalence of major depressive disorders and a validation of the Beck depression inventory among Nigerian adolescents. *European Child & Adolescent Psychiatry, 16*(5), 287–292. https://doi.org/10.1007/s00787-006-0557-0

Amnesty. (2018). Farmer-herder clashes kill 3,600 in Nigeria. Archived from the original on 6 February 2019. Retrieved June 20, 2019.

Atilola, O., Ayinde, O., Emedoh, C., & Oladimeji, O. (2014). State of the Nigerian child—Neglect of child and adolescent mental health: A review. *Paediatrics and International Child Health, 35*, 2046905514Y0000000137. https://doi.org/10.1179/2046905514Y.0000000137

Atilola, O., & Ola, B. (2016). Towards school mental health programmes in Nigeria: Systematic review revealed the need for contextualised and culturally-nuanced research. *Journal of Child & Adolescent Mental Health, 28*(1), 47–70.

Becker, A. E., & Kleinman, A. (2012). An agenda for closing resource gaps in global mental health: Innovation, capacity building, and partnerships. *Harvard Review of Psychiatry, 20*(1), 3–5. https://doi.org/10.3109/10673229.2012.652875

Central Intelligence Agency. (2021). The world factbook: Nigeria. Retrieved from https://www.cia.gov/the-world-factbook/countries/nigeria/#people-and-society

Chinawa, J., Manyike, M., Obu, P. C., Odetunde, O. I., Aniwada, E. C., Ndu, I. K., & Chinawa, A. (2014). Behavioral disorder amongst adolescents attending secondary school in Southeast Nigeria. *Behavioral Neurology, 2014*, 705835. https://doi.org/10.1155/2014/705835

Cortina, M. A., Sodha, A., Fazel, M., & Ramchandani, P. G. (2012). Prevalence of child mental health problems in sub-Saharan Africa: A systematic review. *Archives of Pediatrics & Adolescent Medicine, 166*(3), 276–281. https://doi.org/10.1001/archpediatrics.2011.592

Esan, O., Abdumalik, J., Eaton, J., Kola, L., Fadahunsi, W., & Gureje, O. (2014). Global mental health reforms: Mental health Care in Anglophone West Africa. *Psychiatric Services, 65*(9), 1084–1087.

Ewhrudjakpor, C. (2010). A comparative study of knowledge and attitude of urban and rural dwellers towards vagrant sufferers of schizophrenia in Delta state of Nigeria. *East African Journal of Public Health, 7*(2), 114–119.

Federal Ministry of Health. (2013). *National Policy for mental health services delivery.* Abuja.

Flisher, A. J., Dawes, A., Kafaar, Z., Lund, C., Sorsdahl, K., Myers, B., & Seedat, S. (2012). Child and adolescent mental health in South Africa. *Journal of Child & Adolescent Mental Health, 24*(2), 149–161.

Gureje, O. (2003). Revisiting the National Mental Health Policy for Nigeria. Archives of Ibadan. *Medicine, 4*(1), 2–4.

Gureje, O., Omigbodun, O. O., Gater, R., Acha, R. A., Ikuesan, B. A., & Morris, J. (1994). Psychiatric disorders in a pediatric primary care clinic. *British Journal of Psychiatry, 165,* 527–530.

Hawkins, D. R. (2014). Leeting go: The pathway of Surrender. Hay House Incoporated

Jacob, K. S., Sharan, P., Mirza, I., Garrido-Cumbrera, M., Seedat, S., Mari, J. J., & Sreenivas, V. (2007). Mental health systems in countries: Where are we now? *Lancet, 370*(9592), 1061–1077.

Jegede, R. O., Ohaeri, J. U., Bamgboye, E. A., & Okunade, A. O. (1990). Psychiatric morbidity in a Nigerian general out-patient clinic. *West African Journal Medicine, 9,* 177–186.

Kessler, R. C., Angermeyer, M., Anthony, J. C., Demyttenaere, K., Gasquet, I., Gluzman, S., & Üstün, T. B. (2007). Lifetime prevalence and age-of-onset distributions of mental disorders in the World Health Organization's world mental health survey initiative. *World Psychiatry, 6,* 168–176.

Kharas, H., Hamel, K., & Hofer, M. (2018). Future development: The start of a new poverty narrative. Retrieved 5 Jan, 2020, from https://www.brookings.edu/blog/future-development/2018/06/19/the-start-of-a-new-poverty-narrative/

Lasebikan, V. O., Ejidokun, A., & Coker, O. A. (2012). Prevalence of mental disorders and profile of disablement among primary health care service users in Lagos Island. *Epidemiology Research International, 2012,* 6. https://doi.org/10.1155/2012/357348

Mbamalu, S. (2019). Nigeria has a mental health problem, Aljazeera News

Mwaniki A. (2018). *The 10 most populated countries in Africa.* Retrieved from https://www.worldatlas.com/articles/the-10-most-populated-countries-in-africa.html

Ndetei, D. M., Muthike, J., & Nandoya, E. S. (2017). Kenya's mental health law. *BJ Psych International, 14*(4), 96–97.

Nwaopara, A. U. (2016). Doctor to patient ratio and infrastructure gap in a psychiatric Hospital in Oil Rich Eket, Nigeria. *Journal of Psychiatry, 19,* 2. https://doi.org/10.4172/2378-5756.1000356

Olashore, A. A., Frank-Hatitchki, B., & Ogunwobi, O. (2017). Diagnostic profiles and predictors of treatment outcome among children and adolescents attending a national psychiatric hospital in Botswana. *Child and Adolescent Psychiatry and Mental Health, 11*(1), 8.

Olson, R. P. (2006). Mental Health Systems Compared: Great Britian, Norway, Canada and the United States. Charles C. Thomas Publisher

Omaka, A. C. (2014). Decongesting prisons in Nigeria: The EBSU law clinic model. *International Journal of Clinical Legal Education, 20,* 533.

Omigbodun, O. (2008). Developing child mental health services in resource-poor countries. *International Review of Psychiatry, 20*(3), 225–235.

Owen, J. P., Baig, B., Abbo, C., & Baheretibeb, Y. (2016). Child and adolescent mental health in sub-Saharan Africa: A perspective from clinicians and researchers. *BJPsych International, 13*(2), 45–47.

Patel, V., Flisher, A. J., Hetrick, S., & McGorry, P. (2007). Mental health of young people: A global public-health challenge. *Lancet, 369*(9569), 1302–1313. https://doi.org/10.1016/S0140-6736(07)60368-7

Phalen, P. (2014). Guinea Hospital shows West How to treat Mental Illness without Chains, Humanosphere

Raviola, G., Severe, J., Therosme, T., Oswald, C., Belkin G., Eustache F. E. (2013) The 2010 Haiti Earthquake Response. Psychiatric Clinics of North America 36(3) 431–450. https://doi.org/10. 1016/j.psc.2013.05.006

Reem, M., Ghandour Laura, J., Sherman Catherine, J., Vladutiu Mir, M., Ali Sean, E., Lynch Rebecca, H., Bitsko Stephen, J., Blumberg (2019). Prevalence and Treatment of Depression Anxiety and Conduct Problems in US Children. *The Journal of Pediatrics* 206256–267.e3 https://doi.org/10.1016/j.jpeds.2018.09.021

Sanni, A. A., & Adebayo, F. O. (2014). Nigerian Mental Health Act 2013 assessment: A policy towards modern international standards. *American Academic and Scholarly Research Journal, 6*, 1–13.

Saraceno, B., van Ommeren, M., Batniji, R., Cohen, A., & Gureje, M. J. (2007). Barriers to improvement of mental health services in low-income and middle-income countries. *Global Mental Health, 370*(9593), 1164–1174. https://doi.org/10.1016/S0140-6736(07)61263-X

Saxena, S., Jané-Llopis, E., & Hosman, C. (2006). Prevention of mental and behavioural disorders: Implications for policy and practice. *World Psychiatry, 5*(1), 5–14.

Shackman, J., & Price, B. K. (2013). Mental health capacity building in northern Sierra Leone: Lessons learned and issues raised. *Intervention, 11*(3), 261–275.

Solomon, O. J., Nwankwoala, R., & Ushi, V. (2014). The plight of female prisoners in Nigeria and the dilemma of health rights violations. *Asian Journal of Social Science Humanity, 3*, 152–161.

Suleiman, D. (2016). Mental health disorders in Nigeria: A highly neglected disease, Annals of Nigerian Medicine

Thirunavukarasu, M. (2011). Closing the treatment gap. *Indian Journal of Psychiatry, 53*, 199–201.

Thirunavukarasu, M., & Thirunavukarasu, P. (2010). Training and national deficit of psychiatrists in India - A critical analysis. *Indian Journal of Psychiatry, 52*, 83–88.

Ude, P. U. (2015). Policy analysis on Nigerian Lunacy Act (1958): The need for a new legislation. *Journal of Psychiatry, 19*, 343. https://doi.org/10.4172/2378-5756.1000343

Uwakwe, R., & Otakpor, A. N. (2014). Public mental health – Using the mental health gap action program to put all hands to the pumps. *Frontiers in Public Health, 2*, 33. https://doi.org/10. 3389/fpubh.2014.00033

Weems, C. F., & Overstreet, S. (2008). Child and adolescent mental health research in the context of Hurricane Katrina: An ecological needs-based perspective and introduction to the special section. *Journal of Clinical Child & Adolescent Psychology, 37*(3), 487–494.

Westbrook, A. H. (2011). Mental health legislation and involuntary commitment in Nigeria: A call for reform. *Washington University Global Studies Law Reviw, 10*, 397–418.

WHO-AIMS Report. (2006). *WHO-AIMS Report on mental health system in Nigeria*. WHO and Ministry of Health. Retrieved from https://www.mindbank.info/item/1303

World Health Organization. (2001). *The World Health Report 2001: Mental health: New understanding, new hope*. World Health Organization.

World Health Organization. (2008). *Integrated health services—What and why? Making Health Systems Work*. Technical Brief No. 1, p. 1. Retrieved from https://www.who.int/healthsystems/technical_brief_final.pdf

World Health Organization. (2012). Depression: A global crisis. World Mental Health Day, October 10 2012. World Federation for Mental Health, Occoquan, VA

World Health Organization. (2014). *Mental health: A state of well-being*. Retrieved from http://origin.who.int/features/factfiles/mental_health/en/

World Health Organization. (2018). *Mental health: Strengthening our response*. Retrieved from https://www.who.int/news-room/fact-sheets/detail/mental-health-strengthening-our-response

Yoder, H. N., Tol, W. A., Reis, R., & de Jong, J. T. (2016). Child mental health in Sierra Leone: A survey and exploratory qualitative study. *International Journal of Mental Health Systems, 10* (1), 1–13.

Child and Adolescent Mental Health in Kenya: Do We Need a Child and Adolescent Mental Health Policy?

Muthoni Mathai, Anne Wanjiru Mbwayo, Teresia Mutavi, and David Bukusi

Introduction

Children are the foundation of every society. Children are the parents, teachers, health providers, engineers, economists, artists, etc., and even more important the leaders of tomorrow. When we grow older and engage less in the matters of our societies, it is they who will decide in which direction we go and grow, to the well-being or detriment of our society, our world and some would say our universe. The importance of the mental well-being of children to society is well summarized in this World Health Organization (WHO) quote: "Children are our future. Through well-conceived policy and planning, governments can promote the mental health of children, for the benefit of the child, the family, the community and society" (WHO, 2005). And yet parenting and early childhood development remain one of the least prioritized areas in many low- and middle-income countries (LMICs). Even when education has a high priority, the focus is on crunching numbers in academic subjects. There is more to success in life beyond getting an "A" in mathematics. Examples abound of people who, despite very high academic scores, have not been able to achieve life satisfaction or contribute to their societies positively.

> Njoroge (not his real name), is a 42-year-old Kenyan male. Born and brought up in Nairobi. A child of upper middle class professionals. Njoroge struggled through school, with help of private tutors to supplement the strictly structured school system. He passed and went on to university to study engineering. His problems became more severe, missing classes and delayed submission of work plagued him. He moved from job to job. He had serious problems finishing tasks. He had also started drinking in college and this got worse.

M. Mathai (✉) · A. W. Mbwayo · T. Mutavi
Department of Psychiatry, University of Nairobi, Nairobi, Kenya
e-mail: amuthoni@uonbi.ac.ke

D. Bukusi
Kenyatta National Hospital, Nairobi, Kenya

© Springer Nature Switzerland AG 2022
F. M. Ssewamala et al. (eds.), *Child Behavioral Health in Sub-Saharan Africa*,
https://doi.org/10.1007/978-3-030-83707-5_7

Eventually, he was diagnosed as having adult ADHD with co-morbid Bipolar Mood Disorder and Alcohol dependence.[1]

Indeed, a good percentage of such people, who society would dub as failures, are persons suffering from one type or other of mental illness. Others are people who could not take advantage of the opportunities offered by education because of undetected, undiagnosed behavioural and emotional problems in childhood. WHO reports that one out of four people will be affected by mental illness at some time in their lifetime (WHO, 2001a). Many have their onset in childhood or adolescence, with risk factors progressively piling up from childhood.

With an increasing knowledge on the significance of neuropsychiatric disorders through the life span, WHO reports indicate that 10–20% of children and adolescents are likely to suffer from mental illness with the majority of these having been in adolescence (WHO, n.d.). Depression is of particular significance, rated as being the ninth leading cause of illness and disability in adolescence, and closely linked to suicide in adolescence, which has been reported as the third leading cause of mortality in the age group of 15–19 years (WHO, 2020).

A serious question here is: How often is depression recognized and or diagnosed in this age group and how many children access treatment for depression? Every nation in the world today sets out an educational programme to ensure that children and young people learn the skills they need to achieve their lives' goals in a highly competitive world: achieving their potential, becoming independent and sustaining development and growth of their countries. Every year a large number of children do not meet the set standards. These children are in some countries labelled failures. How many of these are children/youth living with undiagnosed and untreated mental illness. Who is a failure here? Dr. Gro Harlem Brundtland, Director-General of WHO, said, "Mental illness is not a personal failure. In fact, if there is failure, it is to be found in the way we have responded to people with mental and brain disorders" (WHO, 2001b).

Mental disorders in childhood and adolescence are complicated by several psychosocial and environmental factors, a wide treatment gap, and the tendency to heavily impact adult life and achievement of potential if left untreated. The majority of suicides—nearly 79% globally—occur in low- and middle-income countries, which have the lowest resources for the detection and treatment of mental health disorders in all age groups (WHO, 2019). An estimated 46% of Kenya's population live below the poverty line (WHO, 2017).

Stigma remains one of the biggest limiting factors in the management of mental illness globally, affecting LMICs even more. In many sub-Saharan African countries traditional belief systems regarding mental illness as curses, being bewitched, having transgressed against some norms, displeasing the ancestors, etc. still abound.

The high prevalence of mental and neurological disorders in children and youth and the huge treatment gap have dire implications in countries like Kenya and other

---

[1]Case study from Author M.M.

LMICs where children and young people below the age of 25 years make up the bulk of the population.

Kenya is a young country with more than 40% of all Kenyans being children under 18 years, 75% being under 30 years and a median age of 19.7 years (worldpopulationreview, n.d.) (CIA, 2021). During the most recent census (2019) the total population was reported as 47,564,296 million (KNBS, 2019). The future of the country depends on prioritizing and investing heavily on children, on their physical, mental and social well-being and intellectual development.

In this chapter we want to look at how Kenya, through policies and regulations, has a bearing on the mental health and well-being of children and adolescents. We will forward the argument that although mental well-being of children is recognized and extensively covered through several acts of parliaments, policies and both global and regional conventions of which Kenya is a signatory, the lack of a single platform dedicated to the child and adolescent mental health, as a policy document, where these come together, can be a limiting factor in the implementation of mental health strategies for children and adolescence.

Background Information

Kenya: Historical, Sociopolitical and Demographic Profile

Kenya is an Eastern African country that lies on the equator. It borders Uganda to the west, Tanzania to the south and South Sudan, Somalia and Ethiopia to the north. To the East lies the Indian Ocean and the port city of Mombasa.

The country that is now known as Kenya was born in 1920. From 1920 Kenya was to be ruled by the British until 1963 when it got independence. Significant is that this colonial period formed the foundation of the country's modern education system and health services.

The Arabs however were there hundreds of years before this. Introduction of Islam and establishment of Islamic school for children, the Madrassas, continue to be an important influence in the socialization of children wherever Islam is practiced in Kenya.

Kenya's pre- and immediate postcolonial history is steeped in oppression and violence and this has played out negatively on different generations of children from the colonial era to today, predisposing them to ill mental health that has limited the achievement of their full potential as human beings.

Kenya's population was estimated at ten million at independence. Kenya now has a population of 47.6 million. The capital of Kenya, Nairobi, has exploded from a population of 360,000 at independence to become one of the biggest cities in Africa boasting an estimated 4.4 million inhabitants at the last census (KNBS, 2019).

The population structure is well depicted in Fig. 1.

Per this figure, more than a half of Kenyans (approximately 59%) are aged below 24 years and approximately 19 million are children of 14 years and less. How does

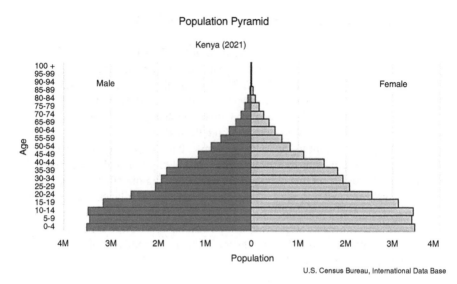

Fig. 1 Kenya population pyramid (CIA, 2021)

this structure play out in real life? School structures planned for 25–30 children 50 years ago now accommodate 70–80 children attended to by one teacher. That children are learning and coming through and getting good grades is an indication of the inherent resilience of children and their capacity to adapt. The children with limitations including behavioural disorders fall out of the system becoming adolescent delinquents constantly in trouble, abusing alcohol and drugs, committing petty crimes and moving on to become disturbed adults. They limp on through life, unfulfilled, never having achieved their potential, being a big burden to their families and the state. What opportunities are we missing by failing to address child and adolescent mental health and social determinants?

A Brief Overview of Health and Mental Health Structure with an Emphasis on Child Health Services

Kenya adapted the bottom-up policy grounded in primary healthcare culminating in the Kenya Essential Package for Health (KEPH) concept, which was adopted in 2005 (MOH, 2006). The health system is based on a hierarchy system with six levels starting at the community level 1 and proceeding upwards; level 2, dispensaries and clinics; level 3, health centres and maternity and nursing homes; level 4, sub-county hospitals and medium-sized private hospitals; level 5, county referral hospitals and large private hospitals; and level 6, national referral hospitals and large private teaching hospitals.

Child and Adolescent Mental Disorders in Kenya: A Review of Local Studies

Children around the world have more things in common than they have differences. The mental well-being of children depends on the same factors. First there is the inherent genetics and predisposing genetic factors, the profiling and influencing of which are advancing but still in experimental stages. One thing that health scientist can do is to determine the genetic make-up of a foetus and its progression to full development or not, an option available in many high-income countries (HIC). Beyond the genetics other factors are much more amenable to our influence. A healthy pregnancy is the first big step towards an infant with a healthy brain. And this is where mental well-being starts—a *healthy brain*. A safe delivery with no foetal injuries or hypoxia, is another step. Appropriate nourishment of the infant and growing child is the next step, providing optimal care, free of diseases and injuries as well as adequate emotional stimulation. The next step is going to school in a healthy educational environment to learn skills that will enable him/her to manage the demands of the modern society and acquire social skills through guided integration and interaction with other children.

Many women living in the LMICs and the inner cities of some of the HIC suffer from poor nutrition, embracing high-caloric poor-nutrient food as well as low-activity lifestyles diminishing chances of favourable pregnancy outcomes. That said, maternal and child health care is offered to all Kenyans for free at the primary healthcare level. And in many areas access is within reach. While modern maternal healthcare is an advantage, the benefits are compromised by individual beliefs, low education and lifestyle disorders. The dark figure behind this is the number of infants who escape death but live on with minimal or moderate brain damage that impacts their cognitive functioning, predisposing them to mental disorders including intellectual disability but also emotional and behavioural disorders.

Children in today's world have the benefit of immunizations and antibiotics and that is a benefit that cannot be underrated. The children in the inner cities start life in overcrowded polluted environment, are poorly nourished and are continuously being assaulted by noise both inside and outside the house. Low-income rural babies have to deal with inadequate and poorly balanced diet, dirty water and smoky houses and in sub-Saharan Africa like Kenya malaria, multiple other tropical infections and HIV/AIDS. Nearly 48.8% of children and adolescents living with HIV/AIDS were found to have psychiatric morbidity in a study in 2012 (Kamau et al., 2012).

A quick walk through the informal settlements of LMICs will show you children barely toddlers, walking out on to alleys or streets filled with cars, motorbikes, donkey carts, wild dogs, heaps of garbage, human waste and staggering and fighting drunks to mention a few (see Fig. 2). They play around pools of filthy water, drinking it and bathing in it and occasionally falling into it, right next to smouldering garbage.

Fig. 2 Korogocho. One of
Nairobi's slums. Picture by
author M.M

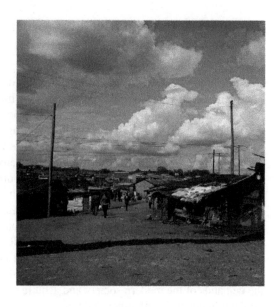

These children go to school in hostile neighbourhoods, with a high level of
violence. They live in the midst of violence: violence at home, violence in school
and violence on the streets. Children in the urban slums often drop out of school after
a few years and rarely get out of the slums. If they survive death in early childhood,
they get caught up in a culture of alcohol and drug abuse if they are boys and early
sex debut and pregnancies and terminations, and STIs, if they are girls. A study by
the authors AM and MM Mbwayo and Mathai (2016) found out that hopelessness
among schoolgoing children was a predictor of conduct problems among
schoolgoing children and adolescents and recommended that there was a need to
look for appropriate strategies to reduce the level of hopelessness as well as the need
for frequent assessments of mental health of children and adolescents in schools.

While children in rural communities may perhaps be better off, poverty there too
limits their potential and confines them to land peasantry like their parents and
grandparents before them, producing barely enough to sustain the family.

While no one is immune to mental illness, poverty does carry high risks of low
mental well-being particularly combined with existence in urban anomic societies.
While the rural families in sub-Saharan Africa are somewhat protected by extended
family and communal support and traditional values, families in the informal
settlements are living in a community where traditional and family values are lost.

The odds are stacked against children from the low- and middle-income countries
and inner cities of some high-income countries. Social economic status is an
important risk factor for mental illness both in childhood and in adulthood and
research shows that poverty and mental illness are increasingly becoming
intertwined (Lund, 2010). However, the human brain carries with it a high degree
of resilience and despite many adverse conditions that children from low social
economic families have to deal with, many grow up to be normal healthy adults to

compete evenly with their more advantaged brothers and sisters from across the economic divide.

The odds of developing mental illness can be reduced through early detection, early diagnosis treatment and follow-up. However, in several LMICs including Kenya, there is little chance of children and adolescents with mental disorders getting treatment at the primary healthcare level or getting to the mental health specialists. In children aged 6–18 years, the prevalence of emotional and behavioural problems was reported to be 27% and 16% for borderline and clinical ranges in central Kenya. This puts the prevalence of mental health problems higher by about a factor of 1.6 in Kenyan children and adolescents when compared to their age mates in high-income countries (Magai et al., 2018).

Evidence from scientific studies indicates that we have a problem that needs serious attention. Ndetei et al. (2016) found the prevalence of psychiatric disorders in Kenyan schools to be as high as 38% with 18% reports of comorbidity. These and other researchers noted that exposure to chronic illness, parental psychopathology, poor parent-child connectedness and poverty among others could be risk factors for mental health problems among children in Kenya.

A Review of Treaties, Conventions, That Advise on Child and Adolescent Well-Being

The Constitution of Kenya 2010

Lasting solutions to the problems of child and adolescent mental health must be anchored in the very framework that governs the running of the country to ensure the maximum well-being of the people. The well-being of the Kenyan people is covered under the Bill of Rights in the Constitution of Kenya. In the Bill of Rights part 3, specific application is dedicated to children and youth among other marginalized persons. Every child has the right to (c) basic nutrition, shelter and healthcare and (d) be protected from abuse, neglect, harmful cultural practices, all forms of violence, inhuman treatment and punishment, and hazardous exploitative labour (Kenya Law, n.d.).

While health is a very broad term, it is also correct to say that this has often been translated to mean physical health ignoring the WHO definition, "A state of complete physical, mental and social well-being and not merely the absence of disease or infirmity" (WHO, 2006). There is a dearth of resources allocated to mental health. The Kenya Government's total expenditure on mental health is 0.01% of total government health expenditure (WHO, 2017). Indeed, there seems to be only one facility in Kenya that has established services in the care of child and adolescent mental health—the Kenyatta National Teaching and Referral Hospital (KNH) in Nairobi. There are about two practicing child psychiatrists in Kenya, and a couple of psychologists. The health of children and youth is covered under the most fundamental document of the country—the constitution. The implementation of this, in terms of rights to mental health, remains a mirage.

The Convention on the Rights of the Child and the African Charter on the Rights and Welfare of the Child Ratified

Kenya is signatory to several global conventions including the Convention on the Rights of the Child in 1990. The African Charter on the Rights and Welfare of the Child (OAU, 1990) is a comprehensive document of the Organization of African Unity (OAU) that shows a thorough reflection on the needs and rights of the African child within the context of the African region with its cultural and ethnic diversity. Four points capture the attention in the preamble:

> *NOTING WITH CONCERN that the situation of most African children, remains critical due to the unique factors of their socio-economic, cultural, traditional and developmental circumstances, natural disasters, armed conflicts, exploitation and hunger, and on account of the child's physical and mental immaturity he/she needs special safeguards and care—* highlighting the challenges that face the African continent, the home of the African child.

The preamble goes on to recognize the highly valued status the child occupies in African traditional societies, and the special physical, mental, moral and social developments of the child that need legal protection.

Each of the 31 articles in part 1 of this charter has some relevance to the mental well-being of the child. These include education, leisure, recreation and cultural activities and a special emphasis on children with challenges. "The right to health", including mental health and spiritual health, whatever the translation is fully captured here. The charter recognizes the adverse prevailing conditions from which children in the continent need to be protected—child labour, child abuse and torture.

Protection against harmful social and cultural practices has particular relevance to the African continent, where there is a diversity of cultural practices, some of which clearly violate the dignity and well-being of the child. Two practices are of particular concern in Kenya: female genital mutilation (FGM) also referred to as female genital cutting (FGC) of girls and child marriages. Kenya has banned the practice of female genital mutilation and marriage of persons below the age of 18 years; however, as has been shown in other countries, it is one thing to make laws; it is another to implement them, given that even some of the administrative personnel responsible for the implementation of a ban are also captives of the same practices.

Kenya is host to an estimated 494,585 refugees and stateless people, with majority of these, 53.7%, from Somalia followed by 24.7% from South Sudan and others from the region UNHCR (UNHCR, 2020). ARTICLE 23: Refugee Children-refers to the rights of children to seek asylum and also to receive appropriate protection and humanitarian assistance. According to the United High Commissioner for Refugees (UNHCR), nearly a half of all asylum seekers/refugees in Kenya are children (UNHCR Kenya, n.d.). The problem of scarcity of schools and teachers in refugee camps is well known; indeed UNHCR in 2016 reported that at a global level 3.7 million of the six million school-age children had no school to go to (UNCHR, 2016).

Among the more controversial articles is ARTICLE 30: Children of Imprisoned Mothers. That prisons in Kenya have opened their doors to children of incarcerated mums, with children up to the age of 4 years, has received positive media coverage; the matter is considered positive mainly from the point of view of mother-child bonding. The issue is however more complex, particularly if you are familiar with the conditions in Kenyan prisons. Cheruiyot (2019) reported what is well known: overcrowding, with mothers sleeping tightly packed together in unhygienic poorly aired cells with unhygienic sanitary facilities. Additionally, mothers share the insufficient food portion with child and children are exposed to the humiliating treatment meted out to the mothers by some guards. Should we believe the stories and images portrayed by the media of prison guards playing with children and the mums in stripes happily walking around with their toddlers? Clearly there is no one simple answer to resolve these issues given that some of these children have no one they can be left with at home, or the level of poverty at home defies child survival. The translation of the charter is that it demands the state to undertake provision of special treatment to expectant mothers and to mothers of infants and young children including (a) a non-custodial sentence, as the first consideration and the establishment of institutions for holding mothers, pregnant or with young babies, surely cannot be met by putting mothers and babies in the common cells with other female prisoners.

This charter and others that Kenya is a party to including the United Nations Convention on the Rights of the Child (UNCRC) have been domesticated through the Children's Act 2001 (GoK, 2001) and the National Children's Policy Kenya of 2010 (GoK, 2010).

The National Children's Policy Kenya

The children's policy (GoK, 2010) is the local framework through which the rights of the child are covered. It notes that the best interest of the child needs to be put into considerations at all times on issues affecting children. Children also need to be respected by upholding their human dignity, accountability, non-discrimination, equity and equality. Services that are required by children need also to be accessible and should have equal participation. Adults also need to take responsibility to protect the rights of children regardless of the individual relationship with the child.

Some of the health needs noted in the policy include provision of quality health services in antenatal and postnatal services throughout a child's life; access to preventive, promotion, curative and rehabilitation services; mitigation on the impact of HIV/AIDS and other childhood diseases; and embrace of reproductive health concerns.

The policy also recognizes that children need protection from physical and psychological abuse, neglect and any other form of exploitation including sale, trafficking or abduction by any person, and as mentioned earlier prohibits harmful traditional practices, specifying female genital mutilation and child marriage.

Although this policy document indicates the need for children to receive the highest attainable standards of health to children, there is no mention of mental health as a unique set of needs among the children. The Kenya Children's Act 2001 recognizes that: "if it appears to the court on evidence of a medical practitioner that a child requires or may benefit from mental treatment, the court when making a probation order against him, may require him to undergo mental treatment at the hand or under the direction of a medical practitioner" (GoK, 2010). This seems to address children who due to some conduct issue have been brought before the court.

The policy serves as a framework to guide the government and other stakeholders in protecting the rights of the children; hence the absence of mental health aspect in the policy is a major gap in the policy document and the implication is that those children in need of mental health services may be overlooked. There is a need to review the policy to include provision of mental health services to children since these are unique services and need to be articulated in the policy.

In the next section, we will be looking at that environment in which a Kenyan child spends a large part of his/her day, and in some cases the longest part of his/her childhood—the school.

Educational Policy and the National School Health Policy 2009

The current Kenya education system evolved from the colonial system of education. This and subsequent adaptations of the system all focused on pre-primary, primary, secondary and post-secondary levels of education. The last one dubbed the 8-4-4 system got criticism for its focus on the achievement of high grades. From anecdotal reports, the heavy workload and the focus on national exams were seen as contributing to high levels of stress among students contributing to widespread school unrest and non-achievement by many learners. The country is now trying out a competency-based curriculum (CBC) since 2018. It is supposed to be child/student centred, and is supposed to provide opportunity to each child to learn and develop based on differing individual competencies. However, it is still in its early stages and the outcomes will become clearer with time.

The education policy in Kenya implies inclusion for all children. According to the Ministry of Education (MoE) Policy Framework for Education, all children should be in school irrespective of their special needs. This is in line with the Basic Education Act which says that all children must be in school (MoE, 2018a, 2018b). To this end, in addition to the regular schools, there are special schools, both at the primary and secondary levels. However, the Ministry acknowledges that these schools are few and only take care of those learners with physical disabilities, for example, hearing and sight problems, leaving out children with behavioural difficulties and learning challenges. It is, however, important to note that the policy is not about setting up special schools but integrating children with special needs in regular schools with additional special-needs teachers. In keeping with this policy and to identify children with special needs, the MoE has developed an assessment tool to assess readiness for children to enter schools:

Kenya School Readiness Assessment Tool (Ksrat)—Target Group—5 Years & Above. This tool assesses basic language and arithmetic, physical disabilities including hearing and sight, concentration and behaviour problems (MoE, 2018a, 2018b). What is missing, however, is a standardized tool to assess children after school entry and during the school lifespan.

In addition to the Education Policy, there is the National School Health Policy, which also targets the health of learners in schools. This policy envisions every school child accessing nutrition and health, with the school and community being the vehicle through which the child accesses these. The policy specifically addresses mental health in schools, where schools are mandated to develop child-friendly environments to promote mental health and provide mental health education and promotion in schools, availing guidance and counselling in schools and ensuring that there is no discrimination of children and staff with mental health problems (GoK, 2009). This is however dependent on the teachers having the skills to detect mental health disorders and take appropriate action. In a study conducted by the authors, to explore teachers' perceptions on mental health in schools, teachers reported that they were able to recognize students who were suffering from some mental health problems from their behaviour, but they lacked the skills and time to intervene (Mbwayo et al., 2020).

A lot of attention has been given to physical disabilities. One could speculate that emotional and behavioural challenges are less easy to identify because they exist in a continuum. However, targeting physical challenges without paying attention to the mental health of the children is like going only part of the way. Indeed, studies have shown that physical disability is associated with emotional and behavioural aspects in children and adolescents (Fauth et al., 2017; Crnic et al., 2004).

Every Kenyan school in compliance with the National School Health Policy is required to have a department of guidance and counselling. The limitation here is that the departments in many schools are not operational, because the teachers have inadequate skills for the tasks; they are overworked and sometimes the school leadership is not interested.

Children experience all kinds of problems, some more traumatic than others, and in many situations, where the child cannot find a solution at home, school can offer an important avenue, if the child finds a friendly and confidential space:

Naliaka (not her real name) came to my office one morning and told me she has a problem that is affecting her and she is not able to concentrate. She was quick to ensure her story was safe with me. This was her story: Although it had happened when she was in class 5-primary 3 years previously, she could remember the events of that evening as if it was yesterday. Her mother had cooked food and she was asked to take it to the grandmother, who lived a few meters from the parents' house. As she headed back home, her much older male cousin, accosted her and raped her. She was threatened not to say anything. The girl never said anything to the mother.[2]

This narration provides a glimpse of the problems that plague children in schools, illustrating one of the highlighted problems, which has serious and long-term

---

[2]Personal story from author A.M., former teacher/clinical psychologist, now lecturer.

physical and mental health effects, those of sexual abuse that are frequently not recognised nor addressed.

In the next section we will go deeper into the problems of sexual abuse by looking at the Sexual Offences Act.

The Sexual Offences Act (SOA)

Research shows that children exposed to sexual abuse or traumatic experiences are likely to develop mental health problems (Mutavi et al., 2017; Mutavi et al., 2018). Sexual abuse and other related traumatic experiences affect and contribute to mental ill health and how both guidance and enforcement of mental health evaluations during the prosecution of the same may lead to better mental health outcomes.

John (not his real name) is 7 years old; the mother works at and lives at an urban residential estate. This is her story:

> One day my son came from outside where he had been playing and told me that a man he didn't know called him took him to some bushes and did to him 'tabia mbaya' (sodomized him) and warned him that if he told his mummy he would kill him. I immediately took him to hospital where the doctor examined him and told me that there was no penetration but that he had ejaculated on him. He was put on PEP (Post Exposure Prophylaxis) and we went home and we were also given some forms. On our way home, John spotted the man and I shouted to people to get hold of him as I ran after him, we eventually caught up with him and took him to the police post. He was set free because there was no evidence. I took John for only two counselling sessions and after he tested HIV negative at six weeks I thought that counselling was a bad reminder to something that he had already forgotten, I remember being called for a support group, but I didn't take him.[3]

This is a common outcome of cases of child sexual abuse. That the cases are dropped because of lack of evidence—whether the doctor who saw this child had collected forensic evidence is not clear, but this does not seem to have been the case. And even in the absence of forensic evidence as is often the case when there is delayed reporting, even years, psychological assessments are now considered valid evidence.

Acts of Parliament and Policies That Touch on Child and Adolescent Mental Health and Well-Being

Kenya Health Policy

The Kenya Health Policy, 2014–2030 (MoH, 2014), is the latest government document conceived as a guideline to the attainment of the highest health standards

---

[3] Case study from author T. M., psychiatric social worker.

in keeping with the constitution and in line with Vision 2030. Vision 2030 is a blueprint for the long-term development agenda that envisions a high quality of life for all Kenyans.

The policy has six objectives and mental health is anchored in objective 2 under the non-communicable diseases.

National Adolescent Sexual and Reproductive Health Policy

Kenya recognizes that adolescents experience specific challenges that have an impact on health and well-being. These include early and unintended pregnancies, unsafe abortion, female genital mutilation (FGM) also referred to as female genital cutting (FGC), child marriages, sexual violence and sexually transmitted infections including HIV. These are areas that also have serious implications on mental health and are very specific to girls, increasing the gender-specific loading to mental disorders in girls particularly internalized disorders—depression and anxiety. These challenges are also addressed in other legislative and legal frameworks, some of which we have already looked at that include the Children's Act (2001), the Sexual Offences Act (2007), Prohibition of FGM (2011), National Youth Policy (2007) and the Marriage Act (2014).

The national adolescent sexual and reproductive policy covers the most important and critical issues around adolescent mental health, in Kenya, including even a paragraph on substance abuse.

Adolescent pregnancy has been identified as the single most important cause for school dropouts among girls. "Crisis as nearly 380,000 Kenyan teenagers become mothers" (Aggrey & Misiko, 2020). Adolescent pregnancy has serious implications for mental health—these include depression, anxiety, loss of self-esteem, loss of educational and later employment opportunities and entry into a hazardous lifestyle for economic survival that includes adolescent prostitution and substance use, which has been implicated in early sexual debut and multiple partners. Additionally, most adolescent pregnancies occur within the context of abuse—sexual abuse, child marriages and other forms of violations that increase the risk of developing mental illness. Clearly a reduction in adolescent pregnancies and support and care, which includes both reproductive health and psychological health, would go a long way in reducing the incidence of mental illness in this age group in girls.

Female genital mutilation has been on the decline and in 2011 the Kenya Government passed a law prohibiting FGM. It is however well known that FGM continues to be prevalent in certain communities and in certain regions like parts of north Kenya, where the prevalence is as high as 98%. Female genital mutilation has been associated with an increased prevalence of mental illness, particularly post-traumatic stress disorder (PTSD). Regina Ndiema, a clinical psychologist master's student at the University of Nairobi, found a PTSD prevalence of 98.7% (13.0% mild, 31.2% moderate and 54.5% severe) among Maasai girls in rescue home after forced FGM in 2008 (Ndiema, 2008).

Child marriage is forbidden through the Marriage Act, where child is any person under the age of 18 years. However, marriage of children is embedded in the traditional cultures of many peoples of Kenya and continues to be practiced particularly in more remote rural areas. An important factor is poverty; girls choose to get married to escape the poverty in their homes, sometimes because they are already pregnant and have no way to sustain a baby and sometimes for the economic benefits in cash or kind that come to the parents as part of the widely practiced dowry/bride price. Early marriages are anecdotally associated with reproductive ill health accruing from biological immaturity as well as increase in intimate partner violence (IPV) often in the context of the power gradient in many such unions. Early marriages in the context of both partners being young also come with many challenges rooted in poverty, lack of opportunity and knowledge about healthcare behaviour that may all contribute towards poor mental health.

The policy also covers environmental conditions such as living in urban slums, being orphaned and being displaced internally or externally—all factors that have implications on both sexual and reproductive health and mental health.

The Kenya Mental Health Act and the Kenya Mental Health Policy: 2015–2030

The Mental Health Act of Kenya (GoK 1989) has its root in the colonial past. It stems from the British Lunacy Act of 1890, from where it travelled to India to become the Indian Lunacy Act of 1912, before arriving in Kenya in 1949, presumably by boat, to become the Mental Treatment Act of 1949. This was the single legislature that was to regulate the treatment of mentally ill people for the next 40 years. While this Act had lost the terminology of lunacy the legacy was to be felt for many years.

After 40 years the Mental Health Treatment Act was seriously outdated and was replaced by the Mental Health Act of 1989. This Act currently provides a legal framework for the detention and care of mentally ill patients in Kenya.

Thirty-one years later, in keeping with global, national developments and the new constitution of 2010, the Act is currently under review—as *the Mental Health (Amendment) Bill* (GoK, 2018). This Act seeks to provide a more humane framework for the provision of mental healthcare incorporating components of individual human rights as well as providing legal direction on responsibilities of the different emerging cadres of human resource involved in the provision of mental health promotion, evaluation and care.

The Kenya Mental Health Policy

The Kenya Mental Health Policy (MoH, 2016) is a document that the mental health fraternity in Kenya are truly proud of. After many years of deliberations from 2015, we now count among the countries with a mental health policy. The policy whose goal is the attainment of the highest standards of mental health for all Kenyans aligns itself with the constitution and the Kenya Health Policy discussed earlier.

The policy highlights the importance of understanding mental health:
"Mental health is a key determinant of overall health and socio-economic development. It influences individual and community outcomes such as healthier lifestyles, better physical health, improved recovery from illness, fewer limitations in daily living, higher education attainment, greater productivity, employment and earnings, better relationships with adults and with children, more social cohesion and engagement and improved quality of life."

The policy identifies what are considered as key barriers to increased access to effective mental health services:

- The absence of mental health from the public health agenda and the implications for funding
- The current organization of mental health services
- Lack of integration within primary care
- Inadequate human resources for mental health
- Lack of public mental health leadership

These are areas that could very well apply to the lack of a child and adolescent mental health policy. All the ten principles of this policy are important to child and adolescent mental health, but of particular interest is number 10, which states: "Policies, plans and services for mental health need to take account of health and social needs at all stages of the life course, including prenatal, infancy, childhood, adolescence, adulthood and older age". It is a clear recognition of the implications of life stages in the development and evolution of mental illness.

One of the most important areas of support to child and adolescent mental health that the policy proposes is under Chaps. 2, 3 and 5—Mental Health Services, under priority action—promotion of mental health:

Promotion of Mental Health: Good mental health of individuals, families, the communities and the society contribute enormously towards investment and development of social capital which is the most important determinant of our health. Mental health promotion should be availed to individuals, families, communities and the society. This will be spearheaded by primary health care team in each county level in partnership with other government sectors, Non-Governmental Organizations, Community Based Organizations, Faith Based Organizations and the private sector. The national government shall be tasked with development of appropriate guidelines. This endeavour of promotion of good mental health should be encouraged throughout the human development life cycle, right from pregnancy to old age.

Advocated strategies include parenting skill education, life skill education programme, training of teachers in mental health promotion and integration of mental health education programmes in all learning institutions.

And finally in Chaps. 2, 3 and 10 the policy addresses directly the mental health needs of children and adolescents under Mental Health and Vulnerable Groups:

"There are certain population groups that are more vulnerable to mental disorders hence the need for targeted mental health interventions for the following groups: a. Children and adolescents Children are often prone to mental disorders either at birth, where there might have been inadequate pre-natal care, or if their environment does not promote care, affection, love, stimulation for cognitive abilities or other emotional and social support. Adolescents face behavioral challenges and exposure or pressure to risky behaviour, such as use of psychoactive substances; make them vulnerable to mental disorders.

With this mention on psychoactive substances, it is important to mention that Kenya has enacted legislature to regulate the sale and use of alcohol and tobacco in the Alcoholic Drinks Control Act 2010 and Tobacco Control Act 2007/2012. The sale and use of alcohol and tobacco and employment in places that deal with these substances are not open to children under the age of 18 years. The two Acts also emphasize the importance of preventive measures through education in the institutions of learning and public.

The Way Forward in Line with Kenya Vision 2030

The *Sustainable Development Goals* (SDGs) (UN, 2020) and the *Millennium Development Goals* (MDGs) (UNDP, 2000) could be said to be the umbrella for Kenya's vision for the near future as the country tries to raise the standards of its citizens to a level that is competitive with other countries.

The call of the SDGs is to ensure that no one is left behind including the world's most vulnerable and marginalized people and this includes the children. Within the SDGs, it is assumed that the government and communities will do their part in ensuring that all the rights of the children are observed as they would lead to good mental health.

The Kenya Vision 2030 is the country's development blueprint covering the period 2008–2030. It aims to transform Kenya into a newly industrializing, "middle-income country providing a high-quality life to all its citizens by the year 2030" (GoK, 2007). The vision has several pillars, among them the "Social Pillar: Investing in the People of Kenya". Under this pillar are two areas namely education and training and the health sector. Education and training: Under this area, the government aims to train highly skilled people who would be competitive in any part of the world. This starts all the way from pre-primary education to university and it is inclusive as it includes even the children with special needs. This would be archived through developing key programmes for learners with special needs. The government has made great strides in an inclusive education to ensure that children with special needs are included (*MoE* 2009). This is also seen in the new competency-based curriculum. The Vision aims for all children to transition from primary school to secondary school; examinations will no longer be a barrier to achieving an education as has been in the past. The Kenya Vision 2030 is a good document that has highlighted the importance of children in our society. However, the crux of the matter is in the implementation. For example, the move to ensure that all children get both a primary and post-primary education has not been complemented with an increase in learning space. There is a lot of overcrowding in the schools and that has implications, like it is difficult for the few teachers to identify children who are struggling with mental health problems.

Summary and Conclusion

Children make up the biggest population group in Kenya and there is no doubt that Kenya is committed to the mental well-being of the children. Kenya, as we have seen, is a signatory to several international conventions that focus on the rights and well-being of children globally and has domesticated these into parliamentary acts and policies. Indeed, the mental health of children and adolescents is thought of and integrated into the other policies that are concerned with the rights and well-being of children.

However, there are limitations in the implementation of the well-thought-out strategies and this is where a policy that picks all the pieces and brings them together would come in. The handicap of not having a guiding policy specific to the management of child and adolescent mental health is the prevailing fragmentation of care. This is not only inefficient, but also expensive. Some functions and roles are duplicated while other important activities fall between the cracks.

A Child and Adolescent Mental Health (CAMH) policy would bring out and highlight all the parts in other policies that concern child mental well-being.

And finally, a CAMH policy would mean that treasury would set aside funds that prioritize and are specific to activities targeting child and adolescent mental well-being.

References

Aggrey, O., Misiko, H. (2020). *Crisis as nearly 380,000 teenagers become mothers*. Daily Nation. Retrieved from https://allafrica.com/stories/202003050665.html

Central Intelligence Agency (CIA). (2021). *The World Factbook: Kenya*. Central Intelligence Agency. Retrieved from https://www.cia.gov/the-world-factbook/countries/kenya/

Cheruiyot J. (2019). An Assessment of the Challenges of Children in Prison with their Mothers: A Case of Langata Women Maximum Prison, Kenya. Interdisciplinary Journal on the African Child Special edition 2019 Vol. 01, Issue 01 Copyright 2019 by Daystar University (School of Human & Social Sciences) and African Institute of Children Studies

Crnic, K., Hoffman, C., Gaze, C., & Edelbrock, C. (2004). Understanding the emergence of behavior problems in young children with developmental delays. *Infants & Young Children, 17*(3), 223–235.

Fauth, R. C., Platt, L., & Parsons, S. (2017). The development of behavior problems among disabled and non-disabled children in England. *Journal of Applied Developmental Psychology, 52*, 46–58.

GoK (1989). Kenya Gazette Supplement No. 90 (acts No. 7) republic of Kenya. Nairobi, 1st Dec 1989

GoK. (2001). *Kenya—Children's Act, 2001 (No. 8 of 2001) (Cap. 141)*. Retrieved from http://www.ilo.org/dyn/natlex/natlex4.detail?p_lang=en&p_isn=61290

GoK. (2007). *Kenya Vision 2030 (Popular Version)*. Retrieved from https://vision2030.go.ke/publication/kenya-vision-2030-popular-version/

GoK. (2009). *National-School-Health-Policy-2009. Kenya.pdf*. Retrieved Sept 10, 2020, from https://www.prb.org/wp-content/uploads/2018/05/National-School-Health-Policy-2009.-without-cover..-Kenya.pdf

GoK. (2010). *The National Children's Policy Kenya, 2010*. Retrieved August 18, 2020, from http://www.childrenscouncil.go.ke/images/documents/Policy_Documents/National-Children-Policy.pdf

GoK. (2018). *Mental Health (Amendment) Bill*. Retrieved on September 10, 2020, from http://www.parliament.go.ke/sites/default/files/2018-12/Mental%20Health%20%28Amendment%29%20Bill%2C%202018.pdf

Kamau, J. W., Kuria, W., Mathai, M., Atwoli, L., & Kangethe, R. (2012). Psychiatric morbidity among HIV-infected children and adolescents in a resource-poor Kenyan urban community. *AIDS Care, 24*(7), 836–842. https://doi.org/10.1080/09540121.2011.644234

Kenya Law. (n.d.). *Constitution of Kenya, 2010*. Retrieved on April 9, 2021 from https://www.constituteproject.org/constitution/Kenya_2010.pdf

KNBS. (2019). *Kenya population and housing census results*. Kenya National Bureau of Statistics. Retrieved from https://www.knbs.or.ke/?p=5621

Lund, C. (2010). Mental health in Africa: Findings from the Mental Health and poverty project. *International Review of Psychiatry, 22*(6), 547–549. https://doi.org/10.3109/09540261.2010.535809

Magai, D. N., Malik, J. A., & Koot, H. M. (2018). Emotional and behavioral problems in children and adolescents in Central Kenya. *Child Psychiatry & Human Development, 49*(4), 659–671. https://doi.org/10.1007/s10578-018-0783-y

Mbwayo, A. W., Mathai, M., Khasakhala, Lincoln, I., Kuria, M. W., & Vander Stoep, A. (2020). Mental health in Kenyan schools: Teachers' perspectives. *Global Social Welfare, 7*(2), 155–163. https://doi.org/10.1007/s40609-019-00153-4

Mbwayo, A. W., & Mathai, M. (2016). Association between hopelessness and conduct problem among school going adolescents in a rural and urban setting in Kenya. *Journal of Child and Adolescent Behaviour, 4*(3), 1–4. https://doi.org/10.4172/2375-4494.1000291

WHO (2017) Mental Health ATLAS. Retrieved from http://www.who.int/mental_health/evidence/atlas/mental_health_atlas_2017/en/

MoE (2009). Specialneedseducationpolicy.pdf. (n.d.). Retrieved July 16, 2020. http://www.gluk.ac.ke/down/specialneedseducationpolicy.pdf

MoE. (2018a). Kenya school readiness assessment tool.

MoE. (2018b). *Sector Policy for Learners and Trainees with Disabilities*. Retrieved August 18, 2020, from https://planipolis.iiep.unesco.org/sites/planipolis/files/ressources/kenya_sector_policy_learners_trainees_disabilities.pdf

MoH. (2006). *Taking the Kenya essential package for health to the community: A strategy for the delivery of level one services*.

MoH. (2014). *Kenya Health Policy 2014–2030*. Retrieved from https://www.google.com/search?client=firefox-b-d&q=Kenya+Health+Policy+2014%E2%80%932030+Published+by%3A+Ministry+of+Health+Afya+House+Cathedral+Road+PO+Box+30016+Nairobi+00100+http%3A%2F%2Fwww.health.go.ke

MoH. (2016). *Kenya Mental Health Policy 2015 to 2030*. Retrieved from http://publications. universalhealth2030.org/ref/e5ab9a205fdbd7c811bb895d09e4f81c#:~:text=The%20Kenya% 20Mental%20Health%20Policyhealth%20systems%20reforms%20in%20Kenya.&text=This% 20includes%20mental%20health.

Mutavi, T., Mathai, M., & Obondo, A. (2017). Post-traumatic stress disorder (PTSD) in sexually abused children and educational status in Kenya: A longitudinal study. *Journal of Child and Adolescent Behavior, 5*, 5.

Mutavi, T., Obondo, A., Kokonya, D., Khasakhala, L., Mbwayo, A., Njiri, F., & Mathai, M. (2018). Incidence of depressive symptoms among sexually abused children in Kenya. *Child and Adolescent Psychiatry and Mental Health, 12*(1), 40.

Ndetei, D. M., Mutiso, V., Musyimi, C., Mokaya, A. G., Anderson, K. K., McKenzie, K., & Musau, A. (2016). The prevalence of mental disorders among upper primary school children in Kenya. *Social Psychiatry and Psychiatric Epidemiology, 51*(1), 63–71. https://doi.org/10.1007/s00127-015-1132-0

Ndiema, R. S. (2008). *Prevalence of post-traumatic stress disorder among Maasai girls who have undergone female genital mutilation as a prerequisite to early marriage in Trans-mara and Kajiado districts-Kenya*, PhD thesis, University of Nairobi.

OAU. (1990). *African charter on the rights and welfare of the child (testimony of OAU)*.

UN. (2020). *The sustainable development goals report 2020*. Retrieved from https://unstats.un.org/sdgs/report/2020/

UNCHR. (2016). *UNHCR reports crisis in refugee education*. UNHCR. Retrieved from https://www.unhcr.org/news/press/2016/9/57d7d6f34/unhcr-reports-crisis-refugee-education.html

UNDP. (2000). *Millennium development goals*. https://www.undp.org/content/undp/en/home/sdgoverview/mdg_goals.html

UNHCR. (2020). *Figures at a glance—UNHCR Kenya*. UNHCR. https://www.unhcr.org/ke/figures-at-a-glance

UNHCR Kenya. (n.d.). *Children*. UNHCR. Retrieved August 18, 2020, from https://www.unhcr.org/ke/children

WHO. (2001a). *Mental health: New understanding, new hope (repr)*. World Health Organization.

WHO. (2001b). *World health report*. World Health Organization. Retrieved from https://www.who.int/whr/2001/media_centre/press_release/en/

WHO. (2005). *Child and adolescent mental health policies and plans*. World Health Organization. Mental Health Policy and Service Guidance Package.

WHO. (2006). Basic documents. In *Constitution of the World Health Organization* (45th ed.). World Health Organization.

WHO. (2017). *Primary health care systems: Case study from Kenya*.

WHO (2019). *Suicide*. Key facts. Retrieved September 10, 2020, from https://www.who.int/news-room/fact-sheets/detail/suicide

WHO. (2020). *Depression*. Retrieved from https://www.who.int/news-room/fact-sheets/detail/depression

WHO. (n.d.). *Child and adolescent mental health*. Retrieved Sept 10, 2020, from http://www.who.int/mental_health/maternal-child/child_adolescent/en/

Worldpopulationreview. (n.d.). *Kenya Population 2020*. Retrieved Sept 10, 2020, from https://worldpopulationreview.com/countries/kenya-population

Towards Entrapment: An Escalating Reality for Children and Adolescents Living with HIV/AIDS in Uganda

James Mugisha and William Byansi

Introduction

In 2004, UNAIDS, UNICEF, and USAID collaborated and authored an influential report titled *Children in the Brink* (UNICEF, 2004). This report is used to set the context of this book chapter. The publication did not only give comprehensive statistics on children orphaned by AIDS and other causes but also gave a framework for understanding the fundamental issues that relate to protection, care, and support for orphaned and vulnerable children (OVC) living in a world plagued by HIV and AIDS. In terms of statistics, the report gave a glaring picture. For example, sub-Saharan Africa (SSA) was reported to have 43.4 million orphans (of all causes) in 2003. During this period, more than 12.3 million children had been orphaned by HIV/AIDS.

The same report labored to provide a framework for the protection, care, and support for OVC. This framework was to be used by national governments to attach resources and also offer both policy and programmatic basis for interventions responding to the growing OVC epidemic. Further, this framework for protection, care, and support of OVC was affirmed by the Global Partners' Forum, with support from UNICEF and other major donors. The weight and value given to this framework raised a lot of hope that children will be removed from what the report referred to as the "brink." It is now over a decade, since this influential report came out of print. However, the plight of children in sub-Saharan Africa is still disheartening. The number of OVC regardless of the cause has remained unacceptably high with

J. Mugisha (✉)
Department of Sociology and Social Administration, Kyambogo University, Kampala, Uganda
e-mail: jmmugi77@hotmail.com

W. Byansi
Brown School, Washington University in St. Louis, St. Louis, MO, USA
e-mail: byansiw@wustl.edu

© Springer Nature Switzerland AG 2022
F. M. Ssewamala et al. (eds.), *Child Behavioral Health in Sub-Saharan Africa*,
https://doi.org/10.1007/978-3-030-83707-5_8

approximately 52 million orphans and 15 million orphaned by HIV and AIDS (UNICEF, 2015). There are glaring structural barriers at family, community, and national levels to allow children escape from the brink.

In this chapter we use examples and other materials from Uganda to demonstrate that the reality of these children is both hazy and obscure. Our claim of obscurity, however, does not serve to undermine the great efforts made by several agencies and national governments in improving the plight of OVC especially those orphaned and/or made vulnerable by HIV/AIDS. Our main concern is the failure of several intervening agencies to take a deeper look into some of the prevailing inequities in the traditional and formal social service systems. Unfortunately, children in such situations are likely to continue investing in unfavorable situations after already devoting too much (psychologically or mentally) in social relations where they live (Katz et al., 2012).

Our general understanding is that OVC, including those made vulnerable by HIV/AIDS, have invested a lot in these social relations while the returns from such relations may, unlikely, contribute to their psychological and mental health development, especially in the short and long term. To researchers, programmers, and practitioners, this should be unacceptable given the expectations that arose when Child at the Brink report was published over 17 years ago (2004).

In writing this chapter, our position is informed by frameworks from positive mental health (PMH). We specifically apply the concept positive mental health to connote high levels of subjective and psychological well-being of an individual (Keyes et al., 2002) and once not achieved, resilience against stressors/mental distress may arise. In many of the families and places where OVC including those made vulnerable by HIV and AIDS live, the context does not offer strong opportunities for PMH. This could partly explain the high prevalence of mental health problems reported by this group and that of their families in sub-Saharan Africa, including Uganda (Cortina et al., 2012; Wamulugwa et al., 2017; Nalugya, 2004). For example, a systematic review by Cortina and colleagues estimated that one in seven children in SSA struggles with a mental health issue (Cortina et al., 2012) and estimates from the WHO indicate the prevalence rates to be even higher than 20% (WHO, 2005). Additionally, in Uganda—one of the poorest countries in SSA—studies indicate that between 12% and 29% of children present mental health symptoms (Nalugya, 2004). Therefore, given the large numbers of children in Uganda, child mental health, if untreated, is a particularly serious concern as it commonly persists through adolescence and adulthood (Belfer, 2008).

Therefore, we make a general claim that current resources that are meant to support PMH need to be carefully examined to avoid entrapment of OVC, including children made vulnerable by HIV/AIDS. Our main focus is on the traditional system of care especially the family in Uganda in the context of HIV/AIDS, though we also make limited focus on the formal sector. The weaknesses in the resource systems create risk factors and these (risk factors) tend to reenforce each other. The remedy would be theoretical and pragmatic models of intervention that can change the plight of children in such circumstances.

We situate our writing in salutogenesis as a theoretical construct/model and its sense of coherence (SOC) to understand the plight of these children with additional reflections from PMH as a general theoretical domain. Within the salutogenic perspective, it is postulated that the SOC construct is an important personal resource that develops during childhood (Margalit, 1998). Within this theoretical construct, children and adolescents with a high SOC may have a good comprehension of most of their contextual conditions, situational demands, and personal experiences (Margalit, 1998). This presupposes that children and adolescents may feel relatively in control of their lives and may possibly consider most of their tasks and participation in age-appropriate activities as meaningful, significant, and worth of investing effort for daily living (Margalit, 1998). As a resource, it could be that when children and adolescents face a stressful situation, they would be able to select in a flexible manner the appropriate strategies to effectively cope with the stressors in their life situation (Margalit, 1998), thus being able to cope and develop coping strategies. Their resilience grows, they will be able to collaborate in productive activities, and they develop healthy social relations and this may enhance the child's resilience and motivation to invest effort to reach both short- and long-term goals (Margalit, 1998).

Methods

The main purpose was to generate people's views that relate to care for OVC, including children made vulnerable by HIV/AIDS. This study is based on the content from published literature from previous projects undertaken in Uganda on OVC and key informant interviews with people working in the field of HIV/AIDS. We conducted an initial review of the content from published literature on OVC in Uganda. This review guided the development of important themes to be covered in the key informant interviews. The themes focused on the management of OVC, changing structure of families, intergenerational trauma, services and support for OVC, and family resources.

Using convenience sampling, ten key informants working in the field of HIV and management of OVC—three senior HIV/AIDS officials from a nongovernmental organization (NGO) that offers HIV counseling and medical services to people infected with and affected by HIV and AIDS, three psychiatrists at a national referral hospital, two social workers at an academic institution, and two caregivers of OVC—were interviewed. These were selected because of their expertise knowledge in the management and care of OVC. Given the COVID-19-related social control measures in Uganda, key informant interviews were done via telephone conversation and each lasted about 30 min.

Data Analysis

Thematic analysis, which involves breaking the text into small units of content and submitting them to descriptive treatments in the analysis process, was used in this study (Braun & Clarke, 2006). Specifically, using the content from published literature and key informant interviews, a qualitative codebook was developed to code the content and responses, respectively. The final codebook included the five primary themes related to HIV and AIDS, caring for OVC, trauma, widow inheritance, and changing family structure. We followed the same steps during analysis to generate emerging themes in the data and subthemes. These were linked to the general categories that were developed and guided the study. The themes, subthemes, and categories were shared out with the co-authors of this book chapter during the research and analysis process. The researcher and co-authors agreed on the meaning systems that had emerged out of the data.

Findings

Changing Family Systems and the "I Am Tired Concept"

Several decades ago, Ankrah (1991) argued that Ugandan families have been resilient at the blunt of HIV/AIDS. However, Mukiza-Gapere and Ntozi (1995) within almost the same period noted that family systems were changing in communities that had been heavily "pounded" by HIV/AIDS. It is a reality in Uganda that many OVC also live with the extended family (Mukiza-Gapere & Ntozi, 1995). Our recent work (Mugisha et al., 2020) among children who have a double burden of HIV and mental distress indicated that some of the children are neglected by their relatives due to the heavy burden of care that they have endured for several years. In such situations, the much-hyped social care system in Uganda manifests socioeconomic stress. In this vein, the voices adduced in this study (Mugisha et al., 2020) indicated a high burden of care and fatigue in the family setting:

> The caregivers normally say 'I am tired, and we are tired' and this is the common trend indeed (PID_02 Health Worker, NGO).

> Over time, you start to get this feeling that when will it ever end and you do not see the end. You also get tired and tired. (PID_10 Caregiver)

One, therefore, wonders how such children who live in fatigued family systems meet both the material and psychological needs. Once families are in a state of psychological fatigue, they are likely to develop emotional distancing as a coping strategy at the detriment of the children they look after (Hubert & Aujoulat, 2018). And, depending on the personality of the child, and other life events that the child goes through, such children are likely to suffer psychological and mental distress. Development of specific interventions becomes vital here. One important strategy is to train such children to deal with this reality of adversity. They could be trained to develop resilience amidst chronic early-life stressors and adversity (Mc Gee et al., 2018).

One vital factor that may play an important role in the development of stress-related resilience is the sense of coherence (SOC). Under this framework, children under adversity may be helped to change the way they view the world (Mc Gee et al., 2018). This facilitates successful coping with stressors (Mc Gee et al., 2018). In essence, they are helped to develop the ability to integrate and balance both positive and negative experiences in order to maintain and develop health and well-being. In such circumstances, they are trained to mobilize internal resources as they face adversity. The sense of coherence becomes the mediator between the child and adversity (Gana, 2001).

To our best knowledge, research using the SOC framework does not exist in Uganda. Yet, such children have to be assessed early in life for appropriate interventions. Social service agencies and academic institutions need to fill in this gap. As observed, continued "wear and tear" is likely to increase susceptibility to stress and mental health problems such as depression, anxiety, and post-traumatic stress disorder (Mc Gee et al., 2018). This wear and tear has to be monitored through functional monitoring systems in places where these children live. SOC tools should be contextually adapted in Uganda and other parts of sub-Saharan Africa for that purpose.

Children in Transient Families

In their work in Masaka district in Uganda, Knizek et al. (2017) established a pattern where orphans were living with different relatives and in several homesteads after a short period of time. The study argued that because of this, such children are characterized by instability and diffuse relationships that provided an insecure basis for secure attachment and emotional support. The study emphasized the view that their past, present, and future psychological and mental health should be of interest to researchers and intervention programs.

> While many of the family members spent the day together for work and meals, they would sleep in different houses. As the family seemed to change form during the 24 h the informants not always knew who to count in their family. (Knizek et al., 2017, p. 4)

As noted above, the above findings indicate a failure by the existing traditional care system to provide avenue for bonding and effective psychological worth for OVCs particularly those orphaned as a direct result of HIV/AIDS. Alternative interventions need to be proposed for such children to meet these needs. A life cycle approach is essential where children are trained to meet their needs using individual as well as group approaches. The beginning is helping these children to appreciate that they are in unique situations and therefore mobilize both internal and external resources to meet this challenge. They could be trained to adopt and manage a life of chaos and find resources for coping (Eriksson, 2017).

Towards Understanding of Intergenerational Trauma

Understanding how parents that have gone through adversity and experienced post-traumatic stress disorder (PTSD) may or may not affect the development and mental health in the offspring is important for communities that have been devasted by HIV/AIDS for decades. The extent of intergeneration trauma has not been well studied in Uganda yet several studies seem to suggest chronicity of PTSD in case negative life events remain unaddressed for a long time (Mugisha et al., 2015). These negative life events may include family-based violence, abject poverty, and civil strife. Related studies indicate an increased level of behavioral disorders, anxiety, and depressive symptoms, as well as post-traumatic stress among offspring of tortured refugee parents suffering from PTSD compared to children with non-traumatized parents (Roth et al., 2014). This calls for early interventions before the onset of chronic trauma. A high sense of coherence is associated with better mental health. As argued, SOC uniquely combines relevant aspects of behavioral, cognitive, and motivational resistance within a child or an individual (Almedom, 2005; Mittelmark et al., 2017). It has an advantage over other resistance factors that may protect an individual from the negative effects of adversity (Almedom, 2005; Mittelmark et al., 2017) and should be nurtured in children that have gone through adversity.

Widow Inheritance

Despite the HIV/AIDS pandemic in Uganda, widow inherence is still a common vice in a number of communities and most widows in Uganda live under deplorable conditions. Under these circumstances, the rights of the widow and her children are always ignored. They are likely to suffer psychological stressors as well as their children. The stressors might be more pronounced in children as they may fail to cope with the demands and dynamics in the new family where they are inherited. The mental distress that is likely to be experienced in the new relationship may affect the treatment seeking for both the mother and the children. Children under this arrangement may also lose out on positive and effective engagements such as play and other freedoms that are vital for normal child growth and development.

> On the surface of it all, widow inheritance is no longer their but in a practical sense, it has only changed form. We see these cases every day. (PID_03 Health Official, NGO)

The sense of coherence is again useful in understanding children that have suffered violence. If not addressed, such children are also likely to undergo personality changes. The women and children that have gone through this violence are likely to have a low sense of coherence (Sitarczyk, 2013). But the same theoretical framework (salutogenesis) can be used to improve their coping and resilience to violence. This will require interventions that can enhance their sense of coherence

(Sitarczyk, 2013). That will take deliberate steps by intervening agencies to train them on how to cope with the violence. A keen interest in studying their personalities as they develop will be essential and if there are any abnormalities, correctional measures should be undertaken. That implies regular employment of culturally validated personality assessment tests.

Revolving-Door Children

It is also a common phenomenon in Uganda to find children oscillate between families and childcare institutions, for example, a child staying with his/her family at night while at the same time spending the day at an orphan/mental health facility. In quite a number of families, this becomes a coping strategy to meet household needs as the family spends less time and resources on such children.

> They drop the child at the hospital during the day and pick the same child at night. They do not want to take on the heavy day care burden. (PID_05 Psychiatrist, National Referral Hospital)

> There are mushrooming child care institutions that are providing day care for orphan children in Uganda today. Though the word care in the real sense is wanting. (PID_07 Social Worker, Academic Institution)

Some of the models of care are hazardous for children who visit these childcare institutions (Walakira et al., 2014).

> For example, there is very limited interaction between the children and adults and among the children themselves. (PID_08 Social Worker, Academic Institution)

Yet, the social service institutions in the country have also kept a blind eye on this reality.

> The weight of government is not easy to feel in these [childcare] matters. Institutions are not supervised and what they do is sometimes dangerous to these children. (PID_08 Social Worker, Academic Institution)

In addition, there are no studies undertaken yet to look at the psychological as well as the mental health status of such children using the SOC scale. One would be interested to know the impact of the childcare models on both preschool and school-attending children orphaned by HIV and AIDS using this framework. It could also be interesting to examine how the size and duration in the orphan care institutions among other variables impact the child's SOC.

In other situations, the family may be running away from stigma associated with HIV, mental illness, or both.

> Stigma for HIV/AIDS is still much despite the several decades of intervention and mental illness makes it worse. (PID_06 Psychiatrist, National Referral Hospital)

A SOC scale and other related instruments could be vital to examine the resilience level of these children in such settings.

Conclusion

As discussed previously, there is a need to re-examine the traditional systems of care since most of them are also at the brink. The social service system in Uganda has been slow in facing this reality and the government has also been slow to head to this wakeup call. New models of thinking should be brought on board. Social service agencies should empower children made vulnerable by HIV/AIDS to face adversity through mobilizing their internal resources but also develop skills to work collaboratively to secure resources outside the family. In the same way, institutions and government need to build adolescent-friendly services that build confidence for adolescents to seek support as well as enhance and improve their physical and mental well-being. In addition, family-strengthening strategies and programs focused on strengths that improve the availability and access to contextual services are important for enhancing the capacity of families and communities to care for orphaned adolescents. Salutogenesis theory becomes vital in such endeavors. It is also important to understand the cultural sensitivity of SOC scale(s) and its key domains in a low-resource context like Uganda. Thus, further research in this area will be vital.

References

Almedom, A. M. (2005). Social capital and mental health: An interdisciplinary review of primary evidence. *Social Science & Medicine, 61*(5), 943–964.

Ankrah, E. M. (1991). AIDS and the social side of health. *Social Science & Medicine, 32*(9), 967–980.

Belfer, M. L. (2008). Child and adolescent mental disorders: The magnitude of the problem across the globe. *Journal of Child Psychology and Psychiatry, 49*(3), 226–236.

Braun, V., & Clarke, V. (2006). Using thematic analysis in psychology. *Qualitative Research in Psychology, 3*(2), 77–101.

Cortina, M. A., Sodha, A., Fazel, M., & Ramchandani, P. G. (2012). Prevalence of child mental health problems in sub-Saharan Africa: A systematic review. *Archives of Pediatrics & Adolescent Medicine, 166*(3), 276–281.

Eriksson, M. (2017). The sense of coherence in the salutogenic model of health. In Mittelmark et al. (Eds.), *The handbook of salutogenesis* (pp. 91–96). Springer.

Gana, K. (2001). Is sense of coherence a mediator between adversity and psychological well-being in adults? *Stress and Health: Journal of the International Society for the Investigation of Stress, 17*(2), 77–83.

Hubert, S., & Aujoulat, I. (2018). Parental burnout: When exhausted mothers open up. *Frontiers in Psychology, 9*, 1021.

Katz, J., Tirone, V., & Schukrafft, M. (2012). Breaking up is hard to do: Psychological entrapment and women's commitment to violent dating relationships. *Violence and Victims, 27*(4), 455–469.

Keyes, C. L., Shmotkin, D., & Ryff, C. D. (2002). Optimizing well-being: The empirical encounter of two traditions. *Journal of Personality and Social Psychology, 82*(6), 1007.

Knizek, B. L., Mugisha, J., Osafo, J., & Kinyanda, E. (2017). Growing up HIV-positive in Uganda: "Psychological immunodeficiency"? A qualitative study. *BMC Psychology, 5*(1), 1–10.

Margalit, M. (1998). Loneliness and coherence among preschool children with learning disabilities. *Journal of Learning Disabilities, 31*(2), 173–180.

Mc Gee, S. L., Höltge, J., Maercker, A., & Thoma, M. V. (2018). Sense of coherence and stress-related resilience: Investigating the mediating and moderating mechanisms in the development of resilience following stress or adversity. *Frontiers in Psychiatry, 9*, 378.

Mittelmark, M. B., Sagy, S., Eriksson, M., Bauer, G. F., Pelikan, J. M., Lindström, B., & Arild Espnes, G. (2017). *The handbook of salutogenesis*. Springer.

Mugisha, J., Kinyanda, E., Osafo, J., Nalukenge, W., & Knizek, B. L. (2020). Health care professionals' perspectives on barriers to treatment seeking for formal health services among orphan children and adolescents with HIV/AIDS and mental distress in a rural district in central, Uganda. *Child and Adolescent Psychiatry and Mental Health, 14*, 1–10.

Mugisha, J., Muyinda, H., Malamba, S., & Kinyanda, E. (2015). Major depressive disorder seven years after the conflict in northern Uganda: Burden, risk factors and impact on outcomes (the Wayo-Nero study). *BMC Psychiatry, 15*(1), 1–12.

Mukiza-Gapere, J., & Ntozi, J. P. (1995). Impact of AIDS on the family and mortality in Uganda. *Health Transition Review, 5*, 191–200.

Nalugya, J. (2004). *Depression amongst secondary school adolescents in Mukono District, Uganda*. Makerere University.

Roth, M., Neuner, F., & Elbert, T. (2014). Transgenerational consequences of PTSD: Risk factors for the mental health of children whose mothers have been exposed to the Rwandan genocide. *International Journal of Mental Health Systems, 8*(1), 1–12.

Sitarczyk, M. (2013). Sense of coherence in women - victims of domestic violence. *Psychiatry and Clinical Psychology, 13*(4), 250–263.

UNICEF. (2004). *Children on the Brink 2004. A joint report of new orphan estimates and a framework for action*. Retrieved from https://www.unicef.org/media/files/cob_layout6-013.pdf

UNICEF. (2015). *State of the world's children 2015 country statistical tables: Uganda statistics*. Retrieved from http://www.unicef.org/infobycountry/uganda_statistics.html

Walakira, E. J., Ochen, E. A., Bukuluki, P., & Alllan, S. (2014). Residential care for abandoned children and their integration into a family-based setting in Uganda: Lessons for policy and programming. *Infant Mental Health Journal, 35*(2), 144–150.

Wamulugwa, J., Kakooza, A., Kitaka, S. B., Nalugya, J., Kaddumukasa, M., Moore, S., . . . Katabira, E. (2017). Prevalence and associated factors of attention deficit hyperactivity disorder (ADHD) among Ugandan children; a cross-sectional study. *Child and Adolescent Psychiatry and Mental Health, 11*(1), 18.

World Health Orginisation (WHO). (2005). *World Health Report*, Geneva.

Part III
Violence and Child Mental Health in Sub-Saharan Africa: Case Examples

The Role of Social Norms: A Case Study of Intimate Partner Violence Among Adolescent Girls in Nigeria

Ilana Seff and Lindsay Stark

Intimate Partner Violence

Intimate partner violence (IPV), defined as any physical, psychological, or sexual violence perpetrated by a current or former intimate partner, poses a threat to women's and girls' rights, safety, and well-being around the globe (World Health Organization, 2013). Nearly one-third of women globally have ever experienced IPV and the likelihood of victimization is particularly elevated in low- and middle-income countries (LMICs) (Butchart & Mikton, 2014). IPV poses a significant threat as young as adolescence; globally, approximately 29.4% of ever-partnered girls aged 15–19 years have faced physical and/or sexual IPV (World Health Organization, 2013). Girls and women in sub-Saharan Africa (SSA) often face even greater risk of IPV, with 37% of ever-partnered women reporting exposure to partner violence in their lifetime (World Health Organization, 2013). Further, risk of IPV in this region often materializes during adolescence, before girls have even entered into a formal union or marriage. In some SSA countries, such as Gabon and Liberia, nearly 20% of ever-married women and girls aged 15–49 years experienced their first incident of IPV prior to marriage (Peterman et al., 2015).

Witnessing IPV has also proven to have negative effects on children. Children exposed to IPV in the household are significantly more likely to exhibit symptoms of post-traumatic stress disorder and mood and anxiety disorders (Levendosky et al., 2013; Wathen & Macmillan, 2013). For example, one study of children aged 6–12 years old whose mothers had experienced IPV in the last year found that the majority of children in the sample had severe adjustment problems, were struggling with respect to psychosocial well-being, or exhibited symptoms of depression (Graham-Bermann et al., 2009). Witnessing IPV as a child is also associated with

I. Seff (✉) · L. Stark
Brown School, Washington University in St. Louis, St. Louis, MO, USA
e-mail: seff@wustl.edu

© Springer Nature Switzerland AG 2022   157
F. M. Ssewamala et al. (eds.), *Child Behavioral Health in Sub-Saharan Africa*,
https://doi.org/10.1007/978-3-030-83707-5_9

increased risk of self-reported alcoholism, drug use, and other risky behaviors, with evidence suggesting a dose-response relationship between frequency of events witnessed and severity of these outcomes later in life (Dube et al., 2002). Women exposed to IPV as children, for instance, were significantly more likely to have had an early sexual debut (defined as sexual debut before age 15) and a greater self-described risk of acquiring AIDS (Hillis et al., 2001). Unsurprisingly, children living in a home with IPV are also themselves more likely to face physical, emotional, or sexual abuse (Holt et al., 2008). One study from Northern Uganda found that mothers' reports of IPV victimization were a strong predictor of aggressive parenting behavior, while another study from SSA estimated that nearly 33% of families in the sample had faced experiences of both IPV and violence against children (Saile et al., 2014), Finally, a wide body of literature demonstrates that children who witness IPV in the home are more likely to experience and perpetrate IPV as adults (Cannon et al., 2009; Ehrensaft et al., 2003; Renner & Slack, 2006).

Of course, directly experiencing IPV also has important health implications for victims, namely, women and girls. In addition to the direct physical injuries sustained by survivors of IPV, research shows that women and girls who have experienced IPV are more likely to develop reproductive health problems, sexually transmitted infections, and induced abortions (Black, 2011; Campbell, 2002; Heise & Garcia-Moreno, 2002). As compared to women and girls who have never been exposed to IPV, survivors are also significantly more likely to exhibit poor mental health outcomes, including depressive symptoms and suicide attempts (Ackard et al., 2007; Devries et al., 2013). Several studies have documented increased alcohol consumption among IPV survivors, though this association likely operates in both directions (Devries et al., 2013). The links between IPV, poor mental health outcomes, and unhealthy coping mechanisms are well documented in the SSA context (Decker et al., 2014; Deyessa et al., 2009; Mapayi et al., 2013; Nduna et al., 2010).

Determinants of IPV

The literature on IPV and its causes has undergone a dramatic expansion in the last few decades. Factors associated with IPV, and violence against women (VAW) and girls more broadly, can be found at multiple sociological levels, and Heise's (1998) widely used ecological framework for the determinants of VAW, adapted from Bronfenbrenner's ecological framework, offers a comprehensive conceptualization of these factors (Bronfenbrenner, 1996; Heise, 1998). This framework helps practitioners and policymakers design more effective prevention strategies to tackle IPV determinants across the social ecology.

The first level of Heise's nested ecological framework focuses on ontogenic, or personal history, factors, and includes elements of an individual's upbringing and personality traits that influence how he or she reacts to external actors, stressors, and situations. The most widely cited ontogenic factors associated with IPV perpetration include having witnessed or experienced violence in childhood (Abramsky et al.,

2011; Jewkes, 2002; Jewkes et al., 2015; Lichter & McCloskey, 2004). The microsystem represents the second level and comprises the interactions a victim or perpetrator has with others (especially those involved in an incident of abuse) as well as the meanings the individual ascribes to those situations. In the case of IPV, for example, the family serves as the microsystem; for an incident of non-partner sexual violence, the microsystem is the immediate setting where the violence takes place. Women in relationships characterized by patriarchal decision-making, marital conflict, and a difference in years of schooling between the couple are more likely to experience IPV (Flake, 2005; Hindin et al., 2008; Jewkes, 2002; Lawoko et al., 2007). The exosystem serves as the third level of the model and comprises formal and informal social structures that interact with and influence the microsystem. Women living in isolation or in families with lower socioeconomic status (SES) typically exhibit greater incidence of IPV victimization (Heise, 1998; Parish et al., 2004; Tang & Lai, 2008).

The fourth and final level of Heise's ecological framework, the macrosystem, includes the wide range of cultural beliefs and values that contribute to factors found at the other three levels of the ecology. While macrosystem factors do not directly contribute to a man's use of IPV, they indirectly influence his likelihood of perpetration through their impact on ontogenic, microsystem, and exosystem factors. Social norms that sustain IPV serve as one of the most widely discussed macrofactors in the literature. For example, social norms supporting male dominance and supremacy will likely influence how gender power dynamics are organized within community structures and households; in turn, as discussed above, women in households that support patriarchal decision-making are then more likely to experience IPV. Similarly, social norms that support patriarchal beliefs (Pallitto & O'Campo, 2005; Parish et al., 2004), rigid gender roles (Pallitto & O'Campo, 2005; Stith et al., 2004), and conceptualizations of masculinity characterized by dominance, toughness, and pride (Heise, 1998) have all been theoretically linked to IPV perpetration. Additionally, incidence of IPV tends to be higher where social norms condone the use of violence as a method of conflict resolution and endorse the use of IPV more specifically (Abramsky et al., 2011; Gage, 2005; Hindin et al., 2008; Khawaja et al., 2008; Koenig et al., 2006).

Labor Participation and Intimate Partner Violence

In recent decades, a growing number of development and poverty reduction policies have included an explicit focus on empowering women and girls economically (Vyas & Watts, 2009). Such policies and programs may take the form of microcredit, financial literacy curriculums, and/or teaching marketable skills. In addition to expanding women's and girls' access to financial capital, these efforts have been shown to improve some outcomes of well-being, such as increased utilization of maternal and antenatal healthcare (Bloom et al., 2001). However, addressing these financial issues in a silo may have unintended consequences as there is mixed

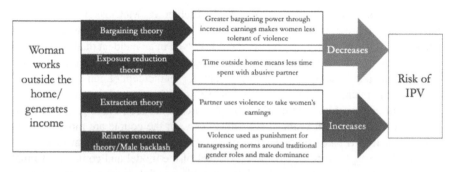

Fig. 1 Working outside the home and IPV risk

evidence on the relationship between women's and girls' labor participation and income generation on the one hand, and exposure to IVP, on the other (Vyas & Watts, 2009).

Two theories are primarily used to explain the pathway between working outside the home and a decreased risk of IPV victimization: bargaining theory and exposure reduction theory (see Fig. 1). Bargaining theory postulates that women and girls who generate their own income become less tolerant of violence through increased financial independence and perceived agency (Farmer & Tiefenthaler, 1997). A qualitative study from Tanzania found, for example, that access to paid work decreased experiences of IPV for many of the women interviewed by minimizing the need to negotiate money from their husbands, a typical trigger of IPV in the study sample (Vyas et al., 2015). Proponents of the second theory, exposure reduction theory, argue that working women and girls decrease their likelihood of IPV victimization simply by spending less time in the home with their abusive partners (Chin, 2012).

In contrast, other studies have found a positive association between women's and girls' working status and IPV. The extraction theory posits that women and girls who earn incomes may face increased risk of IPV if their husbands use violence to seize these earnings (Chin, 2012). The relative resource theory, on the other hand, asserts that an economic power differential within the partnership—for example, if a woman is employed but her husband is not, or if a woman generates a higher income than her partner—may be perceived by the male partner as a challenge to his authority; in response, the theory posits that he may use violence to reassert his dominance (Macmillan & Gartner, 1999; McCloskey, 1996). Stress levels are already elevated when a household's resources are low, but Atkinson et al. (2005) argue that, in settings where men subscribe to traditional gender ideologies, these conditions may lead them to feel especially useless and emasculated (Atkinson et al., 2005). As such, it can be argued that the validity of the relative resource theory varies by setting and depends largely on the strength of traditional gender norms that support a man's role as the patriarch and primary income earner. For example, in a qualitative study from Colombia, where men traditionally hold the decision-making power, women who worked outside the home felt that they experienced more IPV because their husbands were threatened by their wives' transgression of traditional gender norms (Hynes et al., 2016). Similarly, in Bangladesh, where within-household dynamics are characterized by male dominance and decision-making, a study revealed that women's and girls' economic empowerment was accompanied by increased risk of IPV as husbands were opposed to their wives' new autonomy (Schuler et al., 1998).

Investigation of this issue through a social norms lens would allow for the existence of each of these relationships, and assert that the pathway between generating an income outside the home and risk of IPV in a given community is importantly influenced by the normative beliefs and behaviors in that community. Indeed, a systematic review of studies assessing the relationship between female economic empowerment and risk of IPV identified studies finding positive, negative, and nonexistent associations between the two factors (Vyas & Watts, 2009); however, the majority of these studies failed to control for local norms around female empowerment in the analysis, thus potentially diluting the relationship in certain settings. One included study from Bangladesh analyzed the relationship between female economic empowerment and IPV, separately, in both a culturally conservative and less conservative region, and found that measures of empowerment were positively associated with the risk of IPV in the culturally conservative region; the reverse was found to be true—i.e., female empowerment was protective against IPV—in the less conservative region (Koenig et al., 2003). Findings from this study underscore the importance of accounting for norms at a more nuanced level when analyzing the relationship between economic empowerment and IPV for women and girls.

Social Norms and Child Behavioral Health: Understanding the Links

Social norms theory has been substantially developed and revised over the past several decades and has come to play a critical role in how we think about public health policy and interventions, including how we think about child behavioral health outcomes. Social norms, or the implicit rules that regulate human behavior, operate in complex ways to influence individuals' attitudes and behaviors (Bicchieri, 2005). Broadly speaking, a social norm represents what individuals in a given group perceive to be normal, where normal is defined as typical, acceptable, or both (Mackie et al., 2015; Paluck & Ball, 2010). Social norms theorists are particularly interested in not only how individuals define these norms but also how those perceptions inform their own behavior. Such understandings may inform health-related outcomes and hint at ways to change them.

Cialdini and Trost (1998) usefully distinguish between two types of norms, both of which they argue are necessary to sustain a given behavior (Cialdini & Trost, 1998). Descriptive norms are an individual's perceptions of what others do, while injunctive norms reflect an individual's perception of what others *think* that individual *should* do. Research demonstrates that descriptive norms can hold powerful influence over children's and adolescents' health-related behaviors. For example, a wide body of literature shows that college students often overestimate alcohol use among their peers, which in turn leads them to drink more heavily themselves or to assess their own excessive alcohol use as acceptable (Borsari & Carey, 2003; Schultz et al., 2007). Similarly, a study of sixth-grade students in the United States found that the perceived prevalence of smoking among peers was positively associated with smoking initiation (Simons-Morton, 2002). In this case, an individual's behavior is influenced by how *typical* he or she believes the behavior to be among a key peer group. Young people, who are particularly susceptible to peer influence, act in ways to avoid deviating from their perception of "normal" (Halfon & Hochstein, 2002; Steinberg, 2005). Research suggests that an adolescent's perceived prevalence of a behavior among peers may increase the likelihood of engaging in that behavior even when the behavior is typically carried out in private, such as has been shown with risky sexual behavior online (Baumgartner et al., 2010, 2011).

Research also illustrates the sway of injunctive norms on child and adolescent behavioral health. One study on smoking intentions among 11- and 12-year-olds found that children underestimated their friends' disapproval of their smoking behaviors (Zaleski & Aloise-Young, 2013). Further, it was this perceived injunctive norm, as opposed to the actual injunctive norm, that was found to be associated with respondents' likelihood of smoking initiation. Importantly, injunctive norms can also promote the adoption of healthy behaviors, and this relationship can be positively exploited in carefully constructed interventions, as demonstrated in an evaluation of a video-based intervention to reduce child risk-taking behaviors (Morrongiello et al., 2013). In this study, children watched several videos showcasing children engaging in risk-taking behaviors on the playground, such as jumping precariously from one structure to another. Portrayed risk-taking behaviors were accompanied by different verbalizations representing positive and negative injunctive norms around the behavior. Children who watched the video where child actors discouraged and ridiculed the video subject for considering such risky behaviors were significantly less likely to report an intention to engage in risk-taking themselves. Injunctive norms can play a role in adolescents' sexual behavior as well (Fearon et al., 2015). Students aged 12–14 years in Tanzania, for example, were found to be more likely to have reported having had sex if they believed their friends would be less accepting of them if they did not have sex (Kakoko, 2013).

Additionally, of relevance to all social norms frameworks is the central role of the reference group. A reference group refers to a group of individuals for which reciprocal expectations regarding a certain behavior hold for the majority of those in the group (Mackie et al., 2015). Correctly identifying the relevant reference group for a given norm is critical when designing interventions to alter the norm. Illustrative examples can be found in a study on healthy eating and physical activity among high school students that assessed the influence of peer and parent norms on students' intention to carry out these healthy behaviors (Baker et al., 2003). Researchers found that perceived peer norms around healthy eating had a much stronger influence on girls' intentions to eat healthily as compared to parent norms. An intervention promoting healthy behaviors among adolescents might then usefully consider targeting girls' attitudes around healthy eating and making these attitudes public through peer group discussions. Further, a social norm may hold in one reference group and not another. For example, Baker et al. (2003) also found that while perceived peer norms around exercising influenced intention to exercise for boys, no such relationship was found to exist for girls.

Lastly, it is critical to note the importance of attitudes in relation to social norms, as well as to recognize the difference between the two constructs. Unlike a norm, which is externally driven, an attitude is internally and personally motivated and reflects an individual's positive or negative feeling toward a given behavior, person, or relationship (Mackie et al., 2015; Petty & Cacioppo, 1986). While a person's attitude toward a given behavior may be shaped by relevant perceived norms, an individual can—and often does—hold an attitude that differs from the norm (Hogg & Tindale, 2008). However, where social norms sustaining a behavior are strong and perceived sanctions for deviations are grave, an individual may disregard his or her attitudinal disapproval of the behavior when deciding how to act (Mackie et al., 2015; Paluck, 2009; Paluck & Shepherd, 2012). For example, a wide body of literature supports the notion that while many students hold anti-bullying attitudes, these same children rarely speak up against bullying for fear of countering the norm and facing social isolation (Ortega & Mora-Merchan, 1999; Salmivalli & Voeten, 2004; van Goethem et al., 2010).

Social norms have become increasingly relevant in today's discourse around gender identity, roles, and power dynamics, and it is critical that public health practitioners understand how norms might shape male and female identities in ways that influence child and adolescent behavioral health outcomes. Female genital mutilation (FGM), and interventions targeting the eradication of this practice, offer an illustrative example of how attitudes and norms might work to sustain the behavior or lead to its decline over time. FGM is practiced to varying degrees across multiple countries and ethnic groups in sub-Saharan Africa and, unsurprisingly, it is reinforced through a range of different descriptive and injunctive norms. Almost always, the practice is found in communities characterized by patriarchal power dynamics and decision-making; and, in many cases, FGM has historically been used as a way for men to assert power and control over women and their bodies (Mackie, 2009). However, once a practice becomes normative, the initial reasons for its introduction into society may not be the same motivations that sustain the practice. For example, in communities where FGM has been practiced for centuries, parents might opt to have their daughter cut because they endorse the descriptive norm that "everyone else here has their daughter cut—it's just what we do here." Alternatively, parents might perceive negative sanctions (injunctive norms) for failing to have their daughter cut; in such instances, parents might think, "my neighbors will judge me if I don't carry out this practice", or "no one will want to marry my daughter if I don't have her cut." While a mother or father might simultaneously disapprove of the practice (attitude), he or she may feel compelled to comply regardless.

However, interventions that have been thoughtfully designed to leverage the power of social norms have been shown to reduce the incidence of FGM over time. For example, Vaitla et al. (2017) point to Tostan's Community Education Program in Senegal as a successful model of what can be achieved through norms-based programming (Vaitla et al., 2017). The program fostered public discussions of what it means to be a healthy girl in the community, giving rise to definitions that did not include FGM. However, by facilitating these conversations in public, other community members were able to perceive these shifting attitudes and internalize them in such a way that new norms supporting reductions in FGM emerged (Mackie, 2009).

Measuring Social Norms

Social norms are influenced by cultural, political, and economic factors, and their power to influence behavior relies heavily on the types and strength of social ties in a given community (Nayak et al., 2003). Unsurprisingly then, generating reliable and valid measures of social norms is rife with challenges (Cislaghi & Heise, 2016; Mackie et al., 2015). These difficulties not only impact the quality of research related to social norms and health outcomes, but also have direct implications for programming; inaccurate identification of social norms can lead to programs targeting irrelevant norms or reference groups.

Mackie et al. (2015) reviewed 173 studies on the use of social norms in international development and found that only 14% discussed explicit measurement of social norms; the remainder only outlined how social norms theory was employed programmatically. A recent convening of experts in social norms measurement resulted in the identification of two other relevant challenges in measuring social norms (Cislaghi & Heise, 2016). First, there is a need for methods to rapidly identify behaviors under normative influence. This issue echoes one expressed in a call for papers in upcoming special issue of the *Lancet* on gender equality, norms, and health; the call noted a gap in new ways to identify and measure norms in existing datasets. Second, Cislaghi and Heise (2016) noted that many researchers aggregate social norms data to the level of an irrelevant reference group. For example, a researcher might aggregate attitudinal data for some behavior at the community level as a proxy for the community norm, when in fact reciprocal normative expectations might instead hold within religious or ethnic groups (Seff, Under Review). Quick and efficient ways of identifying a relevant reference group for a given norm are critical for ensuring effective targeting of social norms programs.

To date, the majority of research studies attempting to measure social norms utilize qualitative methods; focus group discussions, in-depth interviews, and vignette-based discussions are all popular approaches for exploring normative behaviors and influence in a given reference group (Cislaghi & Heise, 2016). While such methods for measuring norms can help shed light on these issues within small samples, they are time and resource intensive, and not necessarily efficient for measuring a multitude of norms across more heterogeneous settings. This limitation presents a challenge for researchers and practitioners aiming to address social norms on a wider scale, as few adequate quantitative methods exist to identify and measure these constructs. Further, this dearth of quantitative approaches means many large, representative quantitative datasets go unused for examining linkages between social norms and behavioral health outcomes.

In fact, there are myriad datasets that offer nationally representative, rigorously collected information on a wide variety of topics related to health and well-being (see the Living Standards Measurement Study, Multiple Indicator Cluster Survey, Demographic and Health Survey, and Violence Against Children Surveys for a few examples). However, given the difficulty associated with including complex questions on social norms in such surveys, these datasets rarely contain direct insight on norms. Instead, many of these datasets include data on behaviors and attitudes. Intuitively, attitudes are relatively easier to measure than norms; while capturing an attitude depends only on a person's internal preference, measuring a norm requires an individual to reflect on his or her perception of others. Further, individuals are often not even consciously aware of the ways they conceptualize normative and empirical expectations of others and themselves (Forgas, 2016).

As a result, many social norms researchers and policymakers adopt some aggregate measure of attitudes as a proxy for the underlying norms (Haylock et al., 2016). For example, one might construct a community-level variable that represents the average individual-level score on a scale measuring attitudes toward hand-washing; in brief, the researcher might claim that communities with higher scale averages are those where hand-washing or acceptance of hand-washing is normative. However, while some aggregate measures of attitudes *might* reflect the normative thinking and behaviors in a given reference group, this is not a given. Studies show that interventions fostering new attitudes and beliefs, but not addressing the wider norms in the relevant group, often fail to affect sustained change in the targeted behavior (Moosa et al., 2012). As such, an attitude or behavior cannot necessarily serve as a proxy for a norm if the attitude or behavior is not salient and public enough that others in the reference group can perceive and internalize it. More careful thought is needed for how to effectively capture norms using quantitative data, and this chapter utilizes one new approach.

Methods

To explore the topics presented in this chapter, we employ data from the Violence Against Children Survey (VACS) in Nigeria. The VACS is implemented as part of a partnership led by the U.S. Centers for Disease Control and Prevention's Division of Violence Prevention (DVP), along with Together for Girls (TfG) and other bilateral and multilateral entities. The partnership assists LMICs to conduct nationally representative household surveys to generate estimates of violence exposure for children and adolescents. Ultimately, the VACS aims to (1) estimate the national prevalence of sexual violence, physical violence, and emotional violence against males and females; (2) identify risk and protective factors; (3) identify health and well-being consequences; (4) assess disclosure of violence, knowledge, and utilization of services, as well as barriers to accessing services; and (5) identify areas for further research. Surveys also include questions on demographic characteristics, sexual experiences, and knowledge and attitudes toward HIV and HIV testing, among many others (National Population Commission of Nigeria, UNICEF Nigeria, and the U.S. Centers for Disease Control and Prevention, 2016).

Setting

Approximately one-quarter of the female population in Nigeria is comprised of 13- to 24-year-olds, and nearly 29% of girls aged 15–19 years old have already been married or part of a formal union (https://www.unfpa.org/data/adolescent-youth/ NG#). Early relationships and marriage are especially common in certain geographic areas; in some states in the North, nearly 45% of women aged 20–24 years were married before age 15, and more than 80% were married before age 18. Adolescent and young adult relationships are often characterized by inequitable decision-making and power dynamics between genders; 48% of girls aged 15–24 years have a husband or cohabitating partner who is 10 or more years their senior, though there is large variation by state.

To date, there exists minimal evidence about the relationship between female labor participation or income generation and risk of IPV in Nigeria (Vyas & Watts, 2009), and existing studies do not take into account variation in local norms (Okenwa et al., 2009). Nonetheless, IPV is generally accepted in this context. Approximately 40% and 60% of men and women, respectively, believe that IPV is justified in at least one scenario, and 15- to 24-year-olds exhibit nearly 1.5 greater odds of believing that IPV is justified as compared to those 35 years and older (Uthman et al., 2009). Acceptance of IPV among adolescents and young adults is matched by relatively large levels of risk; in one urban setting in Nigeria, 33% of female adolescents aged 15–19 years reported ever experiencing physical or sexual IPV (Decker et al., 2014).

Data

The VACS in Nigeria was implemented in 2014 and utilized a multistage cluster sample design. In the first stage, 353 enumeration areas (EAs), or primary sampling units (PSUs), were randomly selected. Next, 20 respondents were randomly sampled from each EA. All VACS surveys employ a "split sample" approach at the EA level, such that each EA provides either an all-male or all-female sample. Sampling only one gender from a given EA substantially minimizes the likelihood that both a female respondent and her male partner are interviewed, thus protecting both parties' safety and confidentiality. The VACS is not explicitly framed as a violence survey when presented to potential respondents and therefore participants who complete the survey are the only ones in a community who know the actual content of the questionnaire. Both caregiver consent and informed assent were obtained for respondents under 18 years of age; consent was obtained for respondents over 18. The VACS does not collect personally identifying information and interviews are conducted in private spaces when possible.

Variables of Interest

We assessed several self-reported outcomes of interest, including past-year exposure to sexual violence, past-year exposure to physical or sexual IPV, and a few measures of attitudinal acceptance of IPV. Past-year exposure to physical IPV was defined for those that ever had a partner that punched, kicked, whipped, beat, choked, suffocated, tried to drown, burned, or threatened the respondent with a weapon, AND reported that either the first or most recent such incident took place within the last year. Past-year exposure to sexual IPV was defined for those who ever experienced unwanted sexual touching, attempted forced sex, completed forced sex, or coerced sex, AND reported that either the first or the most recent such incident took place within the last year, AND that incident within the last year was perpetrated by an intimate partner. Finally, past-year exposure to sexual violence was defined for those who ever experienced unwanted sexual touching, attempted forced sex, completed forced sex, or coerced sex, AND reported that either the first or the most recent such incident took place within the last year, regardless of the perpetrator.

Various measures of attitudinal acceptance of IPV were constructed from five survey items. Respondents were asked to indicate whether they thought it was "right for a man to beat his wife" in each of the five scenarios: she goes out without telling him, she does not take care of the children, she argues with him, she refuses to have sex with him, or she burns the food. Outcomes of interest used in this analysis included (1) a dichotomous outcome that takes the value of "1" if the respondent agreed with at least one statement, and "0" otherwise, and (2) three dichotomous variables that match the responses given for the three scenarios which might feasibly relate to a woman working outside the home.

The analysis utilized two key predictors of interest, both derived from the same two survey questions. The first predictor, measured at the level of the individual, was defined for those who reported working for pay in the last 7 days AND reported that this work took place outside the family dwelling. We also generated a community-level variable that contains information about the extent to which females engaging in work are normative in that community. Communities were defined at the PSU level and were identified as either those where female labor participation was more normative (progressive communities) or PSUs where female labor participation was not normative (restrictive communities).

Fig. 2 ICC close to 1

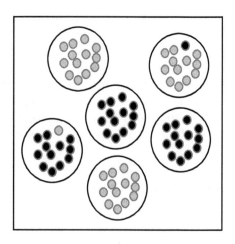

The intraclass correlation coefficient (ICC), an inferential statistic that provides information on how much units within a group—as compared to how much units across groups—resemble each other, with respect to the measurement of interest, was first used to assess the distribution of the average proportion of working females across PSUs. In order to more confidently assert that progressive communities are practically different from restrictive communities, we used the ICC to understand the extent to which female labor participation varied across communities. A very low ICC (e.g., rho = 0.05) would imply that nearly all communities have the same proportion of females engaged in work; in that scenario, it would not be appropriate to classify communities as progressive vs. restrictive. For some characteristics which we expect to be highly clustered across communities in this context, such as whether or not a respondent is Muslim, we would expect an ICC closer to 1. Indeed, a check of this across-community variation confirmed that the ICC for Islam was 0.96 in our sample; each PSU was almost entirely Muslim or not Muslim at all (see Fig. 2 for an example). In contrast, we would expect the proportion of respondents 18 years and younger to be almost the same across every PSU; again, this hypothesis was verified with an ICC of 0.05 in our sample (see Fig. 3).

The ICC for our predictor of interest, female labor participation, was rho = 0.314, suggesting a fairly large level of variation across PSUs. In fact, further assessment revealed that, in two-thirds of PSUs, less than 28% of females were engaged in work. This cutoff of 28% was selected to delineate progressive and restrictive communities.

Analysis

We first compared mean past-year exposure to sexual violence, physical IPV, sexual IPV, and physical or sexual IPV between progressive and restrictive communities. Statistically significant differences between communities were assessed using

Fig. 3 ICC close to 0

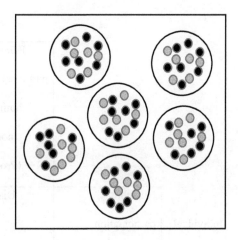

adjusted Wald tests. We then examined whether and how the outcomes of interest were differently affected by an adolescent girl's engagement in labor, depending on the type of community she lived in. Classifying communities as those where female labor participation was more normative and as those where female labor participation was not normative allowed us to examine how a girl's individual behavior influenced her risk of violence depending on the norms in her community (see Fig. 4).

Specifically, we utilized multiple logistic regressions, stratified by community type, to estimate each of the outcomes of interest. Regression models controlled for respondents' labor participation outside the home, marital status, age, and whether or not they had ever attended school. Standard errors were adjusted for complex sampling design and all observations were weighted to be representative of the population of 13- to 24-year-old females in Nigeria. All analyses were conducted using Stata 14.

Findings

Table 1 presents the overall risk of violence for females aged 13–24 years based on the community type. When assessing differences in self-reported exposure to sexual violence in the last 12 months, we find that communities where female labor participation outside the home is more normative (progressive communities) are those where higher proportions of females face sexual violence; the average community-level exposure to past-year sexual violence for females in these communities is 20.4%, compared to 12.6% for restrictive communities. As shown in Table 1, the difference in risk of sexual violence appears to be driven predominantly by sexual violence perpetrated by someone other than an intimate partner. Sexual violence perpetrated by an intimate partner, as well as physical IPV and IPV including both forms of violence, does not occur at different rates across the two

Community level norm

		Females' labor participation outside the home is more normative (Progressive)	Females' labor participation outside the home is NOT normative (Restrictive)
Individual level behavior	NO labor participation outside the home	Discordant	Agreement
	Labor participation outside the home	Agreement	Discordant

Fig. 4 Individual- and community-level labor participation

community types. This finding suggests that adolescent girls who work outside the home are more exposed to other individuals in the community who may perpetrate sexual violence against them.

Next, we estimate females' risk of experiencing sexual violence and IPV depending on both the type of community they live in and their own behavior. Table 2 demonstrates that females who engage in labor outside the home in restrictive communities have significantly higher odds of experiencing IPV compared to females in the community who do not engage in labor outside the home. For example, in communities where female labor participation is not normative, females who participate in labor outside the home have 2.381 greater odds of experiencing physical or sexual IPV. This finding suggests that adolescent girls transgressing the norm around female labor participation may be facing punishment from their intimate partners as a result. In contrast, in communities where norms do not necessarily condemn female labor participation, females who work outside the home are less at risk of facing retribution.

Individual-level labor participation is also associated with differences in females' attitudes toward IPV in these more labor-restrictive communities. For example, in restrictive communities, females who participate in labor outside the home have significantly lower odds of agreeing that it is acceptable for a man to beat his wife if she goes out without telling him (aOR = 0.438) or if she neglects the children (aOR = 0.521). In contrast, individual-level labor participation is not associated with

Table 1 Exposure to violence for females 13–24 years old, by community level of female labor participation outside the home

	Communities where females' labor participation outside the home is more normative (progressive)	Communities where females' labor participation outside the home is not normative (restrictive)	p-Value of difference
Sexual violence (by anyone)	20.4% (2.31)	12.6% (1.75)	0.010*
Sexual violence by a non-intimate partner	17.1% (2.16)	8.0% (1.32)	<0.001***
Intimate partner violence (sexual or physical)	7.3% (1.16)	7.9% (1.50)	0.733
Sexual IPV	3.4% (0.85)	4.5% (0.73)	0.336
Physical IPV	4.6% (0.83)	3.8% (0.81)	0.514
Number of communities	38	81	

Note: Community-level averages were calculated using sampling weights. Standard errors in parentheses have been adjusted for the complex sampling design. Adjusted Wald tests were used to assess significance between the two groups' means. Differences in means are statistically significant at ***p < 0.001, **p < 0.01, and *p < 0.05.

attitudinal acceptance of IPV in progressive communities. These findings imply that the few females who choose to work in restrictive communities may be those that endorse more progressive and gender equitable attitudes. However, our analysis also reveals that these same females face increased risk of IPV, potentially for acting according to these more progressive beliefs.

Links to Child Behavioral Health

As noted earlier in the chapter, experiencing IPV in adolescence has well-documented consequences for mental health during adolescence and lasting well into the life course. The relationship between IPV exposure and mental distress is also evident in the data used for this case study. Using logistic regressions and controlling for age, we find that adolescent girls aged 13–24 years in Nigeria who reported experiencing IPV in the last 12 months had two times greater odds of feeling severe sadness in the last 30 days (P = 0.01), a risk factor for depression, and

Table 2 Predicting exposure to violence and attitudes toward IPV for females 13–24 years old, by community and individual levels of labor participation outside the home

	Communities where females' labor participation outside the home is more normative (progressive communities)	Communities where females' labor participation outside the home is not normative (restrictive communities)
	Labor participation outside home, aOR [95% CI]	Labor participation outside home, aOR [95% CI]
Outcomes	(1b)	(2b)
Sexual violence	0.807	1.368
	[0.559, 1.166]	[0.762, 2.456]
Sexual violence by a non-intimate partner	0.736	1.232
	[0.434, 1.250]	[0.603, 2.517]
IPV (sexual or physical)	0.750	2.381**
	[0.370, 1.521]	[1.292, 4.389]
Sexual IPV	1.268	1.475
	[0.420, 3.834]	[0.750, 2.901]
Physical IPV	0.519	3.222*
	[0.223, 1.204]	[1.326, 7.827]
Attitudinal acceptance of IPV		
Agree with at least one statement around IPV acceptance	1.241	0.745
	[0.854, 1.803]	[0.455, 1.222]
If she goes out without telling him	1.175	0.438*
	[0.695, 1.987]	[0.233, 0.826]
If she neglects the children	1.207	0.521*
	[0.793, 1.835]	[0.304, 0.895]
If she argues with him	1.168	0.923
	[0.791, 1.726]	[0.552, 1.544]

Note: All models are estimated using logistic regressions and control for age, marital status, and having ever attended school. Standard errors are adjusted for complex sampling design. All observations are weighted to be representative of the population. Odds ratios are significant at *p < 0.05, **p < 0.01, and ***p < 0.001.

four times greater odds of suicidal ideation (P < 0.001), as compared to their peers who had not experienced IPV in the last 12 months. Additionally, we find that adolescent girls who reported experiencing IPV in the last 12 months had 1.7 times greater odds of having witnessed IPV in their home before the age of 18. This finding underscores the cyclical and intergenerational nature of IPV, alluding to potential future threats to safety and well-being of children who witnessed the IPV discussed in the previous subsection.

Policy and Program Implications

The findings from this case study offer novel insights into the ways in which the transgression of gender norms might have negative consequences for adolescent girls. Interestingly, overall, girls in more progressive communities faced greater risk of sexual violence by someone other than an intimate partner, presumably by nature of being outside of the home more frequently. One interpretation of this finding might be that staying inside the home and having more restrictive movement are better for adolescent girls' health and safety. However, a more nuanced interpretation might be that along the pathway to gender equality, females may face different kinds of threats to their overall well-being.

This understanding of complex pathways to gender equity is also suggested by the finding that, among adolescent girls living in communities where work outside the home is not normative, those who engage in labor face significantly higher odds of experiencing IPV compared to those who do not engage in labor. The elevated exposure to IPV for working female adolescents in labor-restrictive communities suggests that male partners may be using IPV as a means of punishing girls who have transgressed the norm around work. We also find that adolescent girls who transgress the norm around female labor participation are much less likely to believe that IPV is acceptable. This finding suggests that those who transgress the norm may be particularly progressive with respect to attitudes around gender equity, but that they may simultaneously face greater threats to their well-being for acting on these more progressive attitudes.

These findings underscore the importance of identifying and considering the social and gender norms in a given setting before implementing programs and policies aiming to empower women and girls. Policies and programs that promote behavior counter to the contextual norms run the risk of generating unintended consequences for the very individuals these policies aim to help. Such programs and policies should work to simultaneously address broader gender inequitable norms in order to ensure positive impacts for women and girls in all arenas. For instance, policymakers and practitioners might thoughtfully work with young boys and men to discuss and redefine the concept of "healthy masculinity"; interventions that incorporate such an approach have also been shown to have positive mental health outcomes for boys and men (Peacock & Barker, 2014; Pulerwitz et al., 2015). Stepping Stones, a program that works with men and women, separately, to improve sexual health and behaviors provides another example of an effective approach for engaging men and boys. Stepping Stones uses participatory methods to encourage participants to critically reflect on gender norms, communications skills, and motivations for gender-based violence; an evaluation of the program in South Africa found that male participants were less likely to perpetrate IPV and engage in transactional sex for up to 2 years (Jewkes et al., 2008).

Community-based interventions, the most common type of programming implemented in low- and middle-income countries to reduce intimate partner violence against adolescent girls, perhaps demonstrate the most promising evidence, having been shown to reduce self-reported perpetration of IPV, increase gender equitable attitudes, and increase individuals' likelihood of intervening in a case of IPV (Lundgren & Amin, 2015). Community-based programs engage both men and women and may employ a range of approaches, including community mobilization, peer mentorship, social campaigns, and group dialogues around healthy fatherhood for young men. Our findings hint that these community-wide, gender transformative programs may prove especially beneficial in communities where the rules around gender roles and female labor engagement are particularly rigid. As female empowerment, labor participation, and mobility become more normative over time in a certain setting, women's and girls' individual behaviors will no longer carry the same risk to their safety and well-being (Schuler & Nazneen, 2018).

This study also sheds light on one of the myriad potential sources of mental distress for young females in sub-Saharan Africa. Beyond threats to autonomy and physical well-being experienced by survivors of IPV, our analysis reveals that these young females were also significantly more likely to report symptoms of mental distress. This finding should be considered alongside the budding focus on the range of mental health issues facing adolescents in sub-Saharan Africa, where one systematic review recently estimated that one in seven adolescents bears a mental health burden of some kind (Belfer, 2008). Importantly, evidence from life course studies demonstrates that traumatic exposures during adolescence can fundamentally influence the development of lifelong characteristics and behaviors (Sawyer et al., 2018). It follows that the mental health challenges that might emerge from exposure to IPV are likely to carry into and affect mental health in adulthood, which can in turn have intergenerational effects (Kim-Cohen et al., 2003; Patton et al., 2014).

Options for *treating* mental health issues in sub-Saharan Africa remain alarmingly sparse; recent research found that most countries in the region have only one child psychiatrist for every four million people (Owen et al., 2016). However, the utilization of systemic and coordinated approaches to *prevent* adolescent mental health disorders in sub-Saharan Africa is a small but growing trend, and it is critical that practitioners in this space consider all relevant risk factors and points of entry as the policy landscape continues to grow. For example, policies for suicide prevention conventionally focus on diminishing access to means, but nascent programs in the region have begun targeting psychosocial interventions toward populations with higher-than-average mental distress or corresponding risk factors (O'Connor, 2016). The analysis presented in this chapter suggests that mental health service providers might usefully engage in targeted outreach with young female survivors of IPV in an attempt to prevent mental distress and/or risk of suicide. More broadly, programs working with adolescents in sub-Saharan Africa should thoughtfully consider and address the complex relationships between gender norms, violence, and mental health, in order to break the cycle of violence and improve the safety and well-being of children and adolescents across the region.

Acknowledgements We would like to thank our colleagues who helped make this chapter possible: thanks to Gary Darmstadt, Ann Weber, Ben Cislaghi, and Valerie Meausoone for their invaluable inputs throughout this process; to Greta Massetti and Daniela Ligiero for sharing the data and their expertise; and to Victor Atuchukwu and Dennis Onotu for providing indispensable contextual insights. Lastly, a special thank you to the adolescents and young adults who generously shared their time and experiences for the Violence Against Children Survey.

References

Abramsky, T., Watts, C. H., Garcia-Moreno, C., Devries, K., Kiss, L., Ellsberg, M., Jansen, H. A., & Heise, L. (2011). What factors are associated with recent intimate partner violence? Findings from the WHO multi-country study on women's health and domestic violence. *BMC Public Health, 11*, 109. https://doi.org/10.1186/1471-2458-11-109

Ackard, D. M., Eisenberg, M. E., & Neumark-Sztainer, D. (2007). Long-term impact of adolescent dating violence on the behavioral and psychological health of male and female youth. *The Journal of Pediatrics, 151*(5), 476–481. https://doi.org/10.1016/j.jpeds.2007.04.034

Atkinson, M. P., Greenstein, T. N., & Lang, M. M. (2005). For women, breadwinning can be dangerous: gendered resource theory and wife abuse. *Journal of Marriage and Family, 67*(5), 1137–1148. https://doi.org/10.1111/j.1741-3737.2005.00206.x

Baker, C. W., Little, T. D., & Brownell, K. D. (2003). Predicting adolescent eating and activity behaviors: The role of social norms and personal agency. *Health Psychology, 22*(2), 189–198. https://doi.org/10.1037/0278-6133.22.2.189

Baumgartner, S. E., Valkenburg, P. M., & Peter, J. (2010). Assessing causality in the relationship between adolescents' risky sexual online behavior and their perceptions of this behavior. *Journal of Youth and Adolescence, 39*(10), 1226–1239. https://doi.org/10.1007/s10964-010-9512-y

Baumgartner, S. E., Valkenburg, P. M., & Peter, J. (2011). The influence of descriptive and injunctive peer norms on adolescents' risky sexual online behavior. *Cyberpsychology, Behavior and Social Networking, 14*(12), 753–758. https://doi.org/10.1089/cyber.2010.0510

Belfer, M. L. (2008). Child and adolescent mental disorders: The magnitude of the problem across the globe. *Journal of Child Psychology and Psychiatry, 49*(3), 226–236. https://doi.org/10.1111/j.1469-7610.2007.01855.x

Bicchieri, C. (2005). *The grammar of society: The nature and dynamics of social norms*. Cambridge University Press.

Black, M. (2011). Intimate partner violence and adverse health consequences: implications for clinicians. *American Journal of Lifestyle Medicine, 5*(5), 428–439.

Bloom, S. S., Wypij, D., & Das Gupta, M. (2001). Dimensions of women's autonomy and the influence on maternal health care utilization in a North Indian city. *Demography, 38*(1), 67–78. https://doi.org/10.1353/dem.2001.0001

Borsari, B., & Carey, K. B. (2003). Descriptive and injunctive norms in college drinking: A meta-analytic integration. *Journal of Studies on Alcohol, 64*(3), 331–341.

Bronfenbrenner, U. (1996). *The ecology of human development: Experiments by nature and design*. Harvard University Press.

Butchart, A., & Mikton, C. (2014). *Global status report on violence prevention, 2014*. World Health Organization.

Campbell, J. C. (2002). Health consequences of intimate partner violence. *The Lancet, 359*(9314), 1331–1336. https://doi.org/10.1016/S0140-6736(02)08336-8

Cannon, E. A., Bonomi, A. E., Anderson, M. L., & Rivara, F. P. (2009). The intergenerational transmission of witnessing intimate partner violence. *Archives of Pediatrics & Adolescent Medicine, 163*(8), 706–708. https://doi.org/10.1001/archpediatrics.2009.91

Chin, Y. (2012). Male backlash, bargaining, or exposure reduction?: Women's working status and physical spousal violence in India. *Journal of Population Economics, 25*(1), 175–200.

Cialdini, R., & Trost, M. (1998). Social influence: Social norms, conformity and compliance. In *The handbook of social psychology* (pp. 151–192). McGraw-Hill.

Cislaghi, B., & Heise, L. (2016). Measuring gender-related social norms: Report of a meeting, Baltimore Maryland, June 14–15, 2016. Learning Group on Social Norms and Gender-based Violence of the London School of Hygiene and Tropical Medicine.

Decker, M. R., Peitzmeier, S., Olumide, A., Acharya, R., Ojengbede, O., Covarrubias, L., Gao, E., Cheng, Y., Delany-Moretlwe, S., & Brahmbhatt, H. (2014). Prevalence and health impact of intimate partner violence and non-partner sexual violence among female adolescents aged 15–19 years in vulnerable urban environments: A multi-country study. *Journal of Adolescent Health, 55*(6), S58–S67. https://doi.org/10.1016/j.jadohealth.2014.08.022

Devries, K. M., Mak, J. Y., Bacchus, L. J., Child, J. C., Falder, G., Petzold, M., Astbury, J., & Watts, C. H. (2013). Intimate partner violence and incident depressive symptoms and suicide attempts: A systematic review of longitudinal studies. *PLoS Medicine, 10*(5), e1001439. https://doi.org/10.1371/journal.pmed.1001439

Deyessa, N., Berhane, Y., Alem, A., Ellsberg, M., Emmelin, M., Hogberg, U., & Kullgren, G. (2009). Intimate partner violence and depression among women in rural Ethiopia: A cross-sectional study. *Clinical Practice and Epidemiology in Mental Health, 5*(1), 8. https://doi.org/10.1186/1745-0179-5-8

Dube, S., Anda, R., Felitti, V., Edwards, V., & Williamson, D. (2002). Exposure to abuse, neglect, and household dysfunction among adults who witnessed intimate partner violence as children: Implications for health and social services. *Violence and Victims, 17*(1), 3–17.

Ehrensaft, M. K., Cohen, P., Brown, J., Smailes, E., Chen, H., & Johnson, J. G. (2003). Intergenerational transmission of partner violence: A 20-year prospective study. *Journal of Consulting and Clinical Psychology, 71*(4), 741–753. https://doi.org/10.1037/0022-006X.71.4.741

Farmer, A., & Tiefenthaler, J. (1997). An economic analysis of domestic violence. *Review of Social Economy, 55*(3), 337–358.

Fearon, E., Wiggins, R. D., Pettifor, A. E., & Hargreaves, J. R. (2015). Is the sexual behaviour of young people in sub-Saharan Africa influenced by their peers? A systematic review. *Social Science & Medicine, 146*, 62–74. https://doi.org/10.1016/j.socscimed.2015.09.039

Flake, D. F. (2005). Individual, family, and community risk markers for domestic violence in Peru. *Violence Against Women, 11*(3), 353–373. https://doi.org/10.1177/1077801204272129

Forgas, J. P. (2016). *Social influence: Direct and indirect processes* (1st ed.). Psychology Press. https://doi.org/10.4324/9781315783031

Gage, A. J. (2005). Women's experience of intimate partner violence in Haiti. *Social Science and Medicine, 61*, 343–364.

Graham-Bermann, S. A., Gruber, G., Howell, K. H., & Girz, L. (2009). Factors discriminating among profiles of resilience and psychopathology in children exposed to intimate partner violence (IPV). *Child Abuse & Neglect, 33*(9), 648–660. https://doi.org/10.1016/j.chiabu.2009.01.002

Halfon, N., & Hochstein, M. (2002). Life course health development: An integrated framework for developing health, policy, and research. *Milbank Quarterly, 80*(3), 433–479. https://doi.org/10.1111/1468-0009.00019

Haylock, L., Cornelius, R., Malunga, A., & Mbandazayo, K. (2016). Shifting negative social norms rooted in unequal gender and power relationships to prevent violence against women and girls. *Gender and Development, 24*(2), 231–244. https://doi.org/10.1080/13552074.2016.1194020

Heise, L., & Garcia-Moreno, C. (2002). Violence by intimate partners. In *World report on violence and health* (pp. 87–121). World Health Organization.

Heise, L. L. (1998). Violence against women: An integrated, ecological framework. *Violence Against Women, 4*(3), 262–290. https://doi.org/10.1177/1077801298004003002

Hillis, S. D., Anda, R. F., Felitti, V. J., & Marchbanks, P. A. (2001). Adverse childhood experiences and sexual risk behaviors in women: A retrospective cohort study. *Family Planning Perspectives, 33*(5), 206. https://doi.org/10.2307/2673783

Hindin, M. J., Kishor, S., Ansara, D. L., Nilsson, J. E., Brown, C., Russell, E. B., Khamphakdy-Brown, S., Btoush, R., Haj-Yahia, M. M., & Serbanescu, F. (2008). *Intimate partner violence among couples in 10 DHS countries: Predictors and health outcomes* (Vol. 23). USAID.

Hogg, M. A., & Tindale, S. (2008). *Blackwell handbook of social psychology: Group processes.* Wiley.

Holt, S., Buckley, H., & Whelan, S. (2008). The impact of exposure to domestic violence on children and young people: A review of the literature. *Child Abuse & Neglect, 32*(8), 797–810. https://doi.org/10.1016/j.chiabu.2008.02.004

Hynes, M. E., Sterk, C. E., Hennink, M., Patel, S., DePadilla, L., & Yount, K. M. (2016). Exploring gender norms, agency and intimate partner violence among displaced Colombian women: A qualitative assessment. *Global Public Health, 11*(1–2), 17–33. https://doi.org/10.1080/17441692.2015.1068825

Jewkes, R. (2002). Intimate partner violence: Causes and prevention. *The Lancet, 359*(9315), 1423–1429. https://doi.org/10.1016/S0140-6736(02)08357-5

Jewkes, R., Flood, M., & Lang, J. (2015). From work with men and boys to changes of social norms and reduction of inequities in gender relations: A conceptual shift in prevention of violence against women and girls. *The Lancet, 385*(9977), 1580–1589. https://doi.org/10.1016/S0140-6736(14)61683-4

Jewkes, R., Nduna, M., Levin, J., & Jama, N. (2008). Impact of Stepping Stones on incidence of HIV and HSV-2 and sexual behaviour in rural South Africa: Cluster randomised controlled trial. *BMJ, 337*, a506. https://doi.org/10.1136/bmj.a506

Kakoko, D. C. V. (2013). Reported heterosexual intercourse and related behaviours among primary school pupils in Kinondoni district, Dar es Salaam, Tanzania. *Culture, Health & Sexuality, 15* (2), 235–245. https://doi.org/10.1080/13691058.2012.738829

Khawaja, M., Linos, N., & El-Roueiheb, Z. (2008). Attitudes of men and women towards wife beating: Findings from Palestinian refugee camps in Jordan. *Journal of Family Violence, 23*(3), 211–218. https://doi.org/10.1007/s10896-007-9146-3

Kim-Cohen, J., Caspi, A., Moffitt, T. E., Harrington, H., Milne, B. J., & Poulton, R. (2003). Prior juvenile diagnoses in adults with mental disorder: Developmental follow-back of a prospective-longitudinal cohort. *Archives of General Psychiatry, 60*(7), 709. https://doi.org/10.1001/archpsyc.60.7.709

Koenig, M. A., Ahmed, S., Hossain, M. B., & Khorshed Alam Mozumder, A. B. (2003). Women's status and domestic violence in rural Bangladesh: Individual- and community-level effects. *Demography, 40*(2), 269–288.

Koenig, M. A., Stephenson, R., Ahmed, S., Jejeebhoy, S. J., & Campbell, J. (2006). Individual and contextual determinants of domestic violence in North India. *American Journal of Public Health, 96*(1), 132–138. https://doi.org/10.2105/AJPH.2004.050872

Lawoko, S., Dalal, K., Jiayou, L., & Jansson, B. (2007). Social inequalities in intimate partner violence: A study of women in Kenya. *Violence and Victims, 22*(6), 773–784.

Levendosky, A. A., Bogat, G. A., & Martinez-Torteya, C. (2013). PTSD symptoms in young children exposed to intimate partner violence. *Violence Against Women, 19*(2), 187–201. https://doi.org/10.1177/1077801213476458

Lichter, E. L., & McCloskey, L. A. (2004). The effects of childhood exposure to marital violence on adolescent gender-role beliefs and dating violence. *Psychology of Women Quarterly, 28*(4), 344–357. https://doi.org/10.1111/j.1471-6402.2004.00151.x

Lundgren, R., & Amin, A. (2015). Addressing intimate partner violence and sexual violence among adolescents: Emerging evidence of effectiveness. *The Journal of Adolescent Health: Official Publication of the Society for Adolescent Medicine, 56*, S42–S50. https://doi.org/10.1016/j.jadohealth.2014.08.012

Mackie, G. (2009). Social dynamics of abandonment of harmful practices: A new look at the theory. *Innocenti Working Papers, 2009–06*.

Mackie, G., Moneti, F., Shakya, H., & Denny, E. (2015). *What are social norms? How are they measured?* UNICEF.

Macmillan, R., & Gartner, R. (1999). When she brings home the bacon: Labor-force participation and the risk of spousal violence against women. *Journal of Marriage and the Family, 61*(4), 947. https://doi.org/10.2307/354015

Mapayi, B., Makanjuola, R. O. A., Mosaku, S. K., Adewuya, O. A., Afolabi, O., Aloba, O. O., & Akinsulore, A. (2013). Impact of intimate partner violence on anxiety and depression amongst women in Ile-Ife, Nigeria. *Archives of Women's Mental Health, 16*(1), 11–18. https://doi.org/10.1007/s00737-012-0307-x

McCloskey, L. A. (1996). Socioeconomic and coercive power within the family. *Gender & Society, 10*(4), 449–463. https://doi.org/10.1177/089124396010004006

Moosa, Z., Ahluwalia, K., Bishop, K., Derbyshire, H., Dolata, N., & Donaldson, L. (2012). *A theory of change for tackling violence against women and girls (gender development network)*. DFID.

Morrongiello, B. A., McArthur, B. A., Kane, A., & Fleury, R. (2013). Only kids who are fools would do that!: Peer social norms influence Children's risk-taking decisions. *Journal of Pediatric Psychology, 38*(7), 744–755. https://doi.org/10.1093/jpepsy/jst019

National Population Commission of Nigeria, UNICEF Nigeria, and the U.S. Centers for Disease Control and Prevention. (2016). *Violence against children in Nigeria: Findings from a national survey, 2014*. Abuja, Nigeria: UNICEF.

Nayak, M. B., Byrne, C. A., Martin, M. K., & Abraham, A. G. (2003). Attitudes toward violence against women: A cross-nation study. *Sex Roles, 49*(7), 333–342. https://doi.org/10.1023/A:1025108103617

Nduna, M., Jewkes, R. K., Dunkle, K. L., Shai, N., & Colman, I. (2010). Associations between depressive symptoms, sexual behaviour and relationship characteristics: A prospective cohort study of young women and men in the Eastern Cape, South Africa. *Journal of the International AIDS Society, 13*(1), 44. https://doi.org/10.1186/1758-2652-13-44

O'Connor, R. (2016). *The international handbook of suicide prevention*. Wiley.

Okenwa, L. E., Lawoko, S., & Jansson, B. (2009). Exposure to intimate partner violence amongst women of reproductive age in Lagos, Nigeria: Prevalence and predictors. *Journal of Family Violence, 24*(7), 517–530. https://doi.org/10.1007/s10896-009-9250-7

Ortega, R., & Mora-Merchan, J. (1999). Spain. In *The nature of school bullying. A cross-national perspective* (pp. 157–173). Routledge.

Owen, J. P., Baig, B., Abbo, C., & Baheretibeb, Y. (2016). Child and adolescent mental health in Sub-Saharan Africa: A perspective from clinicians and researchers. *BJPsych International, 13*(2), 45–47.

Pallitto, C. C., & O'Campo, P. (2005). Community level effects of gender inequality on intimate partner violence and unintended pregnancy in Colombia: Testing the feminist perspective. *Social Science & Medicine, 60*(10), 2205–2216. https://doi.org/10.1016/j.socscimed.2004.10.017

Paluck, E. L. (2009). Reducing intergroup prejudice and conflict using the media: A field experiment in Rwanda. *Journal of Personality and Social Psychology, 96*(3), 574–587. https://doi.org/10.1037/a0011989

Paluck, E. L., & Ball, L. (2010). *Social norms marketing aimed at gender based violence: A literature review and critical assessment*. International Rescue Committee.

Paluck, E. L., & Shepherd, H. (2012). The salience of social referents: A field experiment on collective norms and harassment behavior in a school social network. *Journal of Personality and Social Psychology, 103*(6), 899–915. https://doi.org/10.1037/a0030015

Parish, W. L., Wang, T., Laumann, E. O., Pan, S., & Luo, Y. (2004). Intimate partner violence in China: National prevalence, risk factors and associated health problems. *International Family Planning Perspectives, 30*(4), 174–181. https://doi.org/10.1363/ifpp.30.174.04

Patton, G. C., Coffey, C., Romaniuk, H., Mackinnon, A., Carlin, J. B., Degenhardt, L., Olsson, C. A., & Moran, P. (2014). The prognosis of common mental disorders in adolescents: A 14-year prospective cohort study. *The Lancet, 383*(9926), 1404–1411. https://doi.org/10.1016/ S0140-6736(13)62116-9

Peacock, D., & Barker, G. (2014). Working with men and boys to prevent gender-based violence: Principles, lessons learned, and ways forward. *Men and Masculinities, 17*(5), 578–599.

Peterman, A., Bleck, J., & Palermo, T. (2015). Age and intimate partner violence: An analysis of global trends among women experiencing victimization in 30 developing countries. *Journal of Adolescent Health, 57*(6), 624–630. https://doi.org/10.1016/j.jadohealth.2015.08.008

Petty, R., & Cacioppo, J. (1986). *Communication and persuasion: central and peripheral routes to attitude change*. Springer.

Pulerwitz, J., Hughes, L., Mehta, M., & Kidanu, A. (2015). Changing gender norms and reducing intimate partner violence: Results from a quasi-experimental intervention study with young men in Ethiopia. *American Journal of Public Health, 105*(1), 132.

Renner, L. M., & Slack, K. S. (2006). Intimate partner violence and child maltreatment: Understanding intra-and intergenerational connections. *Child Abuse & Neglect, 30*(6), 599–617.

Saile, R., Ertl, V., Neuner, F., & Catani, C. (2014). Does war contribute to family violence against children? Findings from a two-generational multi-informant study in Northern Uganda. *Child Abuse & Neglect, 38*(1), 135–146. https://doi.org/10.1016/j.chiabu.2013.10.007

Salmivalli, C., & Voeten, M. (2004). Connections between attitudes, group norms, and behaviour in bullying situations. *International Journal of Behavioral Development, 28*(3), 246–258. https:// doi.org/10.1080/01650250344000488

Sawyer, S. M., Azzopardi, P. S., Wickremarathne, D., & Patton, G. C. (2018). The age of adolescence. *The Lancet Child & Adolescent Health, 2*(3), 223–228. https://doi.org/10.1016/ S2352-4642(18)30022-1

Schuler, S. R., Hashemi, S. M., & Badal, S. H. (1998). Men's violence against women in rural Bangladesh: Undermined or exacerbated by microcredit programmes? *Development in Practice, 8*(2), 148–157. https://doi.org/10.1080/09614529853774

Schuler, S. R., & Nazneen, S. (2018). Does intimate partner violence decline as women's empowerment becomes normative? Perspectives of Bangladeshi women. *World Development, 101*, 284–292. https://doi.org/10.1016/j.worlddev.2017.09.005

Schultz, P. W., Nolan, J. M., Cialdini, R. B., Goldstein, N. J., & Griskevicius, V. (2007). The constructive, destructive, and reconstructive power of social norms. *Psychological Science, 18* (5), 429–434. https://doi.org/10.1111/j.1467-9280.2007.01917.x

Seff, I. (Under Review). Social norms sustaining interpersonal violence against women and girls: A systematic review of methodologies for proxy measures. Under Review.

Simons-Morton, B. G. (2002). Prospective analysis of peer and parent influences on smoking initiation among early adolescents. *Prevention Science: The Official Journal of the Society for Prevention Research, 3*(4), 275–283.

Steinberg, L. (2005). Cognitive and affective development in adolescence. *Trends in Cognitive Sciences, 9*(2), 69–74. https://doi.org/10.1016/j.tics.2004.12.005

Stith, S. M., Smith, D. B., Penn, C. E., Ward, D. B., & Tritt, D. (2004). Intimate partner physical abuse perpetration and victimization risk factors: A meta-analytic review. *Aggression and Violent Behavior, 10*(1), 65–98. https://doi.org/10.1016/j.avb.2003.09.001

Tang, C. S.-K., & Lai, B. P.-Y. (2008). A review of empirical literature on the prevalence and risk markers of male-on-female intimate partner violence in contemporary China, 1987–2006. *Aggression and Violent Behavior, 13*(1), 10–28. https://doi.org/10.1016/j.avb.2007.06.001

Uthman, O. A., Lawoko, S., & Moradi, T. (2009). Factors associated with attitudes towards intimate partner violence against women: A comparative analysis of 17 sub-Saharan countries. *BMC International Health and Human Rights, 9*(1), 14. https://doi.org/10.1186/1472-698X-9-14

Vaitla, B., Taylor, A., Van Horn, J., & Cislaghi, B. (2017). *Social norms and girls well-being integrating theory, practice, and research*. United Nations Foundation.

van Goethem, A. A. J., Scholte, R. H. J., & Wiers, R. W. (2010). Explicit and implicit bullying attitudes in relation to bullying behavior. *Journal of Abnormal Child Psychology, 38*(6), 829–842. https://doi.org/10.1007/s10802-010-9405-2

Vyas, S., Mbwambo, J., & Heise, L. (2015). Women's paid work and intimate partner violence: Insights from Tanzania. *Feminist Economics, 21*(1), 35–58. https://doi.org/10.1080/13545701.2014.935796

Vyas, S., & Watts, C. (2009). How does economic empowerment affect women's risk of intimate partner violence in low and middle income countries? A systematic review of published evidence. *Journal of International Development, 21*(5), 577–602. https://doi.org/10.1002/jid.1500

Wathen, C. N., & Macmillan, H. L. (2013). Children's exposure to intimate partner violence: Impacts and interventions. *Paediatrics & Child Health, 18*(8), 419–422.

World Health Organization. (2013). *Global and regional estimates of violence against women: Prevalence and health effects of intimate partner violence and non-partner sexual violence.* World Health Organization.

Zaleski, A. C., & Aloise-Young, P. A. (2013). Using peer injunctive norms to predict early adolescent cigarette smoking intentions: Injunctive norms and smoking. *Journal of Applied Social Psychology, 43*, E124–E131. https://doi.org/10.1111/jasp.12080

Current State of Child Behavioral Health: Focus on Violence Against Children in Uganda

Agatha Kafuko, Clare Ahabwe Bangirana, and Timothy Opobo

Acronyms

ACRWC	Africa Charter for the Rights and Welfare of the Child
CRC	Convention on the Rights of the Child
FY	Financial year
GBV	Gender-based violence
GBVMIS	Gender-Based Violence Management Information System
HMIS	Health Management Information System
JLOS	Justice Law and Order Sector
MDG	Millennium Development Goals
NCA	National Children's Authority
NGO	Non-governmental organization
NVACS	National Violence Against Children Survey
OVC	Orphans and other vulnerable children
OVCMIS	Orphans and other Vulnerable Children Management Information System
RCI	Residential care institutions
SDG	Sustainable Development Goals
UN	United Nations
UNCRC	United Nations Convention on the Rights of the Child
UNESCO	United Nations Education, Social and Cultural Organization

A. Kafuko (✉)
Department of Social Work and Social Administration, Makerere University, Kampala, Uganda
e-mail: agatha.kafuko@mak.ac.ug

C. A. Bangirana · T. Opobo
The AfriChild Centre, Kampala, Uganda

© Springer Nature Switzerland AG 2022   181
F. M. Ssewamala et al. (eds.), *Child Behavioral Health in Sub-Saharan Africa*,
https://doi.org/10.1007/978-3-030-83707-5_10

UNICEF   United Nations Children's Fund
VAC   Violence against children
WHO   World Health Organization

Introduction

Uganda's journey has been riddled with social, political, economic and environmental upheavals, including multiple civil wars between 1967 and 2010 (Sejjaaka, 2004). Prior to the ratification of the United Nations Convention on the Rights of the Child (UNCRC) in 1990 and subsequently the African Charter on the Rights and Welfare of the Child (ACRWC), children in Uganda bore the brunt of disruption in Uganda, with limited recourse to their protection (Spitzer & Twikirize, 2013; Cheney, 2005). Child mortality rates were high due to the effects of war and diseases including AIDS. Under-five mortality increased from 180 in 1969 to 205 per 1000 live births in 1988 (Nuwaha & Mukulu, 2009). Children who lost their lives fighting at frontlines in civil wars in Uganda were victims of war, and many were co-opted to fight in wars at the frontline. The impact of HIV and civil wars of the 1980s and 1990s forced to live on the streets, under exploitative conditions of labour and abuse. Some children who remained in their homes, without adult caretakers, became de facto household heads and were forced to fend for themselves and their siblings.

The fortunes of children in Uganda however began to slowly change when the country ratified the United Nations Convention on the Rights of the Child (UNCRC), and subsequently enacted the first ever Children's Statute in 1992. Violent actions such as physical punishment against children that had hitherto been considered to be normal were questioned. The UNCRC makes explicit provisions for four broad categories of rights (United Nations, 1989): the (1) survival rights—including the right to life, nutrition, shelter, an adequate living standard and access to medical service; (2) development rights—including the right to education, play, leisure, cultural activities, access to information and freedom of thought, conscience and religion; (3) protection rights—including protection from all forms of abuse, neglect and exploitation, safeguards for children in the criminal justice system, protection for children in employment, and protection and rehabilitation for children who have suffered exploitation or abuse of any kind; and (4) participation rights—including children's freedom to express opinions, to have a say in matters affecting their own lives, to join associations and to assemble peacefully. The convention altered the lens through which government regarded children, from protecting them against specific ills to a holistic approach that guarantees all rights for all children.

The ratification of the UNCRC resulted in gradual but steady investments in laws, policies and practices that focus on uplifting the status of children in Uganda. As required by the UNCRC, the Government of Uganda was to put in place structures and systems to protect children and ensure that they have their rights fulfilled. Uganda also ratified the African Charter on the Rights and Welfare of the Child (ACRWC) on August 17, 1994. The ACRWC sought to contextualize the UNCRC on the African continent by discouraging customs, traditions, cultural or religious practices that are inconsistent with the rights, duties and obligations of the broad African familial values (Ekundayo, 2015). In addition to these two key frameworks for the protection of children, the country has also embraced various development frameworks such as the Millennium Development Goals (MDGs) and the successor Sustainable Development Goals (SDGs) and/or the Africa Fit for Children, Agenda 2063, among others. The international frameworks have been domesticated at national level through national legislation and policy enactment. As a result, Uganda has a comprehensive legal and policy framework within which an effective child protection system can be constructed. Uganda consolidated all laws related to children into the Child Statute, and later the Children's Act. A national council for children was established to monitor and supervise the state of children.

Despite the significant strides made by Uganda since the 1990s in domesticating the principles set forth by the key international and regional instruments into national laws, the country has encountered challenges in effective enforcement and implementation. The law enforcement seems to contradict the intentions and commitments of the country to uphold the rights of children in totality. Law enforcement has continually been cited as a challenge in implementing the child protection commitments made by the country alongside other systemic and functional bottlenecks including but not limited to resource constraints, technical capacity and political will (Foundation for Human Rights Initiative, 2012; Ministry of Gender, Labour and Social Development, 2020).

A Theoretical Framework for Understanding Violence Against Children in Uganda

This chapter utilizes the World Health Organization (WHO)-recommended ecological framework as a conceptual tool for understanding the drivers and actors in violence against children (VAC). The ecological framework views violence against children as the outcome of complex interaction among factors at the individual, relationship, community and societal levels. At the individual level, personal history and biological factors influence how children behave and increase their likelihood of becoming victims or perpetrators of violence. A child's sex, gender, education level, being a victim of child maltreatment, psychological or personality disorders, alcohol and substance abuse and a history of abuse may influence violence experiences (Fig. 1).

Relationships with family, friends, intimate partners and peers may influence the risks of becoming a victim or perpetrator of violence. For example, having violent friends may influence whether a young person engages in or becomes a victim of

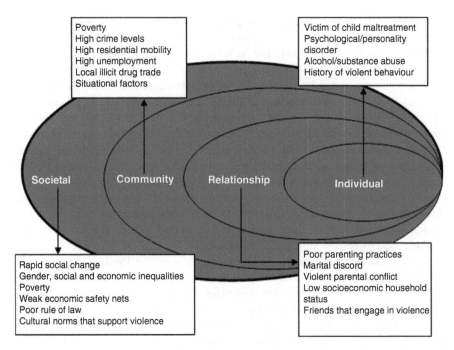

Fig. 1 Ecological framework: examples of risk factors at each level (WHO, 2021). Reprinted from the VPA approach: The ecological framework, World Health Organization, Copyright 2021. Used with permission. https://www.who.int/violenceprevention/approach/ecology/en/

violence. Relationships may also provide support in the context of violence. The communities in which children live and where social relationships occur, such as schools, neighbourhoods and workplaces, influence violence.

Societal including economic and social policies that maintain inequalities, social and cultural norms such as those around male dominance over women, parental dominance over children and cultural norms that endorse violence as an acceptable method to resolve conflicts are factors that may influence occurrence and responses to violence.

The ecological framework treats the interaction between factors at different levels with equal importance to the influence of factors within a single level, and is useful in the identification of strategies to respond to violence against children at the ecological level.

National Perspective on Violence Against Children

In consonance with the global definition, the Uganda Children (Amendment) Act (2016) defines violence as "any form of physical, emotional or mental injury or abuse, neglect, maltreatment and exploitation, including sexual abuse, intentional use of physical force or power, threatened or actual, against an individual which may result in or has a high likelihood of resulting in injury, death, psychological harm, mal-development or deprivation".

Article 19 of the UNCRC stipulates the state's responsibility to protect children from all forms of violence (The United Nations, 1989). This therefore mandates signatory states to put in place a legal and policy framework that ensures safety and protection of children from violence and institutions that oversee it. The UN Committee on the Rights of the Child General Comment[1] 135 provides guidance on the implementation of Article 19. It recognizes the family as the first unit or system of child protection. The General Comment stipulates that violence prevention measures should support parents and caregivers to understand, embrace and implement good child-rearing, based on the knowledge of child rights, child development and techniques for positive discipline in order to support families' capacity to provide children with care in a safe environment.

Twenty-five years after the adoption of the UNCRC, Uganda did not have reliable national data on the prevalence of violence against children. Incidents of various forms of violence were reported in the media, but this did not provide a clear understanding of the magnitude of the problem. The limited data available was from studies conducted by NGOs and was largely thematic, geographically limited in scope and sometimes methodologically questionable (Walakira & Ddumba, 2012). The lack of valid statistics created a lacuna for a trend analysis of violence against children over 30 years. In 2015 however, the Uganda Government conducted the first ever nationally representative quantitative survey on VAC. As shown in Fig. 2, the National Violence Against Children Survey (NVACS) established that over 75% of Ugandan children had experienced violence; almost six in every ten boys and four in every ten girls aged 13–17 years had experienced physical violence in the reference period (Ministry of Gender, Labour and Social Development, 2015). Approximately one in every five boys and girls aged 13–17 years reported that they experienced emotional violence in the same period and about one-quarter of girls and one-tenth of boys had experienced sexual violence in the year preceding the survey (Ministry of Gender, Labour and Social Development, 2015).

The NVACS did not cover certain specific contexts, such as children in refugee settings, children out of the household including street-connected children as well as children living in residential care institutions. As with other national VAC studies, the target was older children (13–24 years of age). To provide more insights into the other contexts, the AfriChild Centre conducted qualitative studies alongside the NVACS on children 0–8 years in the household, street-connected children and children in residential care institutions exploring risk and protective factors for violence against children in these contexts. These studies revealed that children in

---

[1] A General Comment is a treaty body's interpretation of human rights treaty provisions, thematic issues or its methods of work. General comments often seek to clarify the reporting of state parties with respect to certain provisions and suggest approaches to implementing treaty provisions.

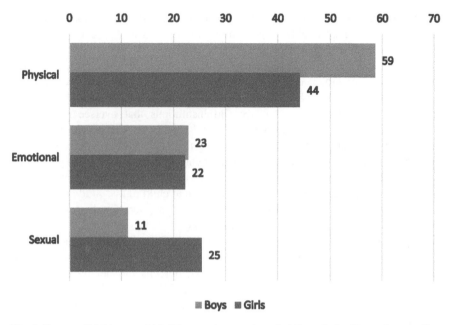

Fig. 2 Percent of children aged 13–17 years who experienced violence in the 12 months preceding the survey, by type of violence. Source: National Violence Against Children Survey (2015)

all contexts continue to experience different forms of violence. It is clear that with this snapshot on the situation of VAC in Uganda, there is still much work to be done to make the country safer for children.

Types of Violence

Violence against children in Uganda manifests itself in diverse forms including but not limited to sexual abuse, corporal punishment, burning, cutting, verbal abuse and child sacrifice. NVACS categorized all maltreatment against children in three major types, namely sexual, physical and emotional violence (Ministry of Gender, Labour and Social Development, 2015).

Violence against children is considered a major human rights violation and public health problem as all three forms of violence have the potential to cause significant short- and long-term health consequences for children. These include injury, sexual and reproductive health problems, unintended pregnancy, increased risk of human immunodeficiency virus (HIV), mental health issues, alcohol and drug abuse, social ostracization and increased incidence of chronic diseases in adulthood (Ministry of Gender, Labour and Social Development, 2015). Those who have experienced childhood violence are more likely to engage in risky behaviours as adolescents and adults, and may be more likely to become perpetrators of violence themselves.

Sexual Violence Against Children

Sexual violence is defined as all forms of sexual abuse and exploitation of children, and encompasses a wide range of acts including attempted and completed non-consensual sex acts, abusive sexual contact and exploitative use of children from sex (Ministry of Gender, Labour and Social Development, 2015). The NVACS explored prevalence of sexual violence along those categories.

Prevalence of sexual violence against children in Uganda is comparable to that of other countries that have conducted NVACS. A comparison of Uganda's prevalence statistics on sexual violence against children with those of other countries that conducted NVACS (Sumner et al., 2015) shows that Uganda has a high level of prevalence of sexual violence against children. Girls are more predisposed to sexual violence compared to boys. Thirty-five percent of girls and 17% of boys reported experiencing sexual violence during their childhoods.

Twenty-five percent of girls and 11% of boys among the children aged 13–17 years reported sexual violence in the year preceding the study (Ministry of Gender, Labour and Social Development, 2015). Neighbours, strangers, relatives, intimate friends, boyfriends and classmates, among others, were cited as the common perpetrators of VAC among boys and girls. Among children with disabilities, girls are more prone to sexual violence as a result of their disabilities (Ministry of Gender, Labour and Social Development and UNICEF Uganda, 2015).

Until recently, much of the research in sub-Saharan Africa has considered boys mainly as perpetrators but not victims (Miller et al., 2018; Adjei & Saewyc, 2017). However, recent studies identify gender as an associated factor for sexual violence (Adjei & Saewyc, 2017). Boys are increasingly experiencing sexual violence although at a lower scale, compared to girls. The parental presence and orphan status of a child are also associated with sexual violence among children (Kidman & Palermo, 2016). The National Violence Against Children Survey reveals that of the 18- to 24-year-old Ugandans that were interviewed, 17% of the boys reported experiencing sexual violence during their childhoods while 11% of the boys aged 13–17 years reported sexual violence in the past year (Ministry of Gender, Labour and Social Development, 2015).

Prior to the NVACS, the annual crime reports produced by the Uganda Police Force provided proxy indicators of the prevalence of child sexual abuse. Over the last 3 years, there have been shifts in the number of child sexual abuse cases that are registered by the police nationwide. In 2019, 13,613 cases were reported compared to 15,366 cases in 2018, indicating a decrease of 11.4%. In 2017, the number of cases reported by policy was 14,985 indicating 2.5% increase (Uganda Police Force, 2019).

Research evidence suggests that sexual violence against children in Uganda is rife within the school setting. A study by the Education Local Expertise Centre Uganda found that seven out of ten pupils in primary schools have ever been sexually abused. The abuse was perpetrated by a male teacher (67%), fellow children (22%), female teachers (5%) and non-teaching staff (6%). In this study, 60% of children who have experienced sexual violence in schools did not report the abuse to any authority (Education Local Expertise Centre Uganda, 2017). When children experience sexual violence, very often they are not able to report to any authorities. Within school settings, children with disability are particularly vulnerable to the risk of sexual violence (Devries et al., 2014).

There are significant associations between sexual violence and behavioral health outcomes for the affected children. Children who experience sexual violence are at risk of post-traumatic stress disorder (Amone P'Olak et al., 2018) and report higher levels of mental distress and suicidal ideation compared to their age mates. They are also more likely to get drunk, smoke, use drugs or intentionally hurt someone else. These children are also more likely to report symptoms of sexually transmitted infections. While mental distress is a universal outcome for both girls and boys who experience sexual violence, it is most likely to be reported by boys. Prevalence of mental distress was higher among boys who reported sexual violence across the different age groups (Ministry of Gender, Labour and Social Development, 2015).

Child Marriage

Child marriage is a harmful traditional practice that is linked to sexual violence against children in Uganda (Ministry of Gender, Labour and Social Development, 2015). The age of sexual consent and marriage in Uganda is legally set at 18 years (Penal Code Act, 2007: Africa Child Policy Forum, 2013). By implication, no person below the age of 18 is expected to be married. More than 10 years ago, Uganda was ranked in ninth place on the list of hotspot countries for child marriage, with 54% of women being married before the age of 18 (Jain & Kurz, 2007). More recent statistics reveal that at least 8.2% of girls aged 13–17 years have ever been married or living as if they are married compared to 1.4% of the boys in the same age group (Ministry of Gender, Labour and Social Development, 2015).

Uganda has over the last 20 years generated information on child marriage through the Demographic and Health Surveys that show a declining trend in early marriage, among females who get married before the age of 15 and 18 years. In 2016, 34% of women aged 20–24 years had gotten married before age 18 and 7% before the age of 15. A summary of evidence in Table 1 shows that the percentage of women aged 20–24 years married before age 15 declined from 9.9% in 2011/2012 to 7% in 2016, while those married before age 18 declined by about 6 percentage points from 39.7% in 2011/2012 to 34% in 2016. However, among the married adolescents, 15–19-year-olds who are married or in union, the percentage remained stagnant at about 20% over the last 10 years.

Child marriage is a widely acceptable norm in many cultures across Uganda. Customary practices are prevalent and take precedence over the legal provisions regarding marriage (Reisen, 2017). The laws banning child marriage are poorly enforced allowing social norms that allow marriages to occur on the onset of puberty to prevail (Diesch & Ntenga, 2016). The drivers of child marriage are deeply rooted

Table 1 Prevalence of child marriage (2000–2015)

	2000/ 2001	2005/ 2006	2011/ 2012	2015/ 2016
Percentage of women aged 20–24 years married before age of 15	15.2	12.3	9.9	7
Percentage of women aged 20–24 years married before age 18	53.9	46.3	39.7	34
Percentage of adolescents (15–19 years old) married or in union	28.9	19.6	20.0	19.9

Source: Uganda Demographic and Health Surveys 2000/2001, 2005/2006, 2011/2012, 2015/2016

in inadequate access to education, poverty and gender and sociocultural norms (Wamimbi, 2018). Child marriage constitutes a gross form of social injustice against children that encumbers their rights to education. Once they marry, children drop out of school, and acquire adult responsibilities.

The introduction of Universal Primary Education in 1997 resulted in increased opportunities for the education of girls (Nishimura et al., 2008). Despite this, negative attitudes towards girls' education still persist. Gender disparities in education in Uganda remain significant and difficult to chance, despite the modest progress resulting from the abolition of school fee payments. Only one out of every four girls is likely to complete the lower secondary educational cycle. Poor families prefer to invest in the education of boys; investment of meagre family resources in a girl's schooling is thought to be a waste, as the latter will eventually get married, and be of little benefit to the family. This is in contrast to the boy children who carry on the family heritage (Wodon et al., 2016). Girls who do not attain higher education are at a greater risk of child marriage and early pregnancy. There is a close linkage between child marriage, associated teenage pregnancy and low education attainment (Wamimbi, 2018). Child marriage is one of the key reasons that lead girls to drop out of school or even to not enrol in secondary school in the first place (Wodon et al., 2016). The proportion of teenagers who start childbearing decreases with increasing levels of education. For example, among girls between the ages of 15 to 19 years, 35% of those with no education had begun childbearing compared to 11% of those who had post-primary education (Uganda Bureau of Statistics, 2016).

Besides the perception that investment in girls' education is a burden, poor families consider their daughters as an asset that can be exchanged for economic benefit. In some communities, marrying girls off early has the potential of generating social and financial benefits for the family. Girls therefore are sometimes viewed as assets which can be exchanged to support families (Wamimbi, 2018). For example, among the Karamojong—one of the poorest communities in Uganda—girls are culturally seen as a source of potential wealth for the household (Wodon et al., 2016). Parents pay little attention to the education of the female children, and prefer to marry them off.

Child marriage in Uganda is associated with poor health outcomes including increased risk for HIV infection, low nutrition status and high maternal mortality

(Rubin et al., 2009). Married women aged 15–24 years are five times more likely to have HIV/AIDS than those who are not married (Ministry of Health and ORC Macro, 2005). Child marriage is closely linked to teenage pregnancies since the young brides are expected to get pregnant soon after they are married (MGLSD 2011). Women who marry early are likely to experience pregnancy complications that lead to death or disability, obstructed labour and obstetric fistula (Bantebya et al., 2014). Adolescent mothers in Uganda are twice as likely to die from pregnancy and delivery complications compared to those who are older, and their babies or children have higher chances of dying (Sekiwunga & Whyte, 2009). Child marriage also impacts the health of children born to young mothers. An analysis on the intergenerational effects of child marriage found that children born to women who marry before age 18 years are at a greater risk of being developmentally off-track and being stunted compared to those whose mothers married later (Efevbera et al., 2017).

Women who marry young are more vulnerable to gender-based violence. The Uganda Demographic and Health Survey (UDHS) 2006 and 2011 indicates a slightly higher proportion of ever-married women who married before the age of 18 years who had ever experienced physical violence since age 15 years compared to those who married at age 18 or older (UBOS & Macro International Inc., 2007; UBOS & ICF, 2012). Girls who marry while young have limited opportunities for decision-making in their households, surrendering their right to their husbands and in-laws. As a consequence, these girls have weaker control over household resources their time, and have more restricted access to information and health services (Parsons et al., 2015). An analysis of UDHS data reveals that women who married before the age of 14 years were less likely to make decisions in their households compared to those who married at the age of 15 or older (Rubin et al., 2009).

Research from elsewhere has shown that children who find themselves entrapped in marriage may suffer from stress and other mental health difficulties (Malak et al., 2020; Parsons et al., 2015; Gage, 2013). In Uganda, the national strategy to end child pregnancy and early marriage recognizes the impact on psychological well-being. It is recognized that girls who marry young enter into informal unions which deny them basic protection and social status leading to isolation and limited access to support structures (Bantebya et al., 2014). However, there is limited research on the mental health consequences of child marriage.

Physical Violence

Physical violence in Uganda is defined by the Ministry of Gender, Labour and Social Development (2015) as the intentional use of physical force, with the potential to cause death, disability, injury or harm. It includes acts such as punching, kicking, whipping, beating with an object, strangulation, suffocation, attempted drowning, burning, and using or threatening with a knife, gun or other weapons. The boys in Uganda are at a higher risk of physical violence compared to girls. According to the

Uganda NVACS (Ministry of Gender, Labour and Social Development, 2015), 59% of girls and 68% of boys aged 18–24 years reported experiencing physical violence during their childhood. Among the younger adolescents aged 13–17 years, 44% of girls and 59% of boys experienced physical violence in the year preceding the study. The reported perpetrators include teachers, parents, other adults in the community and fellow children. Physical violence in Uganda is widely practiced and is considered a normal practice, and an effective tool for enforcing discipline among children to help shape responsible behaviour (Boydell et al., 2017). As a result, caregivers, including parents and teachers, openly embrace physical punishments (Nyakito & Allida, 2018). Children also condone the practice, believing it to be positive for their future welfare (Mulinga, 2012).

Most of the physical violence against children is perpetrated by parents and caregivers. Among the older adolescents, 45% of girls (45.3%) and 49% of boys (48.5%) reported experiencing physical violence by a parent or caregiver (Ministry of Gender, Labour and Social Development, 2015).

Physical Violence in Family and Community Settings

Many parents in Uganda have life experiences that are impacted by violence, from their families, homes and communities. Previous experiences of armed conflict in the different central, western and northern Uganda regions unleashed unprecedented violence in the population. Within the population in northern Uganda for example, research evidence shows that exposure to violence that was characteristic of the 20-year armed conflict that parents were embroiled in as children contributed to their violent tendencies. Violence is therefore intergenerational, as parents who were exposed to traumatic and violent acts perpetrate the same among their children (Saile et al., 2014; Kinyanda et al., 2013).

Evidence indicates that violence meted by parents is sustained by three motivating factors including (1) the need to ensure good behaviour and maintain respectability; (2) establishing household routines and managing resources; and (3) impacting knowledge to empower children and protect them from potential health risks (Boydell et al., 2017). While parents seem to endorse physical violence, they also acknowledge that it can be counterproductive (ibid.).

Physical Violence in School Settings

Violence happens not only in the home but also in schools where physical violence is meted out by teachers, non-teaching staff as well as fellow children. Although physical violence in schools was suspended in 1997 and subsequently banned by the Uganda education ministry in 2006 (Naker & Sekitoleko, 2009), the use of corporal punishment still thrives in some schools in a bid to enforce learning and aid children to attain better grades (Devries et al., 2014; Naker & Sekitoleko, 2009), despite evidence elsewhere that casts doubt on the efficacy of physical punishment in promoting academic performance (Haji & Bali Theodora, 2013). Many teachers, caregivers as well as children view it as a normal and positive practice of child upbringing. As a result, violent disciplinary measures are not necessarily viewed as a violation of children's rights (Gwirayi, 2011).

According to the Ministry of Education and Sports (2015), corporal punishment in schools was at 74.3% for children in government schools and 75.6% for children in private schools. An earlier survey found that 81% of school children experienced physical punishment in school, with 90% reporting that it occurs weekly (ANPPCAN, 2011). Physical violence in schools comes in the form of corporal punishment, harsh physical punishment and bullying.

Despite the justification for the use of physical punishment in school, it has negative consequences for affected children. It destabilizes children, contributes to absenteeism from school (Komakech and Osuu, 2014) and prevents them from completing their school (Komakech and Osuu, 2014; Tukundane et al., 2014). Violence that occurs in the school setting is associated with physical injuries (Devries et al., 2014; Gwirayi, 2011), as well as aggressive and antisocial behaviour. Evidence shows that violence in schools has negative effects including contribution to high attrition rate, poor academic performance and increased school dropout rates and absenteeism (Devries et al., 2014; Ministry of Gender, Labour and Social Development and UNICEF Uganda, 2015).

Emotional Violence

Emotional violence is a pattern of verbal behaviour over time or an isolated incident that is not developmentally appropriate and supportive and that has a high probability of damaging a child's mental health and their mental, spiritual, moral or social development (Ministry of Gender, Labour and Social Development, 2015). Prevalence of emotional abuse is higher among older young people. Emotional violence in Uganda is widely normalized and not recognized as a violation of children's rights in the Ugandan society (Ministry of Gender, Labour and Social Development, 2015). At the heart of most of the emotional abuse experienced by children in Uganda is the cultural expectation of unquestioned submission and obedience to older persons at all times. It is not surprising that most of the emotional violence is perpetrated by parents and other persons charged with responsibility over children.

The National Violence Against Children Survey provides statistics on the prevalence of emotional violence among children in Uganda. Among the 18- to 24-year-olds, one in three reports experiencing emotional violence during their childhood, compared to more than one in five reported among children in the 13- to 17-year-old age group. Thirty-four percent of girls and 36% of boys experienced emotional violence before the age of 18; for the majority of these children (82% girls and 72% boys), emotional violence constituted multiple incidents. More than half of these children reported that the first incident of emotional violence occurred between the ages of 12 and 17 years, an indication that as children experience the turbulent stage of adolescence, they are likely to experience heightened emotional violence from their caretakers. During this stage, children ideally need to receive emotional support from significant others, to help them navigate through. Most of the emotional violence against children occurred in their households and was perpetrated by caretakers including mothers, stepmothers, aunts and uncles as well as fathers (Ministry of Gender, Labour and Social Development, 2015).

Among the younger children in the 13- to 17-year-old age group, the reported prevalence of emotional violence was lower at 22% for both girls and boys. However, similar to the older age group, most of the emotional violence was characterized by multiple incidents, commenced between 12 and 17 years of age, perpetrated by caregivers in the same environment and was characterized by multiple incidents of emotional violence.

Qualitative research in Uganda highlights the nature of emotional violence that is prevalent among street-connected children and those who are separated from their families and live in residential care institutions and streets. Street-connected children experience emotional violence, comprised of verbal abuse, humiliation, stigmatization, social rejection, neglect and being forced to engage in traumatic activities (AfriChild, 2017). Children in Ugandan residential care institutions experience emotional violence from both their caregivers and peers. Mugumya et al. (2017) provide a description of the forms of emotional violence that occur within this context. Caregivers routinely taunt children by reminding them about the circumstances that led them to the institutions. The sad circumstances that separate children who are residents in care institutions are used by caregivers against the children. Children are reminded that they are orphans or come from poor backgrounds. Infractions and mistakes committed by children are punished by incessant reminders about their luck in finding alternative caretaking arrangements in the institutions. Children reported that they are constantly verbally abused and refer to using derogatory words. In addition to this, caregivers are also partial, treating some children in their care differently from others. Some of the hard punishments given to children constituted emotional violence. These included detention for long hours in cramped places, and denial of privileges such as time to play and entertainment.

The credentials of care staff in residential care institutions are reported to be lacking (Mugumya et al., 2017). Most of the staff recruited to directly provide nurturing support to children lack the requisite professional training and skills. This in part, combined with the lack of enforcement of standards, could be the cause of caregiver emotional violence in this context.

The qualitative research in residential care institutions shows that there is a pecking order for emotional violence. A hierarchy of seniority is formed in alignment to the ages of children as they model the behaviour of caretakers. The older children mete abuse to younger ones. Older children were reported to use vulgar language against those younger than them. Gender-based emotional violence was also reported where the boys use body shaming and make fun of the changing physical features of the girls' bodies.

Children reported that these experiences make them sad, are humiliating and make them cry, angry and wish they had other options (Mugumya et al., 2017). Reminders about the circumstances that brought children into residential care institutions make them feel insecure about their places in the institutions. Some of the children reported that they have harboured thoughts of escaping from residential care institutions to take refuge on the streets, believing that it would be a better alternative to enduring the emotional violence by their caregivers. Emotional abuse against children in residential care institutions instils perpetual fear and hinders attachment and development of appropriate relationships with caregivers. Some children reported that they had developed notions of revenge and secretly thought of causing harm to their caregivers in retaliation (Mugumya et al., 2017).

Violence Against Children in Specific Contexts/Environment

While children in all contexts are at risk of violence and associated behavioral outcomes, this section presents the vulnerabilities of children with specific characteristics and those who live in contexts that have the potential of heightening their risks. These include children in residential care institutions, street-connected children, those in contact with the law, children in post-conflict settings and children impacted by HIV/AIDS.

Childcare Institutions

Children in residential care institutions experience different types of violence including exploitative child labour, physical violence, emotional violence as well as sexual violence (AfriChild, 2017). Children in residential care institutions are the most vulnerable, and cannot be supported by their families. While some of these children are orphans, others have parents who are unable or unwilling to take care of them. Children in residential care institutions are subjected to exploitative labour and are assigned tasks that are potentially detrimental to their physical, educational, health and general well-being. The evidence from the narratives of children revealed that younger girls were more likely to be affected. They were often given heavy work, subjected to long hours of work without a break and under the sun and beaten for not working as desired by the caregivers or denied food. Sexual violence was found to exist within the residential care institutions as a form of violence against children with or sometimes without the knowledge of the managers (AfriChild & Webale, 2017).

The narratives of children and key informants indicated that caretakers and fellow children are the main perpetrators and that sometimes abuse cases go unreported. The possibility of girl children being sexually exploited/abused is higher than that of boys. Children noted that caretakers use sticks and pipes when beating them, while others spank, pinch and kick them whenever they make mistakes, big or small (AfriChild, 2017). Not only do they beat them, but they also shout and verbally abuse them, pull their ears, step on them and push them violently or threaten them.

As a consequence, from the beating and threats, some children begin to think about escaping the institutions and others actually run away from the institutions. This presents a paradox in that these institutions where children are supposed to find safety end up exposing them to more violence. The abuse that exists in residential care institutions points to maladministration and lack of supervision by mandated state agencies.

Street-Connected Children

Children outside of family care including child domestic workers opened a window on their worlds of adversity including the forms of violence within the household that pushed them to the street. They also shared their experiences of violence in the streets or in their contexts of domestic work (AfriChild, 2017). Physical violence was documented as one of the most common forms of violence against children both inside and outside of their households. Police and other law enforcement authorities were described by the children as major perpetrators of violence against them in the streets. Incidents of physical violence permeate all aspects of their daily lives and contexts, many times pushing them to the streets and to other exploitative, violent contexts. Psychological violence was documented as the second most prevalent form of violence faced by children outside family care while sexual violence also featured prominently (AfriChild, 2017).

Violence is thus seen as a vicious cycle for many of the street-connected children. These children leave their families due to various hardships that include violence, neglect and poverty. The escape to the streets does not necessarily offer respite, as street life is characterized by deprivation and violence from other street children and state authorities (Dwyer, 2016). Many of the children on the street escape from violence, war, socioeconomic collapse, death of a parent and natural disaster, and end up on the street with little assistance and limited social support, which forces them to resort to scavenging, begging and sleeping in the polluted slums (Dwyer, 2016).

The UNICEF (2015) situation analysis notes that in towns and cities, homeless children (children living on the street) encounter violence from members of the public, urban authorities and sometimes the police, other homeless adults, local government officials and their homeless peers. Walakira and Ddumba (2012) also confirm this by adding that violence among Ugandan street-connected children is endemic, perpetuated by both street-connected children against each other and adults (Walakira et al., 2014). Both male and female children suffer outright abuse from police, from occasional strangers and from each other with boys more frequently physically abused while girls more frequently abused emotionally and sexually.

Children in Contact with the Law

The ever-changing social economic context in Uganda has undoubtedly exposed children to higher levels of vulnerability that many times lead them to conditions that bring them into contact with the law. Children come into contact with the law as either victims of crime, children in need of care and protection, child witnesses or offenders. The type of offenses most children commit as reported in the NVAC survey 2015 and administrative statistics point to general livelihood challenges as well as behavioral problems of adolescent boys. Many child offenders are affected by poverty, and commit minor crimes in a bid to meet their sustenance. The poorly resourced justice system does not provide for assessment to determine the unique circumstances of every individual child, and respond appropriately through social welfare interventions. Some of these children are raised in broken families, that are characterized by economic challenges and dysfunctional social support systems. These cause children to come into contact with the justice system, thereby exposing them to further experiences of violence. Children often find themselves with no support system for counselling or career guidance which explains why many children left school for an alternative way of life.

HIV-Affected Children

Although Uganda has been successful in reducing the prevalence of HIV/AIDS from 18% in the 1990s to the current 5.7% (UAC, 2015), it remains a social, health and economic burden. HIV/AIDS impacts children and their families in Uganda. Children below the age of 15 years account for 11% of the 1.6 million Ugandans living with HIV (UNAIDS, 2017).

Factors at the individual, interactional, community and societal levels heighten risks for HIV infection among adolescents. Young people in Uganda have less than desirable knowledge about HIV. For example, in 2014, only 39% of young women and men aged 15–24 years could correctly identify ways of preventing the sexual transmission of HIV (UNAIDS, 2017). At the personal level, adolescent girls are more vulnerable to HIV infection because their reproductive systems are not fully developed. It is estimated that HIV prevalence is almost four times higher among young women aged 15–24 years than young men of the same age (WHO, 2017) and two-thirds of all new HIV infections in Uganda are found among adolescent girls (UNAIDS, 2017). Adolescent girls in Uganda are more predisposed to gender-based violence including sexual violence and exploitation. This violence is closely associated with HIV infection. Young women who have experienced intimate partner violence are twice more likely to have acquired HIV than women who had not experienced violence (Uganda Aids Commission, 2015). Gender inequality and patriarchal norms also make it difficult for girls and young women to negotiate safe sex. Transactional sex reported by adolescent girls is 24% and cross-generational sex among sexually active adolescent girls in the 10- to 14-year-old age group is 60% (UBOS & ICF, 2018).

With the increased availability of antiretroviral treatment (ART), HIV is no longer a death sentence in Uganda, and those who are infected have the opportunity to access therapy and live productively. Despite this, adolescents grapple with the burden of medication. Although antiretroviral therapy is widely available, statistics show that only 66% of children under 14 years of age are on therapy. More than one-third do not take medication. Sustaining treatment is difficult for young people in the 15- to 19-year-old age group and many of them drop out of care. Studies suggest that stigma, discrimination and disclosure issues, as well as travel and waiting times at clinics, are among the reasons for treatment attrition (Nabukeera-Barungi et al., 2015).

The death of one or both parents due to AIDS led to a phenomenal orphan problem in the country. At the peak of the HIV epidemic in the late 1990s and early 2000s, it was estimated that there were close to 1.5 million orphans and vulnerable children mainly as a result of HIV/AIDS (Barton & Wamai, 1994; Nyakuni, 1996; UNICEF, 2005; The Republic of Uganda. MInistry of Gender, Labour and Social Development, 2004). Previously catered for by the extended families in the face of weak and absent formal foster alternatives, the burgeoning numbers of orphans soon became unmanageable, resulting in a phenomenon of child-headed families. At one time the number of child-headed households was over 32,130 (ChildFund International, 2018). Children in child-headed families experienced psychological effects and reported high levels of anxiety resulting from the compounded insecurity of the absence of adult caregivers (Satzinger et al., 2012).

HIV/AIDS in Uganda carries stigma and children who are affected are subjected to bullying. They also experience a range of mental health difficulties including depression and suicide ideation (Ashaba et al., 2018). Caregivers of HIV-affected children may, however, not be able to identify and recognize symptoms of mental disorder (Nalukenge et al., 2019). This implies that children may not access the requisite support from their caregivers.

Children in the Post-conflict Context

In the period between 1988 and 2007, children living in parts of northern Uganda were victims of armed conflict, and were subjected to various violations including abductions, conscription into armed forces, forced marriages and sexual slavery, and internal displacement. The effects of these experiences continue to impact the well-being of population in the region. The prevalence of post-traumatic stress disorder (PTSD) in war-affected districts of northern Uganda is 12% resulting from exposure to war trauma events, childhood trauma, negative life events, negative coping style and food insecurity (Mugisha et al., 2015).

Children in post-conflict northern Uganda have been reported to have a high prevalence of childhood depressive disorders (Kinyanda et al., 2013), and exposure to war trauma is a predictor of anxiety (Abbo et al., 2013). In this context, the quality of relationships that children had with their caregivers is associated with their mental health. Complex structural factors including poverty and deprivation, stigma, neglect and abuse interact to cause emotional distress for children affected by conflict (Akello et al., 2010). Despite the extreme suffering experienced, children did not openly share their emotional distress and if they do, they risk being met with negative reactions characterized by indignation, condemnation, irritation, disregard and downplaying the significance of their distress. The reactions from others in the social context silence children and hinder them from expressing their distress. Children however share their emotions in spaces where they feel safe.

Risk Factors Associated with Violence Towards Children

Risk factors associated with violence against children can be identified at different socioecological levels. At the level of the individual gender, age and orphanhood status are risk factors (Natukunda et al., 2019). The gender of an individual child is associated with a higher risk to specific forms of violation. Specifically, being a female is a risk factor for sexual violence, while being a male is associated with physical violence. This assertion is consistent with the prevalence of different forms of violation among children of different genders. National statistics of child sexual violence indicate a prevalence of 25% among the females and 11% among the males in the younger age group of 13–17 years. These differences persist among the older adolescents where 35% of females report experiencing sexual violence compared to 17% of males (Ministry of Gender, Labour and Social Development, 2015). Gender as a risk factor for sexual abuse has been variously confirmed by different studies in Uganda (Ninsiima et al., 2020; Natukunda et al., 2019; Muhanguzi, 2011). Statistics on physical violence suggest that boys are more at risk. Among the younger age group of 13–17 years, 59% of boys compared to 44% of girls reported experiencing physical violence. The same trend is observed in the older age group of 18–24 years where 68% of boys compared to 59% of girls reported physical violence. Scholars in Uganda suggest that the gender differences in sexual violence against children are a result of patriarchal community values that hinder boys from opening up regarding sexual abuse (Natukunda et al., 2019). Fear of embarrassment for self and/or family as the most cited reason for service non-use among adolescents reporting past-year sexual abuse in the NVACS was more common among boys (36%) than girls (14%).

The age of the child is also a risk factor for specific forms of violence. Older children and adolescents are more likely to experience all the forms of violence compared to the younger ones.

The parent status of a child (parents alive or dead) has also been found to be associated with violence against children, particularly physical violence and polyvictimization (Natukunda et al., 2019). Orphanhood in Uganda is widely accepted as being closely associated with vulnerability of a child. The orphanhood construct has shaped public policy and practice with interventions being specifically designed for children without parents. This notion, although widely spread, is not universally accepted. There is a school of thought that argues that orphanhood per se is not a risk factor for violation, but rather the quality of caregiver and child relationship. Nonetheless, many orphans in Uganda are subjected to differential treatment by their caregivers that could potentially lead to violation.

Risk Factors at the Caregiver Level

Factors at caregiver level are also responsible for the promotion and prevention of violence against children. Risk factors for physical and emotional violence are prevalent among caregivers who embrace values that are accepting of harsh disciplinary practices (Natukunda et al., 2019). Caregivers who embrace harsh punishment also espouse specific social norms that sustain this behaviour. These norms include the belief that physical violence leads to greater respect for teachers and parents by children, that it is an effective tool for imparting discipline and positive behaviour and that it contributes to improvement in school performance (AfriChild, 2018).

Inadequate monitoring and supervision of children by caregivers are also risk factors for multiple violations against children (Natukunda et al., 2019). Children who are not adequately monitored and supervised by their caregivers were at a higher risk of experiencing multiple forms of abuse. Children who are poorly supervised lack adequate protection and are exposed to inappropriate content in the media (AfriChild, 2018). Moreover, inadequately supervised adolescents may engage in bad behaviour which may lead to harsher disciplining. Other negative parenting practices that increase children's risk to violence are wilful neglect including lack of concern for a child's future, lack of protection, care, neglect of health and poor nutrition and corporal punishment (AfriChild Centre, 2015a, 2015b).

Community Level

A critical factor for violence perpetration is the social norms at the macro level that continually provide a conducive environment for violence to thrive. There is a set of negative social norms that significantly perpetuate and sustain child marriage and sexual and physical violence among children in schools, families and communities with far-reaching consequences on child well-being (AfriChild Centre, 2018). Girls are most likely affected by social norms attributed to child marriage and sexual harassment. These social norms include pressure from society to attain social recognition through acquisition of material possessions that can only be available through sexual transactions, expectation to repay for gifts given by boys and men through sex, tolerance and protection of perpetrators by the community, equating of sexual readiness to physical features (Bantebya et al., 2014; AfriChild, 2018) and acceptance of premarital relationships and sex (Samara, 2010).

All is not gloom, however, with social norms as there are positive sets of social norms that have the potential to enhance prevention of VAC efforts. These include respect of a girl's virginity, respect for girl education and an acknowledgement that it is an avenue for socio-economic transformation. Social norms were found to be driven by deeply rooted values of protection, honour and pride, and reinforced mainly by household economic status, especially for child marriage and sexual harassment. Social norms did not operate in isolation in perpetuating and sustaining violence against children. Along with them were other factors found interacting with social norms to drive violence against children. The other drivers included social factors for example religious ideology and inadequate parenting skills and practices, economic factors, and alcohol and drug abuse.

There has been some positive change in social norms, from harmful ones to protective ones. New social norms are being created and built. For example, increasingly the social norm that child marriage is prestigious is shifting to a new one that marrying off children is shameful. The socio-economic factor underlying child marriage is gradually changing from marrying off a child to receive a dowry to investing in a child's education to secure a better economic future (AfriChild Centre, 2018). The change in social norms has been largely driven by factors including education, mass sensitization on children's rights, civil society advocacy efforts as well as institution and enforcement of child protection legal frameworks (ibid.)

Consequences of Violence Towards Children

Children subjected to violence experience mental distress and other health outcomes. They experience a range of negative behavioral, psychological and cognitive consequences that have the potential to persist over the life course, and influence their quality of life and subsequent parenting choices (Ministry of Gender, Labour and Social Development and UNICEF Uganda, 2015). The notion that in societies where violence is normalized as a tool for enforcing discipline there are no adverse consequences on the population is not supported by evidence in Uganda. Although exposure to the physical violence is the norm in Ugandan schools and families, it has an adverse impact on the mental health of children. Violence from peers and school staff in Uganda is associated with mental health difficulties among schoolgoing children (Clarke et al., 2016; Thumann et al., 2016; Devries et al., 2014). Violence that occurs in the family setting is also associated with mental health difficulties (Ssenyonga et al., 2019).

In the NVACS females and males of different age groups who suffered sexual abuse in childhood reported significantly higher prevalence of mental distress in the past 30 days compared to those who did not report sexual abuse. Among the younger girls, those who reported experiences of sexual abuse in the past 12 months were significantly more likely to report moderate mental distress in the past 30 days

(43.8%) compared to those without a sexual abuse experience (26.5%). More than half of the boys (54%) in the 13- to 17-year-old age group who experienced sexual abuse reported mental distress in the past 30 days, compared to 31% of those who did not experience recent sexual abuse. Among older female adolescents (18–24 years) who experienced sexual abuse in childhood, 20% experienced serious mental distress in the past 30 days compared with 6.8% of those who did not experience sexual abuse. Unwanted pregnancy is another consequence of sexual violence. Twenty-eight percent of females who experienced pressured or physically forced sex prior to age 18 became pregnant as a result. Among males, 50% of those who experienced sexual abuse in childhood experienced moderate mental distress in the past 30 days, compared to 39.1% who did not experience childhood sexual abuse. Overall mental distress, being drunk, smoking cigarettes or chewing tobacco, using substances in the past 30 days, intentional self-harm, contemplation of suicide and attempted suicide are the major mental health outcomes associated with violence against children.

Access to and Utilization of Services Especially Addressing Mental Health

Left unattended to, mental health difficulties that begin in childhood are likely to persist throughout adulthood, and impact individuals' ability to live to their full potential. Moreover, the UNCRC obligates government to ensure provision of appropriate and responsive services. Article 39 of the UNCRC states:

"State parties shall take all appropriate measures to promote physical and psychological recovery and social reintegration of a child victim of: any form of neglect, exploitation, or abuse ... Such recovery and reintegration shall take place in an environment which fosters the health, self-respect and dignity of the child" (United Nations Convention on the Rights of the Child, 1989).

The Uganda Government has made investments in strengthening the child mental health services within the primary healthcare system, through policy and legislation (Ministry of Health, 2010). Uganda's policy action to improve availability and access to mental health services is decentralization and integration within the public health sector (Wakida et al., 2018; Ssebunnya et al., 2018; Mugisha et al., 2016; Kigozi et al., 2010). Inpatient and outpatient mental health services are available in the national referral mental hospital and mental health units and 13 regional referral hospitals. Mental healthcare is also provided at all levels of service delivery, including the general hospitals and health facilities as a component of the minimum healthcare package. These efforts have however not been matched with the appropriate and necessary increased and improved service delivery. For example, the move to decentralize mental health services was not accompanied by centralization of resource allocation and this has a negative impact on the efficiency of service delivery (Ssebunnya et al., 2018).

There is a dearth of child mental health services in Uganda. While children account for 36% of clients who seek for consultation from mental health professionals, only the National Referral Mental Health Hospital has a specialized ward for children and adolescents (Kigozi et al., 2010). Children in Uganda comprise 56% of the total population under the age of 18 years, and 48.7% of these are under the age of 15 years (UBOS, 2016).

In response to child and adolescent mental health challenges in Uganda, the Ministry of Health developed the Child and Adolescent Mental Health (CAMH) to streamline service provision. The National Violence Against Children Survey that assessed the availability of services found that 92% and 65% of health facilities in Uganda provide psychosocial support and mental health screening, respectively, for child survivors of violence (Ministry of Gender, Labour and Social Development, 2019). However, the survey relied on health worker reports; it is not clear whether these services are effective in responding to the specific challenges that children experience. To date, there is no comprehensive assessment of the impact of these guidelines in improving access to and utilization of mental health services for children and adolescents.

Mental health service delivery is hindered by several bottlenecks including limited financial and human resources, inadequate medications and negative attitudes towards persons with mental health difficulties (Kisa et al., 2016).

Mental distress and difficulties in Uganda are poorly understood and largely associated with bad luck or witchcraft. The widely held belief that mental health problems are linked to witchcraft and the supernatural (Okello et al., 2006; Okello et al., 2007; Quinn, 2014) means that many children who need assistance may initially be taken to religious leaders or traditional healers for prayers and exorcism (Quinn, 2014). Conventional mental health services are believed to be beneficial but limited; they are thought to provide temporary respite by way of helping children with mental health difficulties to calm down (Quinn, 2014). The traditional and religious exorcism is seen as effective in dealing with the root cause of mental health difficulties (ibid.) Overall, many people in Uganda are unlikely to seek for mental health services, unless the severity of their condition is considered dire. Mental health-seeking behaviour is constrained by lack of money for transport, stigma (Quinn, 2014), delays due to fear of diagnosis and lack of trust in healthcare system and health workers. Overall, Uganda continues to grapple with the challenge of effective and efficient service delivery in response to violence against children (Ministry of Gender, Labour and Social Development, 2019).

Availability of Services to Respond to Violence Against Children

Children who experience violence receive a range of services to counter the undesirable deleterious consequences and support their recovery. Uganda's continuum of care for violence against children includes a range of services including (1) identification, reporting and referral of children in need; (2) investigation of violations against children; (3) response and support services to violated children (including

Table 2 Percent of probation offices that provide specific VAC response services (multiple response)

Service	Percent
Reintegration of the child survivor into their family or community or resettling	98.0
Investigating cases of abuse and violence against children	97.0
Preparing social inquiry reports about children at risk of harm	97.0
Preparing and directly accompanying survivors for legal proceedings (court)	96.0
Directly providing counselling or psychosocial support to survivors	95.1
Assisting child survivors to access counselling or psychosocial support	94.1
Assisting child survivors to access medical examination report	89.1
Assisting survivors to access legal aid services	88.1
Assisting child survivors to access relevant health services	83.2
Providing therapeutic feeding or food supplements to malnourished children (**If malnourished due to child neglect**)	16.0

Source: Uganda VAC Services Survey Report

counselling, psychosocial support, health, legal aid, educational support and family reintegration for children living outside their families); and (4) documentation, monitoring and follow-up (Ministry of Gender, Labour and Social Development, 2015).

Uganda has made significant progress in providing specific services for children faced with violence. Probation offices offer a range of services in response to violence against children (Ministry of Gender, Labour and Social Development, 2019). The range of services that are provided by probation officers is summarized in Table 2.

Table 2 shows the services that are available in district probation offices. While probation officers offer psychosocial support and counselling services to children, the setting in which these services are provided presents constraints that have the potential to undermine the effectiveness of their efforts. There are inadequate facilities to create a conducive environment in which counselling can happen. Only 40% of probation officers reported that they have a counselling room (Ministry of Gender, Labour and Social Development, 2019). Moreover, these probation officers are not easily accessible to children, as they lack adequate resources to traverse the communities where children live. Children who are likely to access probation services are those who somehow manage to travel to the administrative headquarters where offices are set up. Despite the goodwill of probation officers, the reality is that this office is poorly resourced and underfunded. Probation officers cover a wide jurisdiction, which makes it difficult for them to reach every child that needs services. Offices are usually located at the district headquarters, meaning that children who need services have to incur transport costs. The VAC services survey revealed that on average the district probation office is allocated UGX 7,785,903 (approximately USD 2180) annually. Only about 60% of the allocation is released. With this low level of funding, it is difficult for probation officers to effectively provide services to children.

Survivor support services are extremely limited and uncoordinated. Services are defragmented, and Uganda lacks one-stop service centres for abused children (Ministry of Gender, Labour and Social Development, 2015). As a result, children seeking services are required to visit multiple service providers at different locations. The unavailability of one-stop service centres for children who experience violence means that they need to be referred to various service points. This notwithstanding, there is no clearly defined referral pathway or universal case management framework for abused children. The actions taken in handling the child abuse cases generally depend on the range of accessible services available within the community and the level of awareness of the person seeking the service or handling the case (Ministry of Gender, Labour and Social Development, 2015).

In Uganda, there are limited opportunities for screening for violence against children in schools, hospitals and communities. As a consequence, there is limited referral, with the exception of incidents where an affected child and their caregiver (s) voluntarily seek services. Most service delivery points rely on client walk-in to enrol survivors into services (Ministry of Gender, Labour and Social Development, 2019). The challenge to client walk-in is the low service-seeking behaviour of survivors of violence as reported in the NVAC survey 2015, where many children who experienced abuse did not know of a place to report; many of those who knew did not report the abuse due to minimization of the abuse incident, and fear of repercussions (Ministry of Gender, Labour and Social Development, 2015).

To ensure availability of data for service provision and decision-making, Uganda has introduced multiple information systems including the Orphans and Other Vulnerable Children Management Information System (OVCMIS), the Gender-Based Violence Information Management System (GBVIMS) and the Health Management Information System (HMIS). However, there is lack of evidence to suggest that the data generated from these systems is useful for service provision for children affected by violence. For example, the Gender-Based Violence Information Management System (GBVIMS) is not connected or harmonized with state departments of police, prosecution and judiciary, who have the primary mandate to respond to violence. It is also not harmonized with the Health Management Information System.

Financing of VAC-Focused Agencies

Government is the most common source of funding in government agencies, while donors are the most frequent source of NGO funding. The national average budget allocated and disbursed from the district local government to each probation or labour office is insufficient considering the number of cases they handle. A unit cost analysis used in the VACS (Ministry of Gender, Labour and Social Development, 2019) found that the local government funding allocated to a probation office was enough to handle approximately 18 VAC cases, yet the average case load for probation offices was 323 in FY 2017/2018. Similarly, the allocated local government funding to a labour office was enough to handle approximately 10 child labour cases, yet the average case load for labour offices was 89 cases in FY 2017/2018.

Non-governmental organizations spend more on VAC services than district local governments. In the 2017/2018 financial year, non-governmental organizations spent an average of Uganda shillings 140 million (approximately $40,000) on the provision of services to affected children. This was ten times higher than the expenditure of local governments which spent Uganda shillings 13.7 million (approximately $4000). Majority of the district probation offices (87%) and labour offices (85%) reported failing to provide some services due to funding gaps. On the other hand, non-state service providers largely rely on foreign donor funding, which is not sustainable in the long run.

Survivors of violence and their families have to pay user fees to access services. While services for response are in place, the burden most times falls on the survivors of violence and their families to access these services, through direct and indirect charges. Some of these which have to be paid for include HIV tests and post-exposure prophylaxis (PEP) which are free in nearly all the health facilities but often have to be paid for by the state. Contrary to the official policy, some police stations impose fees on survivors for the transportation of accused persons to the police station, photocopying or printing of police forms 3A and 24A, facilitating police officers during inquiries or investigations and facilitating police officers during prosecution.

Human Resource Capacity of VAC-Focused Agencies

Notably, the major offices have staff that are trained and equipped with in-service training in each of the areas of child protection; applicable laws and duty bearers; child protection training using the National Child Protection Curriculum; and management of VAC cases. However, this does not apply to all and there are still pockets of vacant positions and staff that have not been adequately trained.

While success has been registered with the establishment of several information management systems aimed to enhance coordination of access and utilization of various services in the country including the GBVMIS and the OVCMIS, there are still pockets of gaps in information and coordination. A case in point is the fact that information on some of the Health Sector Strategic and Investment Plan (HSSIP) indicators, such as nationally aggregated data on the level of access to mental health services by young people, is not currently available (Uganda Child Rights NGO Network 2014). There are still gaps in the provision of adolescent-sensitive mental health counselling services and making them known and accessible to adolescents which the Convention on the Rights of the Child recommended for strengthening.

Conclusion and Recommendations

The evidence from Uganda shows that violence mostly occurs in the household, schools and community, in spaces where children are supposed to feel safe, perpetrated by persons supposed to protect them. Utilizing the WHO-recommended ecological framework is thus a critical tool in understanding the drivers and actors in VAC and therefore generating specific solutions that involve tackling social norms and attitude change for the prevention of violence against children. The Government of Uganda should prioritize strengthening of child protection mechanisms right from household, community and subnational to national level to ensure that children are protected from risks that execrate violence.

A harmonized and coordinated information management system that enables early detection of risk, monitoring and tracking of children at risk of violence will go a long way in harnessing the efforts of government in fighting against VAC. Regular data collection is critical to early detection, risk mapping and prevention interventions. Therefore, a starting point for improvements in information management will be to harmonize the existing information management systems for a more coordinated effort.

Coordination remains a critical feature of an effective national child protection system. As such, a central government coordination mechanism bringing together central government departments, different provinces, central and local levels and civil society is recommended to consolidate the gains made thus far in protecting Uganda's children. Ideally this should be within the mandate of National Children Authority (which is legally provided for but functionally not in place yet), to coordinate all matters pertaining to child protection and advocating for children's issues within all government departments considering the multidimensional nature of violence against children. In the absence of a functional NCA, an interim structure such as the National Child Protection working group should be strengthened to play the coordination role.

Children are central to prevention and response to VAC efforts. Therefore, scaling up of child rights awareness and child empowerment is another critical measure that will fast track the country's efforts to prevent and respond to VAC. The list of modalities on how this can be done is endless including explicit awareness-raising campaigns, embracing technology and use of both mainstream mass media and social media in the fight against VAC.

In addition to promoting positive parenting, it is critical to align policy and practice for effective violence prevention particularly strengthening supportive child protection systems at community level to complement initiatives at household level because children operate both at household and community levels. Hence, a supportive and responsive child protection system including informal child protection actors at community level is essential. The family or the household being the primary platform both for nurturing and protection of children as well as ensuring safety, well-being and development of vulnerable children must be part of the child protection efforts. Similarly, at the community level exist a number of child protection actors including extended family members, clan/traditional leaders, schools, police, community development officers, probation and social welfare officers, local councillors, child protection committees and children's groups. Harnessing synergies between these various actors is essential for a concerted violence prevention effort.

While it is important to implement formal social welfare programmes and social policies for improved child well-being, addressing the deeply rooted and imbedded social norms will lead to the realization of child rights and sustainable well-being of children. A framework that starts with social norms diagnosis, followed by building evidence for measurement and eventually community dialogue and action, will be important to bring about social norm change.

Uganda's several commitments to the protection and promotion of the rights of children are reflected in its robust national legal, policy and institutional framework, including the nascent child policy (2020) which is a successor to the national OVC policy, the Child Labour Policy. This can in part explain the remarkable strides the country has made in ensuring protection of children. Statistics on prevalence and access to services however point to gaps in this framework. There are still a multiplicity of systemic and functional bottlenecks affecting the system and thereby curtailing the progress demonstrated in domesticating the commitments. A critical examination of the legal, policy and institutional framework for child protection reveals lack of a comprehensive and harmonized reporting and feedback mechanism for information flow on offences of violence against children. There is need for a streamlined framework which will facilitate a harmonized and coordinated effort to ensure protection of children from violence.

Despite the robust legal and policy framework, implementation and enforcement continue to be constrained. Notable is the absence of a comprehensive child protection policy specifically addressing issues pertinent to children's well-being. Also notably absent in the existing framework are policy interventions targeting the root causes and the deep vulnerabilities to violence among children in different contexts.

The place of research cannot be overemphasized. More research should be conducted to continuously avail current and up-to-date evidence on the prevalence, trends and emerging issues in the ever-changing context of violence against children. Longitudinal studies, studies on the social constructs of violence, mental health outcomes as well as studies that document the economic, social and political burden of VAC in the long run will provide the much-needed evidence for the government to prioritize child protection efforts and invest in the required services.

References

Abbo, C., Kinyanda, E., Kizza, R. B., et al. (2013). Prevalence, comorbidity and predictors of anxiety disorders in children and adolescents in rural North-Eastern Uganda. *Child and Adolescent Psychiatry and Mental Health, 7*, 21. https://doi.org/10.1186/1753-2000-7-21

Adjei, J., & Saewyc, E. (2017). Boys are not exempt: Sexual exploitation of adolescents in sub-Saharan Africa. *Child Abuse & Neglect, 65*, 14–23. https://doi.org/10.1016/j.chiabu.2017.01.001

AfriChild Centre. (2015a). *Investing in Ugandan children: A response to Uganda's National Development Plan II*. The Centre of Excellence for the Study of the African Child.

AfriChild Centre. (2015b). *Tying loose ends and promoting exchange of information between the National Strategic Program Plan of interventions for orphans and other vulnerable children; and the Child Justice System in Uganda*. AfriChild.

AfriChild Centre. (2017). *Window on the world of violence against children outside of family Care in Uganda: Pushing the limits of child participation in research and policy-making through youth-driven participatory action research (YPAR)*. AfriChild.

AfriChild Centre. (2018). *Understanding the role of social norms to prevent and respond to violence against children in Uganda*. UNICEF.

AfriChild Centre, & Webale, T. B. (2017). *National Scoping Study on Appropriate Juvenile Justice Models for Uganda*. PILAC.

Akello, G., Reis, R., & Richters, A. (2010). Silencing distressed children in the context of war in northern Uganda: An analysis of its dynamics and its health consequences. *Social Science & Medicine, 71*(2), 213–220. https://doi.org/10.1016/j.socscimed.2010.03.030

ANPPCAN, U. (2011) Baseline Survey to Assess Violence against Children in Arua, Apac, Kitgum, Mukono, and Rakai Districts. Uganda: ANPPCAN

Amone-P'Olak, K., Elklit, A., & Dokkedahl, S. B. (2018). PTSD, mental illness, and care among survivors of sexual violence in Northern Uganda: Findings from the WAYS study. *Psychological trauma: theory, research, practice and policy, 10*(3), 282–289. https://doi.org/10.1037/tra0000295

Ashaba, S., Cooper-Vince, C., Maling, S., Rukundo, G. Z., Akena, D., & Tsai, A. C. (2018). Internalized HIV stigma, bullying, major depressive disorder, and high-risk suicidality among HIV-positive adolescents in rural Uganda. *Global Mental Health, 5*, e22. https://doi.org/10.1017/gmh.2018.15

Bantebya, G. K., Muhanguzi, K. F., & Watson, C. (2014). *Adolescent girls and gender justice: Changes and continuity in social norms and practices around marriage and education in Uganda*. ODI.

Barton, T., & Wamai, G. (1994) Equity and vulnerability: a situation analysis of women, adolescents and children in Uganda, Kampala, Uganda: Government of Uganda/Uganda National Council for Children.

Boydell, N., Nalukenge, W., Siu, G., et al. (2017). How mothers in poverty explain their use of corporal punishment: A qualitative study in Kampala, Uganda. *The European Journal of Development Research, 29*, 999–1016. https://doi.org/10.1057/s41287-017-0104-5

Cheney, K. E. (2005). 'Our children have only known war': children's experiences and the uses of childhood in northern Uganda. *Children's Geographies, 3*(1), 23–45. https://doi.org/10.1080/14733280500037133

ChildFund, Plan, Save the Children, World Vision, Teres des Hommes, SOS Villages. (2018). Thirty Years of implementing the conventions on the rights of children in Uganda: Progress and persisting challenges, 2018.

Clarke K, Patalay P, Allen E, et al. (2016). Patterns and predictors of violence against children in Uganda: a latent class analysis. *BMJ Open, 6*, e010443. https://doi.org/10.1136/bmjopen-2015-010443

Damien, Mbikyo Mulinga (2012). Attitudes of Stakeholders Towards Physical Punishment on Pupils of International and National Schools in Kampala District, Uganda. *World Journal of Education, 2*, 96–116.

Devries, K. M., Child, J. C., Allen, E., Walakira, E., Parkes, J., & Naker, D. (2014). School violence, mental health, and educational performance in Uganda. *Pediatrics, 133*(1), e129–e137. https://doi.org/10.1542/peds.2013-2007

Diesch, A. & Ntenga, M. (2016). Child marriage. *Result of poverty. Development + cooperation*, 17/06/2016.

Dwyer, M. (2016). *Iganga street children: Community Development Project (2016)*. MA IDS Thesis Projects. 54. https://digitalcommons.csp.edu/cgi/viewcontent.cgi?article=1011& context=cup_commons_grad_ids

Efevbera, Y., Bhabha, J., Farmer, P. E., & Fink, G. (2017). Girl child marriage as a risk factor for early childhood development and stunting. *Social Science & Medicine, 185*, 91–101. https://doi.org/10.1016/j.socscimed.2017.05.027

Ekundayo, O. (2015). *Does the African Charter on the Rights and Welfare of the Child (ACRWC) only underlines and repeats the convention on the Rights of the Child (CRC)'s Provisions?: Examining the similarities and the differences between the ACRWC and the CRC.*

Foundation for Human Rights Initiative. (2012). *A review of law and policy to prevent and remedy violence against children in police and pre-trial detention in Uganda*. Penal Reform International.

Gage, A. J. (2013). Association of child marriage with suicidal thoughts and attempts among adolescent girls in Ethiopia. *Journal of Adolescent Health, 52*, 654–656. https://doi.org/10.1016/j.jadohealth.2012.12.007

Gwirayi, P. (2011). Functions served by corporal punishment: Adolescent perspectives. *Journal of Psychology in Africa, 21*, 121–124.

Haji, H. A., & Bali Theodora, A. L. (2013). Assessing the effects of corporal punishment on primary school Pupils' academic performance and discipline in Unguja, Zanzibar. *International Journal of Education and Research, 1*(12).

Jain, S., & Kurz, K. (2007). *New insights on preventing child marriage. A Global Analysis of Factors and Programmes*. International Center for Research on Women.

Kidman, R., & Palermo, T.M. (2016). The relationship between parental presence and child sexual violence: Evidence from thirteen countries in sub-Saharan Africa. *Child abuse & neglect, 51*, 172–80.

Kigozi, F., Ssebunnya, J., Kizza, D. et al. (2010). An overview of Uganda's mental health care system: results from an assessment using the world health organization's assessment instrument for mental health systems (WHO-AIMS). *Int J Ment Health Syst 4*, 1. https://doi.org/10.1186/1752-4458-4-1

Kinyanda, E., Kizza, R., Abbo, C., et al. (2013). Prevalence and risk factors of depression in childhood and adolescence as seen in 4 districts of North-Eastern Uganda. *BMC International Health and Human Rights, 13*, 19–19.

Kisa, R., Baingana, F., Kajungu, R. et al. (2016). Pathways and access to mental health care services by persons living with severe mental disorders and epilepsy in Uganda, Liberia and Nepal: a qualitative study. BMC Psychiatry 16, 305. https://doi.org/10.1186/s12888-016-1008-1

Komakech, R. A., & Osuu, J. R. (2014). Students' Absenteeism: A Silent Killer Of Universal Secondary Education (USE) In Uganda. *International Journal of Education and Research, 2*(10)

Malak, M. Z., Al-amer, R. M., Khalifeh, A. H., & Jacoub, S. M. (2020). Evaluation of psychological reactions among teenage married girls in Palestinian refugee camps in Jordan. *Social Psychiatry and Psychiatric Epidemiology, 56*(2), 229–236. https://doi.org/10.1007/s00127-020-01917-6

Miller, J., Smith, E., Caldwell, L., Mathews, C., & Wegner, L. (2018). Boys are victims, too: The influence of perpetrators' age and gender in sexual coercion against boys. *Journal of Interpersonal Violence, 36*(7–8), NP3409–NP3432. https://doi.org/10.1177/0886260518775752

Ministry of Gender, Labour and Social Development. (2015). *Violence against children in Uganda: Findings from a National Survey, 2015*. UNICEF.

Ministry of Gender, Labour and Social Development. (2019). The Uganda VAC Services Survey 2018: Availability of Services for Preventing and Responding to Violence against Children in Uganda.

Ministry of Health and ORC Macro. (2005). *Uganda HIV sero – behavioral survey 2004–2005.* MOH and ORC Macro.

Ministry of Gender Labour and Social Development (2020). National Child Policy. Government of Uganda

Ministry of Gender, Labour and Social Development and UNICEF Uganda (2015) Situational Analysis of Children in Uganda.

Mugisha, J., Muyinda, H., Wandiembe, P., & Kinyanda, E. (2015). Prevalence and factors associated with Posttraumatic Stress Disorder seven years after the conflict in three districts in northern Uganda (The Wayo-Nero Study). *BMC psychiatry, 15*, 170. https://doi.org/10.1186/s12888-015-0551-5

Mugisha, J., Ssebunnya, J. & Kigozi, F.N. Towards understanding governance issues in integration of mental health into primary health care in Uganda. Int J Ment Health Syst 10, 25 (2016). https://doi.org/10.1186/s13033-016-0057-7

Mugumya, F., Ritterbusch, A., Boothby, N., Wanican, J., Opobo, T., Nyende, N., Meyer, S., & Bangiran, C. (2017) Qualitative Study of Risks and Protective Factors for Violence against Children living in Residential Care Institutions (RCIs) in Uganda. The AfriChild Centre: Uganda-Kampala

Muhanguzi, F. K. (2011). Gender and sexual vulnerability of young women in Africa: Experiences of young girls in secondary schools in Uganda. *Culture, Health & Sexuality, 13*(6), 713–725. https://doi.org/10.1080/13691058.2011.571290

Nabukeera-Barungi, N., Elyanu, P., Asire, B., Katurbee, C., Lukabwe, I., Namusoke, E., et al. (2015). Adherence to antiretroviral therapy and retention in care for adolescents living with HIV from 10 districts in Uganda. *BMC Infectious Diseases, 15*, 520.

Naker, D., Sekitoleko, D. (2009). *Positive discipline: Creating a good school environment without corporal punishment.* Raising Voices.

Nalukenge, W., Martin, F., Seeley, J., & Kinyanda, E. (2019). Knowledge and causal attributions for mental disorders in HIV-positive children and adolescents: Results from rural and urban Uganda. *Psychology, Health & Medicine, 24*(1), 21–26. https://doi.org/10.1080/13548506.2018.1467021

Natukunda, H. P. M., Mubiri, P., Cluver, L. D., Ddumba-Nyanzi, I., Bukenya, B., & Walakira, E. J. (2019). Which factors are associated with adolescent reports of experiencing various forms of abuse at the family level in post-conflict northern uganda? *Journal of Interpersonal Violence.* https://doi.org/10.1177/0886260519888526

Ninsiima, A. B., Michielsen, K., Kemigisha, E., Nyakato, V. N., Leye, E., & Coene, G. (2020). Poverty, gender and reproductive justice. A qualitative study among adolescent girls in Western Uganda. *Culture, Health & Sexuality, 22*, 65–79. https://doi.org/10.1080/13691058.2019.1660406

Nishimura, M., Yamano, T., & Sasaoka, Y. (2008). Impacts of the universal education policy on education attainment and private costs in rural Uganda. *International Journal of Educational Development, 28*, 161–175. https://doi.org/10.1016/j.ijedudev.2006.09.017

Nuwaha, F., & Mukulu, A. (2009). Trends in under-five mortality in Uganda 1954-2000: Can millennium development goals be met? *African Health Sciences, 9*(2), 125–128.

Nyakito, C., & Allida, D. (2018). "Spare the rod and spoil the child" - is corporal punishment morally and legally justified in Ugandan secondary schools? A case of Gulu District. *Baraton Interdisciplinary Research Journal, 8*, 1–10.

Nyakuni, Z., & Barton T. G. (1996). Equity and vulnerability : a situation analysis of women, adolescents and children in Uganda: 1996 statistical update. Government of Uganda and National Council for Children

Okello, E. S., & Neema, S. (2007). Explanatory Models and Help-Seeking Behavior: Pathways to Psychiatric Care Among Patients Admitted for Depression in Mulago Hospital, Kampala, Uganda. *Qualitative Health Research, 17*(1), 14–25. https://doi.org/10.1177/1049732306296433

Okello, E. S., & Musisi, S. (2006). Depression as a clan illness (eByekika): An indigenous model of psychotic depression among the Baganda of Uganda. *Journal World Cultural Psychiatry Research Review, 1*(2), 60–73.

Parsons, J., Edmeades, J., Kes, A., Petroni, S., Sexton, M., & Wodon, Q. (2015). Economic impacts of child marriage: A review of the literature. *The Review of Faith & International Affairs, 13*(3), 12–22. https://doi.org/10.1080/15570274.2015.1075757

Quinn, N., & Knifton, L. (2014). Beliefs, stigma and discrimination associated with mental health problems in Uganda: Implications for theory and practice. *International Journal of Social Psychiatry, 60*(6), 554–561. https://doi.org/10.1177/0020764013504559

Reisen, M. (2017). *Early Child Marriage, Sexual Practices and Trafficking of the Girl Child in Uganda.* Europe External Policy Advisors.

Rubin, D., Green, C. P., & Mukuria, A. (2009). *Addressing early marriage in Uganda.* Futures Group, Health Policy Initiative.

Saile, R., Ertl, V., Neuner, F., & Catani, C. (2014). Does war contribute to family violence against children? Findings from a two-generational multi-informant study in northern Uganda. *Child Abuse and Neglect, 38,* 135–146. https://doi.org/10.1016/j.chiabu.2013.10.007

Samara, S. (2010). Something-for-something love: the motivations of young women in Uganda. *Journal of Health Organization and Management, 24*(5), 512–519. https://doi.org/10.1108/14777261011070538

Satzinger, F., Kipp, W., & Rubaale, T. (2012). Ugandan HIV/AIDS orphans in charge of their households speak out: a study of their health-related worries. *Global Public Health, 7*(4), 420–431. https://doi.org/10.1080/17441690903339652

Sejjaaka, S. (2004). A political and economic history of Uganda, 1962–2002. In *International businesses and the challenges of poverty in the developing world* (pp. 98–110). Springer. https://doi.org/10.1057/9780230522503_6

Sekiwunga, R., & Whyte, S. R. (2009). Poor parenting: Teenagers' views on adolescent pregnancies in eastern Uganda. *African Journal of Reproductive Health, 13*(4), 113–127.

Spitzer, H., & Twikirize, J. (2013). War-affected children in northern Uganda: No easy path to normality. *International Social Work, 56,* 67–79. https://doi.org/10.1177/0020872812459067

Ssebunnya, J., Kangere, S., Mugisha, J. et al. (2018). Potential strategies for sustainably financing mental health care in Uganda. *Int J Ment Health Syst, 12,* 74. https://doi.org/10.1186/s13033-018-0252-9

Ssenyonga, J., Muwonge, C. M., & Hecker, T. (2019). Prevalence of family violence and mental health and their relation to peer victimization: A representative study of adolescent students in Southwestern Uganda. *Child Abuse & Neglect, 98,* https://doi.org/10.1016/j.chiabu.2019.104194.

Sumner, S. A., Mercy, A. A., Saul, J., Motsa-Nzuza, N., Kwesigabo, G., Buluma, R., Marcelin, L. H., Lina, H., Shawa, M., Moloney-Kitts, M., Kilbane, T., Sommarin, C., Ligiero, D. P., Brookmeyer, K., Chiang, L., Lea, V., Lee, J., Kress, H., Hillis, S. D., & Centers for Disease Control and Prevention (CDC) (2015). Prevalence of sexual violence against children and use of social services - seven countries, 2007-2013. MMWR. *Morbidity and mortality weekly report, 64*(21), 565–569.

The African Child Policy Forum. (2013). http://www.africanchildforum.org

The Republic of Uganda, Ministry of Gender, Labour and Social Development. (2004). *National orphans and vulnerable children policy.*

Thumann, B. F., Nur, U., Naker, D. et al. (2016). Primary school students' mental health in Uganda and its association with school violence, connectedness, and school characteristics: a cross-sectional study. *BMC Public Health 16,* 662. https://doi.org/10.1186/s12889-016-3351-z

Tukundane, C., Zeelen, J., Minnaert, A., & Kanyandago, P. (2014). 'I felt very bad, I had self-rejection': Narratives of exclusion and marginalisation among early school leavers in Uganda. *Journal of Youth Studies, 17*(4), 475–491. https://doi-org.libproxy.wustl.edu/10.1080/13676261.2013.830703

UAC. (2015). 'An AIDS Free Uganda, My Responsibility: Documents for the National HIV and AIDS Response, 2015/2016–2019/2020'.

Uganda Bureau of Statistics. (2016). *The National Population and Housing Census 2014 – Main report.* .

Uganda Bureau of Statistics (UBOS) and ICF. (2018). *Uganda demographic and health survey 2016*. UBOS and ICF.

Uganda Bureau of Statistics (UBOS) and ICF International Inc. (2012). *Uganda demographic and health survey 2011*. ICF International.

Uganda Bureau of Statistics and Macro International Inc. (2007). *Uganda demographic and health survey 2006*. UBOS and Macro International.

Uganda Child Rights NGO Network. (2014). *Accountability for children's rights. A review of the effectiveness of child rights monitoring and accountability mechanisms in Uganda*. UCRNN.

Uganda Children (Amendment) Act. (2016). Retrieved from https://www.ilo.org/dyn/natlex/docs/ELECTRONIC/104395/127307/F-171961747/UGA104395.pdf

Uganda Police Force. (2019). *Annual Crime Report, 2019*.

Uganda: The Penal Code (Amendment) Act, 2007 [Uganda], Act 8 of 2007, 17 August 2007

UNAIDS. (2017). 'UNAIDS DATA 2017' [pdf] although the percentage of young men with this knowledge rose from 39.3% in 2011 to 42.3% in 2104, it fell among young women during this time, from 38.6% to 35.7%.UAC (2015) '2014 Uganda HIV and AIDS Country Progress Report' [pdf].

United Nations Convention on the Rights of the Child. (1989). https://www.ohchr.org/en/professionalinterest/pages/crc.aspx

Wakida, E. K., Obua, C., Rukundo, G. Z. et al. (2018). Barriers and facilitators to the integration of mental health services into primary healthcare: a qualitative study among Ugandan primary care providers using the COM-B framework. *BMC Health Serv Res 18*, 890. https://doi.org/10.1186/s12913-018-3684-7

Walakira, E. J., & Ddumba, I. N. (2012). *Violence against children in Uganda: A decade of research and practice, 2002–2012*. Ministry of Gender Labour and Social Development and UNICEF.

Walakira, E. J., Nyanzi, D., Lishan, S., & Baizerman, M. (2014). No place is safe: Violence against and among children and youth in street situations in Uganda. *Vulnerable Children and Youth Studies, 9*(4), 332–340. https://doi.org/10.1080/17450128.2014.934750

Wamimbi, W. R. (2018). *Understanding social norms to prevent and respond to violence against Children*. https://www.africhild.or.ug/downloads/understanding-social-norms-to-preventand-respond-to-violence-against-children-in-uganda/

WHO/Uganda Ministry of Health. (2017). 'The Uganda Population-Based HIV Impact Assessment 2016-17' [pdf].

Wodon, Q., Nguyen, M. C., & Tsimpo, C. (2016). Child marriage, education, and agency in Uganda. *Feminist Economics, 22*(1), 54–79. https://doi.org/10.1080/13545701.2015.1102020

World Health Organization. (2021). *Violence Prevention Alliance: The VPA Approach*. https://www.who.int/violenceprevention/approach/ecology/en/

Determinants of Intergenerational Trauma Transmission: A Case of the Survivors of the 1994 Genocide Against Tutsi in Rwanda

Célestin Mutuyimana, Vincent Sezibera, and Cindi Cassady

Introduction

Post-traumatic stress disorder (PTSD) is a trauma- and stress-related disorder found worldwide. People may develop PTSD after exposure to actual or threatened death, serious injury, or sexual violence either as direct exposure, witnessing, in person, the event(s) as it occurred to others, learning that the traumatic event(s) occurred to a close family member or close friend, or experiencing repeated or extreme exposure to aversive details of the traumatic event(s) (APA, 2013). Estimates of the lifetime prevalence of PTSD vary considerably according to social background and country of residence, ranging from 1.3% to 12.2% (Karam et al., 2014).

Although it is natural to feel afraid during and after a traumatic situation and everyone will experience a range of reactions after trauma, most people will recover from those symptoms naturally. Those who continue to experience problems may be diagnosed with PTSD. People who have PTSD may feel stressed or frightened even when they are no longer in danger. A cluster of symptoms including a feeling of re-experiencing, avoidance, arousal and reactivity, and problems with cognition and mood usually follow within 3 months of the traumatic incident, but may begin later. Symptoms must last more than a month and be severe enough to interfere with functioning in relationships or work in order to consider a diagnosis of PTSD. The course of the illness varies from person to person. Some people recover within 6 months, while others have symptoms that last much longer. In some people, the condition becomes chronic (Lee et al., 2015). Not everyone who lives through a

C. Mutuyimana · V. Sezibera (✉)
Center for Mental Health, College of Medicine and Health Sciences, University of Rwanda, Kigali, Rwanda
e-mail: vsezibera@gmail.com

C. Cassady
Department of Clinical Psychology, University of Kibungo, Kibungo, Rwanda

© Springer Nature Switzerland AG 2022
F. M. Ssewamala et al. (eds.), *Child Behavioral Health in Sub-Saharan Africa*,
https://doi.org/10.1007/978-3-030-83707-5_11

dangerous event develops PTSD. In fact, most will recover quickly without intervention. Many factors play a part in whether a person will develop PTSD.

Risk factors make a person more likely to develop PTSD. These include getting hurt; seeing people hurt or killed; childhood trauma; feeling horror, helplessness, or extreme fear; having little or no social support after the event; dealing with extra stress after the event, such as loss of a loved one, pain and injury, or loss of a job or home; and having a history of mental illness or substance abuse. Other factors, called resilience factors, can help reduce the risk of developing the disorder. Some of these risk and resilience factors are present before the traumatic event and others become important during or after the traumatic event (Wimalawansa, 2014).

The 1994 Genocide against the Tutsi was a major traumatic event experienced by all Rwandans; more than one million Tutsi were brutally killed. During the genocide, victims struggled to have hope to survive or to find any possible meaning in life. Neighbors went after neighbors with guns, machetes, or sticks searching house by house for people to kill. Stealing property, marauding, murder, and sexual violence were common throughout the country (Straus, 2004). The daily living conditions became very critical with the continuous rainy season occurring throughout the 100 days of the genocide and most victims lost their sense of hope (Straus, 2004). Those who survived continued to experience psychological torture as they received messages of the death of their parents and siblings and the loss of their home and livestock. Survivors and their descendants as the targeted group experienced 12 major traumatic events on average (Rieder & Elbert, 2013).

Currently 26 years after the 1994 Genocide, survivors continue to manifest high rates of mental health problems due to the unfathomable horrors and dehumanizing violence that they personally experienced or witnessed. Most survivors have no social support system as their families were killed, their property was destroyed, livestock was stolen or killed, and a pervasive sense of fear and mistrust existed within the community. Studies have indicated that PTSD is the most prevalent diagnosis among the survivors of the Genocide against the Tutsi (Pham et al., 2004). Study findings indicate that highly traumatized groups, including holocaust survivors, Armenian Genocide survivors, Cambodian survivors, and Genocide against the Tutsi survivors, may either experience various psychopathologies which have notable indirect effects on their offspring (Kellerman, 2001; Perroud et al., 2014) or integrate their trauma and become resilient and successful (Roth et al., 2014).

Research has demonstrated that trauma can be intergenerationally transmitted, which has led to further studies being conducted on the 1994 Genocide against the Tutsi survivors (Perroud et al., 2014). Low resilience scores among the 1994 Genocide survivors are associated with complex post-traumatic stress disorders and intergenerational trauma among their offspring (Shriraa et al., 2019).

In this chapter we discuss the transmission of trauma, models of transmission, intersection of PTSD in parents and parent-infant attachment, determinants of the PTSD transmission within the Rwandan context, possible pathways of child traumatization in post-genocide Rwanda, conclusions, and further perspectives.

Transgenerational Trauma

A multitude of terms describing trauma transmission have been used by various authors (Kellerman, 2001). Albeck (1993) suggested that it is preferable to use the term "intergenerational aspects of trauma" instead of "trauma transmission." Bowers and Yehuda (2016) prefer the term "intergenerational transmission of stress in humans" because severe stress exposure in a parent can result in mental disorders such as depression, anxiety, or PTSD that may be a risk factor for a number of adverse outcomes, including psychopathology in offspring. In accordance with the generational interchange specifically from parent to child, the transmission process is defined as either *transgenerational* (Baum, 2012; Felsen, 1998), *intergenerational* (Sigal & Weinfeld, 1992), *multigenerational* (Danieli, 1998), or *cross-generational* (Lowin, 1983). Kellerman (2001) indicated that as trauma was invariably passed on from one or both of the parents, "*parental*" transmission would perhaps be the most adequate term. However, common sense tells us that whatever traumatic experiences caregivers endured during childhood or as an adult, they are likely to have a profound influence on the well-being of their offspring (Yehuda & Bierer, 2008).

Literature on the transmission of Holocaust trauma (Schwartz et al., 1994; Felsen, 1998) has further differentiated between "direct and specific" transmission, a mental syndrome in the survivor parent which leads *directly* to the same *specific* syndrome in the child and "indirect and general" transmission, a disorder in the parent which makes the parent unable to function as a parent which *indirectly* leads to a *general* sense of deprivation in the child.

While such differentiation seems to be valid, it confuses aspects of the process of transmission (Kellerman, 2001); hence it is important to differentiate the content of transmission and the models of transmission.

Research on the offspring of Holocaust survivors compared to offspring of the general population with emotional problems demonstrated that the Holocaust offspring had distinct difficulties in coping with stress and demonstrated a higher vulnerability to PTSD than the offspring of the general population with emotional problems (Kellerman, 2001). The problems were centered on four areas (Kellerman, 1999):

1. Self-esteem: Impaired self-esteem with persistent overidentification with their parents' status and a need to be superachievers to compensate for what their parents left behind. This small group felt that they needed to represent the six million who had died during the Holocaust, a challenging and daunting responsibility.
2. Cognition: Through their parents' storytelling of the magnitude and horrors of the Holocaust, the offspring of Holocaust survivors developed a catastrophic expectancy or fear of another Holocaust occurring, were constantly preoccupied with death, and experienced stress upon exposure to stimuli that symbolized the Holocaust.

3. Affectivity: The offspring of Holocaust survivors felt a sense of unresolved mourning for their parents. Hence they experienced extreme anxiety, nightmares, and frequent dysphoric mood.
4. Interpersonal functioning: The clinicians and researchers observed interpersonal functioning by interacting with the offspring of Holocaust survivors. They noticed exaggerated family attachments, dependency or exaggerated independence, and difficulties entering into intimate relationships and handling interpersonal conflicts.

Models of Trauma Transmission

The effects of traumatic events may extend to persons who are not directly exposed to the actual traumatic event, but who live with or are close to those directly affected by the event. Research and clinical observation prove that family members including children, friends, caregivers, as well as therapists are likely to become the victims of trauma transmission (Rosenheck & Nathan, 1985). A range of terminologies have been used in the literature to characterize this phenomenon of trauma transmission. McCann and Pearlman (1990) called it vicarious trauma when there are emotional, physical, and spiritual transformations experienced by people (e.g., therapists, researchers, social workers, lawyers) working with traumatized persons. Showalter (2010) called it compassion fatigue when there is a feeling of empathy for the person struck by suffering or misfortune and sharing his/her sorrow and grief.

Other terms used for this type of trauma include co-victimization (Hartsough & Myers, 1985), indirect victimization (McCann & Pearlman, 1990), traumatic counter-transfer (Herman, 1992), and contact victimization (Courtois, 1988). Transgenerational trauma is used specifically when the trauma consequences are present in the offspring of traumatized people (Dekel & Goldblatt, 2008).

Trauma transmission from parents to offspring is a result of biopsychosocial factors. Several studies found that PTSD-affected subjects have significant intrapersonal and interpersonal suffering within their families. Unhealthy family functioning in areas such as affective responsiveness, problem-solving, conflict, family cohesion, marital adjustment, and offspring maltreatment is a psychosocial mechanism of PTSD transmission (Lehrner & Yehuda, 2018; Ahmadzadeh & Malekian, 2004). The parent's own trauma is capable of disorganizing healthy attachment between children and parents and can contribute to the development of trauma in the children (Hartsough & Myers, 1985; Dekel & Goldblatt, 2008).

Biological factors focus on the epigenetic transmission changes that do not involve alterations in the DNA sequence, but affect gene activity and expression. The DNA sequences remain intact while the process by which information from a gene is used in the synthesis of a functional gene product is affected (McFarlane, 2009, Perroud et al., 2014). Evidence studies explaining the mechanism of transgenerational transmission of trauma with epigenetics have been suggesting that heritable changes in gene expression can be made as a result of environmental stress or major emotional trauma (Meaney & Szyf, 2005). Parents can pass on such acquired characteristics just like genetic characteristics (Kellermann, 2013). Even though the ways of transmission have been highlighted by different researchers, it is still a challenge to discover how trauma is harming the lives of the people who were not directly exposed to the traumatic event and may not even have been born yet. Kellerman (2001) describes trauma transmission in this way: "In the same way as heat, light, sound, and electricity can be invisibly carried from a transmitter to a receiver; it is possible that unconscious experiences can also be transmitted from parents to their children through some complex process of extra-sensory communication."

Kellerman's (2001) Holocaust transmission study revealed four major theoretical models to understanding trauma transmission: (1) psychodynamic, (2) sociocultural, (3) family system, and (4) biological models of transmission.

1. *Psychodynamic and relational model:* According to the research done on the Holocaust, emotions that could not be consciously experienced by the first generation are passed down to the second generation (Kellerman, 2001). Thus, the child unconsciously absorbs the repressed and insufficiently worked-through Holocaust experiences of survivor parents. Research conducted with the children of Vietnam Veterans indicated that parents with PTSD involuntarily have difficulty containing their emotions, and their attempts to mitigate the pain lead to massive use of projection mechanisms, where severe emotions such as persecution, aggression, shame, and guilt are split and projected onto their children (Kellerman, 2001). As a result, children may identify with the projected parts of their father's emotions and perceive his experiences and feelings as their own (Dekel & Goldblatt, 2008).

2. *Sociocultural and socialization models:* Sociocultural theories of transmission focus on the passing down of social norms and beliefs from generation to generation. The theory suggests that offspring of survivors form their own images through their parents' childrearing behavior, like their various prohibitions, taboos, and fears. Studies indicate that physically abused children often grow up to be child abusers themselves (Blumberg, 1977), and that teenage motherhood and early marriage seem to be passed on from mothers to their daughters. As pointed out by Bandura (1977), children learn things vicariously by observing and imitating their parents; thus, children of Holocaust survivors may be assumed to have taken upon themselves some of the behaviors and emotional characteristics of their parents. In comparison with psychoanalytic theories that focus on unconscious and indirect influences, social learning theories emphasize conscious and direct effects of parents on their children. In much of this literature, Holocaust survivors have been described as inadequate parents. Their multiple losses were assumed to create childrearing problems around both attachment and detachment. For example, overt messages conveyed by Holocaust survivor parents such as "Be careful" and "Don't trust anybody!" were assumed to have left their indelible marks. The exaggerated worries of such anxious parents may have conveyed a sense of an impending danger that the child may have absorbed (Kellerman, 2001).

3. *Biological or genetic models:* These models are based on the presumption that there may be a genetic and/or a biochemical predisposition to the etiology of trauma transmission. Considerable research on trauma transmission through epigenetics has confirmed the hypothesis of this model (Kellermann, 2013; Perroud et al., 2014).

In an attempt to investigate such assumptions, Yehuda et al. (2000) found that low cortisol levels were significantly associated with both PTSD in parents and lifetime PTSD in offspring, whereas having a current psychiatric diagnosis other than PTSD was relatively, but nonsignificantly, associated with higher cortisol levels. Offspring with both parental PTSD and lifetime PTSD had the lowest cortisol levels of all study groups. They conclude: "Parental PTSD, a putative risk factor for PTSD, appears to be associated with low cortisol levels in offspring, even in the absence of lifetime PTSD in the offspring." The findings suggest that low cortisol levels in PTSD may constitute a vulnerability marker related to parental PTSD as well as a state-related characteristic associated with acute or chronic PTSD symptoms.

Recent study indicated that children of Holocaust survivors with PTSD have lower rates of methylation and one type of epigenetic mechanism in a particular stress-related glucocorticoid receptor, the GR-1F, than children of survivors who did not have PTSD (Yehuda et al., 2014).

4. *Family system and communication models:* The traumatized family is designated as a close-fitting system and lives in isolation, as if on an island (Danieli, 1998). The children communicate only with their own parents and siblings and with other survivors. They all try to shield their painful experiences. The more pathological families are described as tight little islands in which children came into contact only with their own parents, with their siblings, and with other survivors. In such highly closed systems parents are fully committed to their children and children are overly concerned with their parents' welfare, both trying to shield the other from painful experiences (Klein-Parker, 1988). Unconscious and conscious transmission of parental traumatization always takes place in a certain family environment, which is assumed to have a major impact on the children (Kellerman, 2001). According to family systems and communication theoretical models, inadequate psychological parenting by the traumatized mother can have a detrimental effect on the development and well-being of the children (Field et al., 2013). Traumatic experiences can also interfere with one's positive childrearing behavior and lead to maladaptive parenting (Ammerman et al., 2012). Less family cohesion and greater family conflict are reported in families with a traumatized parent (Davidson & Mellor, 2012).

Parents with PTSD have major difficulties in providing an adequate maturational environment for their children. Parental avoidance and psychic numbing can result in emotional and physical withdrawal from the children (Ruscio et al., 2002).

Often survivors may trivialize their children's daily needs or issues in comparison to their own trauma, and react in neglectful or insensitive ways. As mothers fail to maintain an adequate level of responsiveness toward the children, children are likely to feel unprotected and insecure (Juni, 2016). Symptoms of hypervigilance of the survivors which may result in angry outburst or hostility may be misunderstood and frightening to the children. Finally, survivors may be overprotective and constantly fear for their children's safety, consequently making it difficult for their children to develop a sense of self-efficacy and autonomy (Field et al., 2013).

Trauma Associated with the Genocide in Rwanda and Possible Pathways of Child Traumatization

During the 1994 Genocide against the Tutsi, there were three groups exposed to the effects of the genocide within the Rwandan population: (1) genocide survivors—those who were targeted by the perpetrators; (2) in-country non-targeted group—those who were in country during the genocide but not targeted; and (3) 1959 returnees—those who were refugees and living outside the country during the genocide but who may have had members of their family targeted. A comparative study of PTSD prevalence among these groups of Rwandan parents and their offspring 25 years after the genocide showed that 30.2% of the population among all three groups met the criteria for having significant symptoms of PTSD (Mutuyimana et al., 2019).

The average prevalence of PTSD in parents among the three groups was 43.8%, while the prevalence among the offspring was 16.5% (Mutuyimana et al., 2019). The likelihood of having PTSD in the sample was associated with the mothers' survival category (survivors, in-country non-targeted, and 1959 returnees). The likelihood of parents having PTSD was 75% lower for the in-country non-targeted group than the survivor group and 70% lower for the 1959 returnees group than for the survivors. Furthermore, the likelihood of the offspring having PTSD was associated with their mothers' survival status.

The odds of experiencing PTSD were 66% lower for the offspring born to in-country non-targeted mothers compared to the offspring born to survivors and 73% lower for the offspring born to 1959 returnee mothers compared to the offspring born to survivors.

The data indicated that the mother's survival status, survivor, 1959 returnee, or in-country non-targeted, influenced their offspring's development of PTSD, whereas the level or degree of trauma experienced by the mother (high, moderate, or low) did not significantly impact the development of PTSD among their children. Based on the results, we find that there may be a relationship between the parents' PTSD and the PTSD of their offspring. The survivor mother category manifested the highest percentage of PTSD development within their offspring. Hence, we were interested in examining possible pathways of offspring traumatization and what the content was that got transmitted to the group of survivors.

Possible Pathways of Offspring Traumatization Post-genocide and Transmitted Content Within the Genocide Survivors

The effects of the Genocide against the Tutsi and its aftermath on individuals, families, communities, and Rwanda have been elaborated upon by numerous researchers (Schindler, 2010; Berckmoes et al., 2017). The transmission of trauma to the next generation is one of the consequences of the Genocide against the Tutsi. When we discuss the transmission of trauma, a number of questions are raised. What exactly is transmitted related to trauma? What are the mechanisms of transmission? Which children are more vulnerable to the transmission of PTSD distress in the family? To answer these questions, qualitative data have been collected from 30 dyads of mother's survivors and their offspring with significant symptoms of PTSD as indicated by the score of PCL-5 for mothers and UCLA-4 index for offspring, during the research of PTSD prevalence of mothers and their offspring (Mutuyimana et al., 2019). The mothers' age varied from 45 to 62 years while the age for offspring varied from 18 to 24 years. A thematic analysis of the mothers' interviews showed that they experienced and witnessed many traumatizing events during the genocide and later suffered from many psychological, physical, social, and economic consequences of the past violence. They emphatically expressed how strongly the past experiences continued to shape their present lives and affect the relationship between their children and them. The offspring of the survivor mothers also shared how the past traumatic experiences of their mothers affected their psychosocial living conditions.

Transmitted Content

Results of this study revealed that although considerable research has addressed the pathways of trauma transmission rather than the content transmitted, reports from genocide survivors and their offspring show the content of the intergenerational legacies. The thematic content was grouped into the following categories:

Longing: The unresolved trauma of the parents was often present in their offspring. They often longed to feel a sense of connection to their unknown, deceased family members. As they listened over time to the stories, the children held onto the information provided to them about their relatives. They were left with a sense that their relatives were psychosocially, emotionally, and economically strong. The children learned that many of their parents continue to feel close to the persons that died and they felt a yearning to know the people that had been lost to them.

Feeling of emptiness: In the Rwandan context, raising a child in a family surrounded by loved ones, parents, relations, friends, and grandparents, helps them to be an individual who is self-assured and affirmative and has a strong sense of self and self-esteem. This was not the case for the offspring of the survivors of the

Genocide against Tutsi. They were born without models of their relatives and community, leading them to ask their parents about their Tutsi identity. They desired to know the exact genealogy of their parents and were often left feeling empty and uncertain about them when their questions were not or could not be answered.

Heart wounds: Offspring of survivors assimilated the trauma of their parents by the process of identification. For the offspring, life was full of continuous psycho-social, economic, and emotional pain which never seemed to end. This created a feeling of hopelessness for the future as it had for their parents. They felt that they cannot abandon their parents in their daily psychological suffering and felt a sense of guilt and responsibility to help their parents overcome their struggle, while being indirectly affected as well.

Mechanisms of Transmission in the Context of Genocide Against Tutsi Survivors

Attachment and Storytelling

Through storytelling, parent-child relationships, and environment in which the children are raised, children indirectly gained an idea of the trauma experienced by their parents. Many parents displayed psycho-emotional symptoms related to PTSD or depression, and their children struggled to understand what was wrong with their parents because the parents did not disclose the reason for their strange or even frightening behaviors. When parents did not provide any explanation for their emotional symptoms, their children often tried to make sense of their parents' behaviors or even imitated their parents' behaviors and attitudes. Some parents shared too many details about the trauma they experienced, which indirectly caused their children to experience their parents' trauma. The nature and vulnerability of a child's symptoms were influenced by the parent-child relationship and environment in which they lived.

We looked at each of these three aspects and their relationship to the transmission of trauma in the offspring of genocide survivor mothers, in-country non-targeted mothers, and 1959 returnee mothers.

The stories children were exposed to by their mothers were influenced by the type of parent-child relationship found in the family. "Hesitant" parents were those who had extremely traumatic experiences which they thought were unnecessary to share with their children. Hesitant parents reported often feeling pressured to share their traumatic experiences with their children who asked about the past and some thought that if they shared with their children, their children's own emotional and behavioral problems might be resolved. However, many parents experienced PTSD flashbacks when they recounted their stories with their children who continued to struggle to understand their parent's emotional and cognitive distress. Repeatedly witnessing parental distress can be frightening and emotionally traumatizing for children who do not understand their parent's emotional disturbance. Offspring of hesitant parents developed anxiety because they learned from their parents that the world is a dangerous place. Children whose parents manifest symptoms of trauma are likely to develop maladaptive thinking and behavior as a direct result of being exposed to their parents' psychopathology (Schwartz et al., 1994).

"Disclosure" parents or relatives were those who provided all the details of the traumatic history to their children without taking into consideration the age or emotional maturity of the children. In-depth interviews revealed that this type of parent was strongly attached to their children and monitored them closely.

As a result of the parent sharing their traumatic stories with their children, the children tended to overidentify with their parent, became parentified, and tried to please their parent and take responsibility for their parent's emotional disturbance or PTSD symptoms. It is in this group that we found frequent symptoms of trauma hyper-arousal, flashbacks, nightmares, and unresolved trauma symptoms among offspring because they were indirectly exposed to and assimilated many of their parent's symptoms. The children wished to help their parents become psychologically stable but they lacked the maturity and ability to help their parents to heal.

The group of "silent parents" were those who were overwhelmed by their traumatic experiences. They were unable to talk about their past and were quiet and emotionally distant with their children and family members. They had insecure attachments with their children and as a result, the children exhibited behavior disorders, tended to isolate themselves, and had a loss of interest in things.

Several studies indicate that maternal PTSD may negatively impact the mother–infant relationship and maternal PTSD symptoms have been associated with greater impairment in mothers' prenatal attachment. Interviews with mothers with PTSD revealed that they interacted with their children in a detached manner and the children felt rejected, uninvolved, or overprotected as a result. Mothers exhibited a range of insensitive caregiving behaviors predictive of insecure attachment with their children such as distorted, inflexible, and negative mental representations of their children (Schechter & Willheim, 2009).

Through interviews with the survivors' offspring, we found that parental story-telling increased the level of internalization of traumatic events and recalling of the event that their parents experienced.

One of the children stated, "Every time that I saw my mother changing her mood, I felt very, very sad at the level I can't explain to you. When I was a little child, I questioned little about my mother's experience. She loves me very much, but she tried to hide the reality around her traumatic experience .... When I saw her mood change I am full of fear thinking that it can happen again, nightmares increases and others ..."

Within the hesitant parent group, one parent noted, "Currently, it is not easy to express my sadness in the presence of my children.

When I feel uncomfortable I try my best to find other ways to deal with my emotions so my children will not continue to suffer from my chronic disease."

"Storytelling is shaped by the environment." In addition to what the children learned, observed, and imitated from their parents, the environment in which the child lived may be one of the factors that shaped the child's trauma due to different memories and living conditions that the child encountered. We found that offspring who lived in genocide survivor settlements and single orphans without social support were more likely to manifest symptoms of trauma. Additionally, parents reported that within their children, they found four categories: (1) those who were really close to them and manifested the symptoms of PTSD by imitating what their parents were doing (imitators); (2) those who thought deeply and carefully about what happened to their parents and finally became traumatized (reflectors); (3) those who directly became detached from social or emotional involvement with the parents and were always shocked by the parents' attitudes including harsh punishment (withdrawers); and (4) those who tended to cope effectively with their parent's trauma because they were distant from their parents and had no time to understand the reason of their symptoms.

Parents reported, *"After the genocide we were dispersed in different regions of the country. Then later, the government of Rwanda helped us to live together in a survivor settlement. The place is inhabited only by Genocide against Tutsi survivors even though we have in country non-targeted and some 1959 returnees as our neighbors. Most of our children who were born after the genocide used to ask us the same question, 'Why do we live here and why are we called 1994 genocide survivors?' We are obliged to explain to them until their curiosity is satisfied, but these explanations make us feel upset and it like revisiting our past. We find it is the same for our children."*

One child reported, *"I am always uncomfortable when I hear [the] saying that I live in a 1994 genocide survivor settlement. Even though this term is used frequently in the meetings, at school, during the discussion with other young people, however, it hurts my heart. I wish our residences could stop being called like that. I always feel sorrow when I see people proudly telling us that we live in genocide survivor settlements. We know that we live there not because of happiness or choice but because of our unique and horrible history. I sometimes worry that we can be attacked by the killers and killed all at once and this fear is in my dreams most of the time."*

Parenting Styles

We examined how parenting styles are affected by PTSD symptoms which in turn affected their children's life. Parenting behaviors and family environment are powerful determinants of physical and mental health outcomes over the life span (Brockman et al., 2016). In Kinyarwanda, the proverb "Uburere buruta ubuvuke" means "the parenting style is more effective than personality." When children have positive relationships with caring adults, they have better health outcomes over time even when they encounter adverse circumstances or when bad things happen.

Parents with PTSD report more parenting and child behavior problems, lower parenting satisfaction, more family violence, and poorer parent-child relationships than parents without PTSD (Leen-Feldner et al., 2011). Parents in our study admitted, "*I know how my children wish to play, socialize with me, but I don't have any interest in this world. I let them go by themselves and stay at home alone.*"

Each specific PTSD symptom cluster has its own consequences for parenting. The more a parent has PTSD symptoms, the more their parenting style is affected. These parental attitudes have a great impact on their children who will also exhibit trauma-related symptoms.

Emotional Avoidance and Numbing

Among parents with emotional numbing, we have identified several characteristics in their interactions with their children: low parenting satisfaction, increased parent-child aggression, disengagement from the parent-child relationship, difficulty displaying warmth and empathy toward their children, and increased likelihood of identifying emotional and behavioral concerns in their children. When the children attempt to understand their parent's reaction to them, they describe it as an "overwhelming situation." They struggled to justify their parent's dysfunctional parenting and they explained, "*Tubona biturenze tukabyakira tukabana nabyo,*" we are overwhelmed by the situation and we calm down. We become vulnerable and we find that perhaps sorrow is a style of life, "Hari *igihe ngirango kubabara nibwo buryo bwiza bwo kubaho.*" For the children, there is a need to accept that they will continue to experience psychological and social pain without hope of their situation changing or their future improving.

Recent studies indicated that PTSD in parents has been associated with less positive engagement with their children, increased withdrawal, and greater avoidance of distress (Brockman et al., 2016). Disengagement and loss of interest are characteristics of parents with avoidance and numbing symptoms. They have lost interest in activities that they used to enjoy and they serve as a reminder of good memories that will never happen again.

Some parents recounted that memories of their childhood and events during their adolescent years that were supposed to be good memories were also marred by remembering traumatic events that had happened, such as being sexually abused by their peers while at a picnic. These parents found themselves becoming overprotective of their children because of their own past history of trauma. Parents also reported that visiting the genocide memorial sites together with their children was a painful reminder of the past and many decided to stop visiting.

Other mothers became numb and unsociable and distanced themselves from family and friends because of physical injuries, health conditions such as chronic disease, and having disabilities related to the genocide and they found that life had become meaningless. When asked about her current situation, one mother responded:

"Currently I have no taste of life. My body has been damaged by rape. I am suffering from HIV/AIDS. Where can I find happiness? Really everything in my life is a reminder to what (....), even the neglect of our children is a reminder of how we really obeyed our parents who no longer exist, and nowadays children are full of carelessness 'Imiteto'. They neither obey and nor recognize the role of parents (.....) so I don't have time to negotiate with them." "They change day to day without apparent reason, they have impaired communication and we are nothing in front of them. But I used to tell them every day that they should trust no one."

Children were deeply affected by their parents' behavior. They expressed feeling sad and hurt because they felt that their parents did not care for them and they were anxious and confused about why their parents were showing emotionally distant behavior. Some were frightened because they did not understand the cause of their parents' symptoms. Others felt frustrated, resentful, or angry and did not want to hear about their parents' problems anymore because the parents were unable or unwilling to communicate with them in a healthy manner. Some children expressed feeling that their mother blamed them for her problems and they resented feeling that she refused to discuss with them why she had PTSD symptoms.

Children reported that after some time, they gave up trying to communicate with their parent, were pessimistic because they felt that there was nothing positive about their relationship with their mother, and felt incapable about making their own decisions. A child shared: *"Since my birth up to now, I didn't see my parents being happy. I didn't benefit from their care or attention. Even in our home, we can't find a positive mood at all, then I find that this is the style of life. I decided it is better to stay calm, to decrease communication, and help myself. Maybe it is that living style that makes people describe me as a traumatized person."*

Another child said, *"When I analyze the behavior of my parents, I revisit my activities again and again because maybe it is related to my misbehavior. I am very confused about what happened to them. I continue my life as it is. I have a fear of talking with my mum but I feel always that I am slowly being attacked by the heart pain and I don't understand the reason."*

The emotional numbing and avoidance exhibited by the parents were due to chronic "unhealed heart wounds" or "intimba," which led to feeling hard-hearted, ungrateful, and uncertain toward other people, including their own children. Due to many difficulties with living conditions, severe trauma, and a lack of social support, the parents became unable to show warmth and/or interest in their children. No activity or creativity on the part of the children was recognized as positive and children felt that they must be the one to initiate engagement with their parents.

One child described the pain she felt when she thought about her relationship with her parents: *"I don't know if my parents really love me. Their temperament is very inconsistent. Whatever I do, it is considered meaningless even if it may contribute to the best interest of the entire family. I am very shocked by the ingratitude of my parents. It breaks my heart having parents who don't appreciate my efforts in household activities, school performance, and relationship with others. They don't value anything I do. Hence, I am suffering from chronic heart wounds and even me, I can't appreciate the efforts of anybody."*

Children saw their parents like "a tree," to mean very unresponsive, hard-hearted, incapable of being moved to pity or tenderness, and unfeeling. Parents tended to be preoccupied with their own problems and were insensitive to their children's needs. *A child reported, "My parents have no pity. It seems they suffer too much to care about us and cover our needs. It is like they have no time for us and they are busy."*

Parents and close relatives display a lack of trust in the children, which provoked feelings of uncertainty, insecurity, and a deep sense of sadness in the children when they realized that the family has lost trust in them. They did not feel safe or protected and hid their emotional vulnerability, often becoming depressed or traumatized.

One child stated: *"I am nothing in front of my parent and our relatives. 'ndi ruvumwa, icyohe, ikirara ntacyo nakora ngo bakizere' All my daily life is under pressure and controlled by my parents and relatives. My heart is really broken because I have no one with whom I can share my psychological pain. I used to hear people saying that my maternal grandfather was a kind man, and he died during the genocide, hence several times I regret for not having him near me. I wish he could be back and use his kindness to help me."*

Alterations in Arousal and Reactivity

Research shows that parental anger is related to increased parenting stress and unhappiness, which in turn provoke negative and ambiguous child behaviors (Pidgeon & Sanders, 2009). It has also been shown that survivors with PTSD frequently have insomnia related to hyper-arousal symptoms.

Chronic lack of sleep provokes irritability and even chronic headaches, thus making the parent's tolerance level low. Parents' difficulty with concentration, managing fear, shame, guilt,,, and anger all contribute to their lack of self-control and harsh punishment of their children (Leen-Feldner et al., 2011).

The majority of children in the study stated that their parents punished them harshly. The parents provided explanation for the strict parenting and harsh punishment like they were worried that their children would lose values and discipline that were the culture of their lost family member. This was especially true for widows who were single parents. Parents stated that they needed their children to grow up quickly and become decision makers in spite of their young age. They wanted their children to become good role models in their neighborhood so that they could not be looked down upon because they were orphans. Harsh punishment was also related to parental intolerance of typical child and adolescent behaviors and a lack of management of such behaviors. The parents stated that they could not manage their children's behavior without harsh punishment and strict control over their children. Interestingly, some parents explained that they used harsh punishment as an attempt to forcibly transform the children into the lost family member. They believed that lost family members are always alive in their children. For others, children had no value, and they considered them as not lasting long in the world because a traumatic event could happen at any time and kill them suddenly.

A mother explained her perspective, *"Really the children have no great value. Yes, we know there is a need of giving birth but I believe that there is no hope to be with them until the end of my life. I am not supportive to their noise when they are playing, I sometimes feel attacked, and hence I am in continuous misunderstanding with them."*

Parents frequently told their children that they had no value and physically and verbally abused them. As a result, the children felt worthless and saw themselves as having no value within the family or community. These children exhibited poor school performance, poor attachment to family, inadequate social skills, chronic symptoms of trauma, and acting out behaviors.

The parents and community considered these children as unimportant and often they were told, "You will achieve nothing in your life." In turn, the children learned to depend only on themselves and did not consult their parents for help with decision-making. This resulted in parents condemning the children as having a rebellious and liberal attitude.

"Since I was ten years old, I lived alone with my paternal aunt because my parents were much traumatized and were incapable of caring for me. My maternal aunt was also traumatized even up until now but at least she has financial means to take care of me. She used to mistreat me, ignore my request and she provided me every time harsh punishment and no any other support she provided to me. Due to such maternal aunt attitudes I used to do all household activities but I cut down any kind of communication with her. I couldn't even told her the basics needs like clothes, school materials. To cut down communication induced my paternal aunt always said, 'Children were those who were exterminated I know that nowadays children will never help us as we wish. They couldn't accept parents' guidance which is the reason why I have no time to lose for them' one child reported."

Negative Alterations in Cognitions and Mood

The relationship between parents and their children is directly affected by the parents' negative beliefs and expectations about themselves and their feelings that they do not deserve the love of their children. They were constantly frustrated because they felt the need to be good parents but did not have the capacity to fulfill their responsibilities.

Feeling alienated from others (detachment, estrangement) and constricted affect (inability to experience positive emotions, numbing) made parents feel absent with their children.

Parents reported that they felt they participate in their own life and in the life of their children as if they were living in an empty shell and not living in the present. They were locked in their emotional past of intolerable heartache.

The parents yearned for the family members who were killed during the genocide and believed that *"none can be more important and successful than our lost people."* In-depth discussions with the children revealed that their parents gave more importance to the deceased family members and consequently they were raised with emotional pain and traumatic grief for relatives they never knew. They stated that they felt that they had an "empty family." They learned from their parents that they would never measure up to the deceased family members who had been idealized. They had a need to know more details about what happened during the genocide or the war. The children have extreme feelings of nostalgia, sentimental longing, or wistful affection for the lost family members. They felt obliged to want to know those lost family members and stated, "*We will never forget them, their strength is ours and we will try to fill in the vacuum.*" However, some children did not know what happened to their parents. They explained that the genocide was a mystery, and it was an extraordinary and incomprehensible event. "*We know that genocide has happened, however until now no one was able to tell me really how it was.*"

According to the results found in the study, we suggest that trauma transmission among genocide survivors may be related to problems with parenting and attachment styles, both of which are impacted by parents' symptoms of PTSD (see Fig. 1). Secondly, while the parent's PTSD was not enough to cause trauma in the children, it interacted with environmental factors which exacerbated children's trauma symptoms.

Conclusion

A significant number of survivors of the Genocide against Tutsi are suffering from PTSD and other trauma-related difficulties such as depression, traumatic grief, and anxiety disorders (Munyandamutsa et al., 2012; Mutuyimana et al., 2019), all of which have a significant impact on parenting (Brockman et al., 2016). More specifically, PTSD symptoms affect parent-child attachment and bonding, parental communication styles, and coping strategies in addition to feelings of hopelessness about the future. Several studies identified promising mechanisms through which PTSD symptoms may influence specific parenting difficulties. Brockman et al. (2016) found that while PTSD symptoms influenced parental distress avoidance, higher experiential avoidance was associated with less positive engagement with children.

The work of Sherman et al. (2015) delineated several ways in which PTSD symptoms may directly influence parent-child functioning by implicating communication as a problem area and by linking specific symptoms of PTSD to areas of difficulty.

Decades of research shows that parents with mental illness, including PTSD, are more likely to utilize ineffective behaviors in parenting young children. Research suggests that PTSD negatively impacts myriad parenting outcomes, including parenting satisfaction, parental engagement, and quality of parent-child relationships. In particular, these findings have begun to elucidate how parental PTSD might increase the risk of maladaptive parenting behaviors in the context of discipline encounters to ultimately negatively impact child outcomes (Sherman et al., 2015).

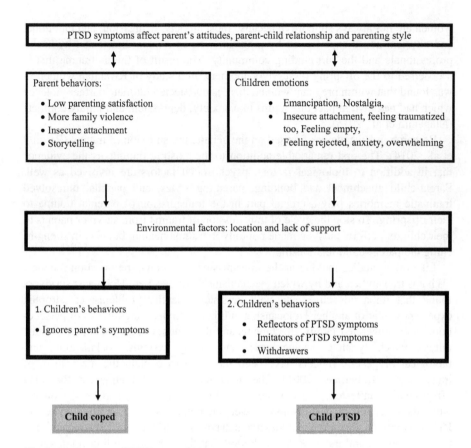

Fig. 1 Mechanisms of PTSD transmission process

The living conditions of the survivors which were derived from the experiences of genocidal violence, torture, and its aftermath affected the child-parent relationship. Parents demonstrated several styles of parenting: they closed themselves off emotionally to their children because of some fatalistic fear of being hurt when their child would die because of an expected catastrophe. They also distanced themselves from their children because of their suffering and lack of ability to trust or to have positive feelings for anyone including their own children. Factors such as environmental stress, maternal anxiety, bereavement and loss, intimate partner violence, and exposure to acute disasters all have an impact on the pregnant mother's health and ultimately upon the normal development of the fetus.

Family distress causes problems in the relationship between adults that are, in turn, linked to less effective parenting—a complex notion that involves insufficient surveillance, lack of control over the child's behavior, lack of warmth and support, inconsistency, and displays of aggression or hostility by parents or older siblings (McClelland, 2000). The attitudes of the community toward traumatized pregnant women are not always supportive because most anxiety, depression, and emotional and physical abuse experienced by pregnant women remain undetected by health professionals and the surrounding community. The result of this is trauma that is transferred to the offspring of survivor mothers. In a study of Rwandan women, it was found that within pregnant women there is undetected intimate partner violence which had negative impact on victims like anxiety, depression, and family conflicts (Ntaganira et al., 2015).

Research in Rwanda has focused on the genetic transmission of trauma (Perroud et al., 2014). The first remarkable addition to the existing findings is the evidence that in addition to biological factors, psychosocial factors are involved as well. Parent-child attachment and bonding, parenting styles, and parents' unresolved traumatic memories play a crucial part in the transmission of parental trauma to their offspring. To stop the cycle of transmission of trauma from survivor parents to their children, efforts must be made not only in trauma healing but also in strengthening the parent-child relationship.

Like other studies looking at the transmission of trauma, the question remains, "What is transmitted and by which mechanisms?" Studies with Holocaust survivors found that impaired self-esteem with persistent identity problems, catastrophic expectancy, fear of another Holocaust, annihilation anxiety, nightmares of persecution, and exaggerated family attachments and dependency were the contents transmitted. Psychodynamic, sociocultural, and family systems, socialization, and biological or genetic models have been theorized to explain the mechanism of transmission (Kellerman, 2001). The inherited legacy of trauma for Rwandan offspring is manifested as a longing, a feeling of emptiness, and heart wounds, while the mechanisms of transmission were attachment styles, parenting style, and PTSD symptoms. Parenting attitudes and behaviors contribute to PTSD transmission to their children and increase the likelihood that their children will develop symptoms of PTSD (Babcock Fenerci et al., 2016).

Certain parenting attitudes and behaviors might add additional variance in predicting the intergenerational transmission of trauma-related distress, especially given that such attitudes and behaviors have been conceptualized as contributing to the overall parent-child relationship (Gerard, 1994). Among mothers with PTSD their relationship with their offspring followed one of the three types of parenting styles: silent parents, disclosure parents, and hesitant parents. Their children responded to these parenting styles in one of the four ways: children who withdrew, children who ignored their parents' destructive and demeaning comments and actions, children who imitated their parents' emotional and psychological dysfunction, and children who reflected on their situation and relationship with their parents. In spite of a significant percentage of victims of the Genocide against Tutsi who developed PTSD, not all victims developed PTSD and not all children assimilated PTSD from their parents.

The group of children who ignored their parents' and relatives' negative and destructive comments and behaviors were best able to cope effectively with the difficult parent-child relationship, lack of attachment, and inadequate parental management.

As we have seen the harmful effects of trauma affecting an entire group of the general population, there is a need to stop the cycle and become better adept at providing early emotional and psychosocial support to victims of trauma and to assist parents in raising emotionally and psychologically healthy offspring in spite of the parent's PTSD. There is also a need to determine if resilience in children is also transferred in a similar or different way as trauma.

References

Ahmadzadeh, G. H., & Malekian, A. (2004). Aggression, anxiety, and social development in adolescent children of war veterans with PTSD versus those of non-veterans. *Journal of Research in Medical Sciences: The Official Journal of Isfahan University of Medical Sciences, 9*(5), 231–234.

Albeck, H. J. (1993). Intergenerational consequences of trauma reframing taps in treatment theory: A second generation perspectives. In M. O. Williams & J. F. Sommer (Eds.), *Handbook of post traumatic therapy*. Greenwood Press.

American Psychiatric Association. (2013). *Diagnostic and statistical manual of mental disorders* (5th ed.). American Psychiatric Association.

Ammerman, R. T., Putnam, F. W., Chard, K. M., Stevens, J., & Van Ginkel, J. B. (2012). PTSD in depressed mothers in home visitation. *Psychol Trauma, 4*, a0023062.

Babcock Fenerci, R. L., Chu, A. T., & DePrince, A. P. (2016). Intergenerational transmission of trauma-related distress: Maternal betrayal trauma, Parenting Attitudes, and Behaviors. *Journal of Aggression, Maltreatment & Trauma, 25*(4), 382–399. https://doi.org/10.1080/10926771.2015.1129655

Bandura, A. (1977). *Social learning theory*. Prentice-Hall.

Baum, R. (2012). Trans-generational trauma and repetition in the body: The groove of the wound. *An International Journal for Theory, Research and Practice, 8*, 34–42.

Berckmoes, L. H., Eichelsheim, V., Rutayisire, T., Richters, A., & Hola, B. (2017). How legacies of genocide are transmitted in the family environment: A qualitative study of two generations in Rwanda. *Societies, 7*, 24. https://doi.org/10.3390/soc7030024

Blumberg. (1977). Treatment of the abused child and the child abuser. *American Journal of Psychotherapy, 31*, 204–215.

Bowers, M. E., & Yehuda, R. (2016). Intergenerational transmission of stress in humans. *Neuropsychopharmacology, 41*, 232–244.

Brockman, C., Snyder, J., Gewirtz, A., Gird, S. R., Quattlebaum, J., Schmidt, N., et al. (2016). Relationship of service members' deployment trauma, PTSD symptoms, and experiential avoidance to post deployment family reengagement. *Journal of Family Psychology, 30*, 52–62. https://doi.org/10.1037/fam0000152

Courtois, C. (1988). *Healing the incest wound: Adult survivors in therapy*. W.W. Norton & Company.

Danieli, Y. (Ed.). (1998). *International handbook of multigenerational legacies of trauma*. Plenum.

Davidson, A. C., & Mellor, D. J. (2012). The adjustment of children of Australian Vietnam veterans: Is there evidence for the transgenerational transmission of the effects of war related trauma? *The Australian and New Zealand Journal of Psychiatry, 35*, 345–351.

Dekel, R., & Goldblatt, H. (2008). Is there intergenerational transmission of trauma? The case of combat veterans' children. *American Journal of Orthopsychiatry, 78*, 281–289.

Felsen, I. (1998). Trans-generational transmission effects of holocaust: The North America research perspective. In Y. Danieli (Ed.), *International handbooks of multigenerational legacies of trauma*. Plenum.

Field, N. P., Muong, S., & Sochanvimean, V. (2013). Parental styles in the intergenerational transmission of trauma stemming from the Khmer rouge regime in Cambodia. *American Journal of Orthopsychiatry, 83*, 483–494.

Gerard, A. B. (1994). *Parent–child relationship inventory (PCRI) manual*. WPS.

Hartsough, D. M., & Myers, D. G. (1985). *Disaster work and mental health: Prevention and control of stress among workers*. National Institute of Mental Health.

Herman, J. (1992). Trauma and recovery. New York: Basic books. Jacobsen, L. K., Sweeney, C. G., & Racusin, G. R. (1993). Group psycho-therapy for children of fathers with PTSD: Evidence of psychopathology emerging in the group process. *Journal of Child and Adolescent Group Therapy, 3*, 103–120.

Juni, S. (2016). Second-generation Holocaust survivors: Psychological, theological, and moral challenges. *Journal of Trauma & Dissociation, 17*, 97–111.

Karam, E. G., Friedman, M. J., Hill, E. D., et al. (2014). Cumulative traumas and risk thresh olds: 12-month PTSD in the world mental health (WMH) surveys. *Depression and Anxiety, 31*, 130.

Kellerman, N. P. F. (1999). *Bibliography: Children of holocaust survivors*. AMCHA, the National Israeli Center for psychosocial support of Holocaust survivors and second generation, Jerusalem. http://www.judymeschel.com/coshpsych.htm

Kellerman, N. P. F. (2001). Perceived parental rearing behaviors in children of Holocaust survivors. *Israel Journal of Psychiatry, 38*(1), 58–68.

Kellermann, N. P. (2013). Epigenetic transmission of holocaust trauma: Can nightmares be inherited. *The Israel Journal of Psychiatry and Related Sciences, 50*, 33–39.

Klein-Parker, F. (1988). Dominant attitudes of adult children of holocaust survivors toward their parents. In J. P. Wilson, Z. Harel, & B. Kahana (Eds.), *The plenum series on stress and coping. Human adaptation to extreme stress: From the Holocaust to Vietnam* (pp. 193–218). Plenum Press.

Lee, D. J., Warner, C. H., & Hoge, C. W. (2015). Posttraumatic stress disorder screening in the U.S. military and VA populations. In *Posttraumatic stress disorder and related diseases in combat veterans* (pp. 13–26). Springer.

Leen-Feldner, E. W., Feldner, M. T., Bunaciu, L., & Blumenthal, H. (2011). Associations between parental posttraumatic stress disorder and both offspring internalizing problems and parental aggression within the National Comorbidity Survey-Replication. *Journal of Anxiety Disorders, 25*, 169–175.

Lehrner, A., & Yehuda, R. (2018). Cultural trauma and epigenetic inheritance. *Development and Psychopathology, 30*(5), 1763–1777. https://doi.org/10.1017/S0954579418001153

Lowin, R.G. (1983). Cross-generational transmission of pathology in Jewish families of Holocaust survivors. California School of Professional Psychology, San Diego. Dissertation Abstracts International, 44, 3533.

McCann, L., & Pearlman, L. A. (1990). Vicarious traumatization: A framework for understanding the psychological effects of working with victims. *Journal of Traumatic Stress, 3*, 131–149.

McClelland, A. (2000). *Impacts of poverty on children, brotherhood comment, Brotherhood of St Laurence*. Scientific Research.

Meaney, M. J., & Szyf, M. (2005). Environmental programming of stress responses through DNA methylation: Life at the interface between a dynamic environment and a fixed genome. *Dialogues in Clinical Neuroscience, 7*, 103–123.

Munyandamutsa, N., Nkubamugisha, M. P., Gex-Fabry, M., & Eytan, A. (2012). Mental and physical health in Rwanda 14 years after the genocide. *Social Psychiatry and Psychiatric Epidemiology, 47*(11), 1753–1756. https://doi.org/10.1007/s00127-012-0494-912

Mutuyimana, C., Sezibera, V., Nsabimana, E., et al. (2019). PTSD prevalence among resident mothers and their offspring in Rwanda 25 years after the 1994 genocide against the Tutsi. *BMC Psychol, 7*, 84. https://doi.org/10.1186/s40359-019-0362-4

Ntaganira, J., et al. (2015). Intimate partner violence among pregnant women in Rwanda. *BMC Women's Health, 8*, 17. https://doi.org/10.1186/1472-6874-8-17

Perroud, N., Rutembesa, E., Paoloni-Giacobino, A., Mutabaruka, J., Mutesi, L., Stenz, L., Malafosse, A., & Karege, F. (2014). The Tutsi genocide and transgenerational transmission of maternal stress: Epigenetics and biology of the HPA Axis. *The World Journal of Biological Psychiatry, 15*, 334–345.

Pham, P. N., Weinstein, H. M., & Longman, T. (2004). Trauma and PTSD symptoms in Rwanda: Implications for attitudes toward justice and reconciliation. *JAMA, 292*, 602–612.

Pidgeon, A. M., & Sanders, M. R. (2009). Attributions, parental anger and risk of maltreatment. *International Journal of Child Health and Human Development, 2*, 57–69.

Rieder, H., & Elbert, T. (2013). Rwanda-lasting imprints of a genocide: trauma, mental health and Psychosocial conditions in survivors, former prisoners and their children. *Conflict and Health, 7*, 6.

Rosenheck, R., & Nathan, P. (1985). Secondary traumatization in children of Vietnam veterans. *Hospital and Community Psychiatry, 5*, 538–539.

Roth, M., Neuner, F., & Elbert, T. (2014). Transgenerational consequences of PTSD: Risk factors for the mental health of children whose mothers have been exposed to the Rwandan genocide. *International Journal of Mental Health Systems, 8*, 12.

Ruscio, A. M., Weathers, F. W., King, L. A., & King, D. W. (2002). Male war zone veterans' perceived relationships with their children: The importance of emotional numbing. *Journal of Traumatic Stress, 15*, 351–357.

Schechter, D.S., & Willheim, E. (2009). Disturbances of attachment and parental psychopathology in early childhood. *Child and Adolescent Psychiatric Clinics of North America, 18*(3), 665–687.

Schindler, K. (2010). *Who does what in a household dafter genocide? Evidence from Rwanda.* German Institute for Economic Research.

Schwartz, S., Dohrenwend, B. P., & Levav, I. (1994). Non-genetic familial transmission of psychiatric disorders? Evidence from children of Holocaust survivors. *Journal of Health and Social Behavior, 35*, 385–403.

Sherman, M. D., Larsen, J., Straits-Troster, K., Erbes, C., & Tassey, J. (2015). Veteran–child communication about parental PTSD: A mixed methods pilot study. *Journal of Family Psychology, 29*, 595–603. https://doi.org/10.1037/fam0000124

Showalter S. E. (2010). Compassion fatigue: what is it? Why does it matter? Recognizing the symptoms, acknowledging the impact, developing the tools to prevent compassion fatigue, and strengthen the professional already suffering from the effects. *The American Journal of Hospice & Palliative Care, 27*(4), 239–242. https://doi.org/10.1177/1049909109354096

Shriraa, A., Mollova, B., & Mudahogora, C. (2019). Complex PTSD and intergenerational transmission of distress and resilience among Tutsi genocide survivors and their offspring: A preliminary report. *Psychiatry Research, 271*, 121–123.

Sigal, J., & Weinfeld, M. (1992). *Trauma and rebirth: Intergenerational effects of Holocaust.* Praeger. https://doi.org/10.2307/2076314

Straus, S. (2004). How many perpetrators were there in the Rwandan genocide? An estimate. *Journal of Genocide Research, 6*(1), 85–98. https://doi.org/10.1080/1462352042000194728

Yehuda, R., & Bierer, L. M. (2008). Transgenerational transmission of cortisol and PTSD risk. *Progress in Brain Research, 167*, 121–135. https://doi.org/10.1016/S0079-6123(07)67009-5

Wimalawansa, S. J. (2014). Causes and risk factors for posttraumatic stress disorder: The importance of right diagnosis and treatment. *Asian Journal of Medical Sciences, 5*(2), 1.

Yehuda, R., Bierer, L. M., Schmeidler, J., Aferiat, D. H., Breslau, I., & Dolan, S. (2000). Low cortisol and risk for PTSD in adult offspring of Holocaust survivors. *American Journal of Psychiatry, 157*(8), 1252–1259.

Yehuda, R., et al. (2014). Influences of maternal and paternal PTSD on epigenetic regulation of the glucocorticoid receptor gene in Holocaust survivor offspring. *American Journal of Psychiatry, 171*(8), 872–880.

Part IV
Poverty and Child Mental Health: Case Examples

Food Insecurity, Malnutrition, and Child Developmental and Behavioral Outcomes in Ghana

Lois Aryee, Emmanuel A. Gyimah, Melissa Chapnick, and Lora Iannotti

Introduction

The second Sustainable Development Goal (SDG 2) seeks to "end hunger, achieve food security and improved nutrition and promote sustainable agriculture" by 2030 (United Nations Statistics Division [UNSD], n.d.). Instead of disaggregating the various areas, SDG 2 combines hunger, food security, nutrition, and sustainable agriculture in an attempt to encourage stakeholders to adopt an integrated and holistic approach when taking action. In addition to the 2030 Agenda, the United Nations (UN) launched the United Nations Decade of Action on Nutrition (2016–2025). These initiatives demonstrate commitment on the part of the international community to eradicate hunger, prevent all forms of malnutrition worldwide, and achieve food security.

Although global food insecurity and undernourishment saw a steady decline between 2000 and 2015, data from the most recent years suggest rising prevalence globally, especially in sub-Saharan Africa (Food and Agriculture Organization (FAO), 2017; Food and Agriculture Organization (FAO), 2018b). In Ghana, an estimated 5% of the population, representing roughly 1.2 million people, are food insecure, and approximately two million people are at risk of becoming food insecure (Hjelm & Dasori, 2012).

In this chapter, we first present an overview of the related problems and determinants of food insecurity and malnutrition, both globally and in the context of Ghana. We then examine the consequences of food insecurity and malnutrition on child health, development, and behavioral outcomes in the country. The chapter concludes with a discussion of policy, programming, and research solutions implemented to date to confront issues of malnutrition and food insecurity in Ghana.

L. Aryee · E. A. Gyimah · M. Chapnick · L. Iannotti (✉)
Brown School, Washington University in St. Louis, St. Louis, MO, USA
e-mail: liannotti@wustl.edu

© Springer Nature Switzerland AG 2022
F. M. Ssewamala et al. (eds.), *Child Behavioral Health in Sub-Saharan Africa*,
https://doi.org/10.1007/978-3-030-83707-5_12

The Problem

Food Insecurity and Malnutrition: Definitions. The concept of *food security* has evolved over the years. When it emerged in the mid-1970s, during the global food crisis, its initial focus was on food supply, that is, ensuring food availability and, to an extent, price stability of basic food at national and international levels (Clay, 2002). However, its definition has expanded to include physical, social, and economic access to sufficient, safe, and nutritious food that meets dietary needs and food preferences, enabling one to live an active and healthy life (World Food Summit [WFS], 1996). Moreover, food security is a multidimensional phenomenon, encompassing food *availability, access, utilization,* and *stability* (Table 1).[1]

Food insecurity measures are usually indirect. Measurements are based on food balance sheets, surveys of household income and expenditure, individual intake surveys, nutritional outcomes/status (using anthropometric surveys), and people's perception of hunger and food insecurity using qualitative methods (Napoli et al., 2011). The Food and Agriculture Organization's (FAO) traditional indicator used to measure hunger and food insecurity is the prevalence of undernourishment, which captures the share of undernourished people in the world population (Food and Agriculture Organization (FAO), 2018b). Recently, this measure has been combined with the prevalence of severe food insecurity, estimated from data collected using the Food Insecurity Experience Scale (FIES). FIES is a direct interview tool that measures the ability of adult individuals worldwide to access food (FAO, 2017).

Table 1 Dimensions of food security (FAO, 2008)

Availability	There has to be adequate quantities of food of suitable quality that is obtained through either imports, domestic production, or food aid on a consistent basis.
Access	Individuals need to have sufficient resources to acquire available nutritionally adequate and safe foods. They should not have to resort to socially unacceptable ways in order to acquire food. Access covers physical, social, and economic dimensions
Utilization	Utilization conceptualizes the way the body obtains and uses nutrients in food consumed. Utilization encompasses not only the consumption of nutritious food but also covers food processing and storage, diversity of diet, adequate sanitation and health services, good feeding practices, and distribution of food within the household, among others. This dimension considers the nonfood aspect of food security
Stability	The concept of stability refers to the fact that at *all times*, a population, household, or individual must have access to adequate food. Acute or recurring emergencies (such as adverse weather conditions, rising food prices, unemployment, and political instability) should not affect access and availability to food

Source: Food and Agriculture Organization of the United Nations, 2008, An Introduction to the Basic Concepts of Food Security, http://www.fao.org/3/al936e/al936e.pdf. Used with permission

---

[1] Food and Agriculture Organization [FAO], 2008

Table 2 Forms of malnutrition (WHO, 2010, , 2018b, , 2018c)

Stunting	Length/height-for-age Z score less than 2 standard deviations below the WHO Child Growth Standards median Chronic form of undernutrition
Wasting	Weight-for-height Z score less than 2 standard deviations below the WHO Child Growth Standards median Acute form of undernutrition Usually indicates recent and severe weight loss
Underweight	Weight-for-age Z score less than 2 standard deviations below the WHO Child Growth Standards median An underweight child may be stunted, wasted, or both.
Nutrient-related malnutrition	Inadequate intake or excess of micronutrients (vitamins and minerals) In global health, iodine, iron, and vitamin A are the most important because deficiencies in these micronutrients represent a major threat to health and development of populations worldwide, most especially for children and women in low-income countries.
Overweight and obesity	Accumulation of abnormal or excess fat that affects health For children, age needs to be considered when defining overweight and obesity. For children under 5 years of age: 1. Overweight is weight-for-height greater than 2 standard deviations above WHO Child Growth Standards median. 2. Obesity is weight-for-height greater than 3 standard deviations above the WHO Child Growth Standards median. For children aged between 5 and 19 years: 1. Overweight is weight-for-height greater than 1 standard deviation above the WHO Growth Reference median. 2. Obesity is weight-for-height greater than 2 standard deviations above the WHO Growth Reference median

Malnutrition is generally included within the *utilization* dimension of food security. We elaborate further on the condition due to its consequences for child development and behavioral health. Malnutrition refers to deficiencies, excesses, or imbalances in a person's intake of energy and/or nutrients (World Health Organization (WHO), 2018b). It is an umbrella term for three groups of conditions (Table 2)[2]: 1. **undernutrition**—includes stunting (low height-for-age), wasting (low weight-for-height), and underweight (low weight-for-age); 2. **micronutrient-related malnutrition**—includes micronutrient deficiencies or micronutrient excess; and 3. **overweight, obesity, and diet-related noncommunicable diseases** (such as some cancers, diabetes, heart diseases, and stroke) (WHO, 2010; , 2018b; , 2018c).

Global Trends. Globally, there was a steady decline in the prevalence of undernourishment from 14.5% in 2005 to 10.6% in 2015. However, the global prevalence has been increasing since 2016 and reached 10.9% in 2017 (Food and Agriculture Organization (FAO), 2018b). Estimates show that the absolute number of undernourished people in the world was around 821 million in 2017, an increase from

---

[2]World Health Organization [WHO], 2010, 2018c, 2018b

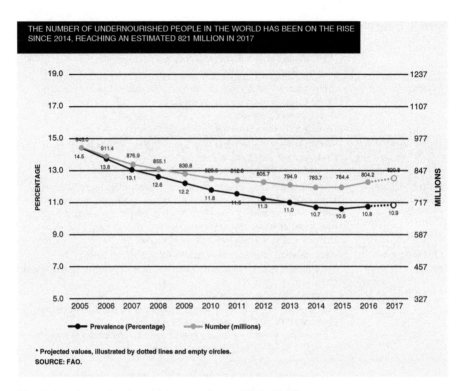

Fig. 1 Prevalence of undernourishment estimates (FAO, 2018b)

804 million in 2016 (Food and Agriculture Organization (FAO), 2018b) (Fig. 1).[3] In the same year, Africa had the highest prevalence of undernourishment, with almost 21% of the population—over 256 million Africans—affected by undernourishment (Food and Agriculture Organization (FAO), 2018b). The situation in sub-Saharan Africa was even more dire; an estimated one out of five people in the region may have experienced chronic food deprivation in 2017, representing 23.2% of the population (Food and Agriculture Organization (FAO), 2018b). Western Africa saw a significant increase in the prevalence of undernourishment from 12.8% in 2016 to 15.1% in 2017. This has been attributed to factors such as droughts, rising food prices, and an almost stagnant growth of real per capita gross domestic product (GDP) (Food and Agriculture Organization (FAO), 2018b).

Using data based on FIES, the Food and Agriculture Organization (FAO) (2018b) estimates that in 2017, 10.2% of the world's population was exposed to severe food insecurity, corresponding to approximately 770 million people. Regional data varied, ranging from 1.4% in Northern America and Europe to almost 30% in Africa (Fig. 2).[4] Africa had the highest prevalence of food insecurity (29.8%) and number

[3] Food and Agriculture Organization [FAO], 2018b
[4] Food and Agriculture Organization [FAO], 2018b

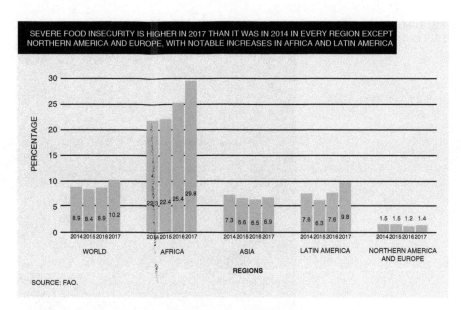

Fig. 2 Global prevalence of severe food insecurity (FAO, 2018b)

of people experiencing severe food insecurity (374.9 million), followed by Asia (6.9% and 311.9 million).

Global estimates from UNICEF, WHO, and the World Bank (2018) indicate that in 2017, among children under age five, 150.8 million (22.2%) were stunted, 50.5 million (7.5%) were wasted or acutely malnourished (very low weight-for-height), and 38.3 million were overweight, with Africa and Asia bearing the greatest burden of all forms of malnutrition. For stunting, in absolute numbers, Asia exceeded all regions with 83.6 million stunted children, followed by Africa (58.7 million), Latin America and the Caribbean (5.1 million), and Oceania and Northern America (0.5 million each). Trends indicate a decreasing number and percentage of young children stunted globally, down from 198.4 million (32.7%) in 2000. However, Africa is the only region where the absolute number of stunted children has increased. Of the 50.5 million children under age 5 who were wasted, 16.4 million of them were severely wasted. More than half of all wasted children in the world live in Asia (35 million), followed by Africa (13.8 million), Latin America and the Caribbean (0.7 million), and Oceania (0.1 million).

The Situation in Ghana. Ghana is located along the Gulf of Guinea in West Africa and shares its borders with Burkina Faso in the north, Togo to the east, and Cote d'Ivoire to the west. As of 2017, Ghana's population was approximately 28.83 million, with an annual growth rate of 2.2% (World Bank, 2018). The per capita gross domestic product (GDP) was 1663.2 USD in 2017, and the GDP per capita growth is 5.7% (World Bank, 2018). Prior to 2019, Ghana was divided into ten

Fig. 3 Map of Ghana (The DHS Program, 2017)

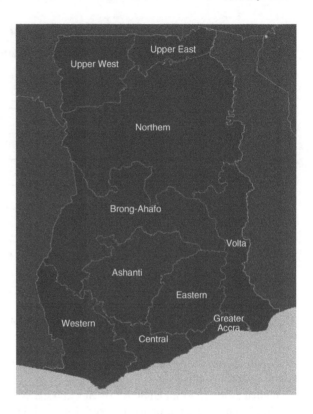

regions: Greater Accra, Brong Ahafo, Ashanti, Western, Central, Eastern, Volta, Northern, Upper East, and Upper West Regions.[5] Although Ghana currently has 16 regions, regional data and references cited in this chapter used data from the ten former administrative regions (Fig. 3).[6]

Prevalence, Trends, Disparities. Despite great strides made to reduce poverty and promote economic development in Ghana, food insecurity and malnutrition remain a challenge. An estimated two million Ghanaians are at risk of being food insecure, and half a million people of this population are located in the three northern regions—Northern, Upper East, and Upper West Regions. The remaining 1.5 million live in the other seven regions, with the largest being in Brong Ahafo (11%), followed by Ashanti (10%), Eastern (8%), and Volta (7%) regions (Hjelm & Dasori, 2012).

An estimated 5% of Ghana's population, representing roughly 1.2 million people, are food insecure (Hjelm & Dasori, 2012). Regional disparities exist within the country, with the three northern regions having the greatest burden of food-insecure

---

[5] A referendum in December 2019 led to divisions of the Brong Ahafo, Northern, Western, and Volta regions, leading to the creation of six new regions. See *Figure 3* for pre-2019 administrative map of Ghana.

[6] The DHS Program, 2017

households. The Upper East region has the highest proportion of food-insecure households, with an estimated 28% of their population being either moderately or severely food insecure (Hjelm & Dasori, 2012). In the Upper West and Northern regions, the prevalence of food-insecure households is 16% and 10%, respectively (Hjelm & Dasori, 2012). The combined absolute number of people who are food insecure in the three regions is approximately more than 680,000 people (Hjelm & Dasori, 2012). A study that explored months of adequate household food provisioning,[7] a measure used to characterize food insecurity in areas that rely mostly on subsistence farming for household consumption, found that farmer households in sampled communities in Northern Ghana[8] experienced between 3 and 7 months of food-insecure periods. The Upper East experienced the longest food shortage period of 6 months, with the Northern and Upper West regions following closely with 5 months of food shortage (Quaye, 2008). According to Ghana's 2014 Demographic and Health Survey Report, 19% of children under the age of 5 were stunted, 5% were wasted, and 11% were underweight (Ghana Statistical Service [GSS], Ghana Health Service [GHS],, & ICF International, 2015). Although there has been an overall declining trend in the percentage of children under 5 years who are stunted, wasted, and underweight, levels of child undernutrition still remain high in Ghana. The proportion of stunted children decreased from 35% in 2003 to 19% in 2014, while the prevalence of childhood wasting decreased from 8% in 2003 to 5% in 2014. For underweight children, the prevalence decreased from 18% in 2003 to 11% in 2014 (GSS et al., 2015) (Fig. 4).[9] Indeed, Ghana has made progress in reducing the prevalence of child undernutrition. However, past childhood stunting in the country affects the current adult population. In 2012, Ghana's National Development Planning Commission (2016) estimated that nearly 5.5 million Ghanaian adults, representing 37% of adults aged 15–64, were stunted before the age of 5. They further estimated that past child undernutrition and related mortalities resulted in approximately $2.6 billion in productivity losses—about 6.4% of the national GDP at the time—during the same year.

Significant regional disparities exist in the prevalence of child undernutrition. For instance, the prevalence of stunting in the Northern Region is 33%, compared to 10% in the Greater Accra Region (Fig. 5).[10] The proportion of wasted children ranges from 3% in the Volta region to 9% in the Upper East Region. Underweight prevalence ranges from 6% in the Brong Ahafo Region to 20% in the Northern Region.

Micronutrient deficiencies in vitamin A, iron, and iodine also remain significant public health challenges in the country, primarily affecting young children and

---

[7] Months of adequate household food provisioning refer to the time between stock depletion and the next harvest (Bilinsky & Swindale, 2010).

[8] Northern Ghana is the collective name for the three Northern regions: Upper East, Upper West, and Northern regions.

[9] Ghana Statistical Service (GSS), Ghana Health Service (GHS), and ICF International, 2015

[10] Adapted from Amoaful (2016)

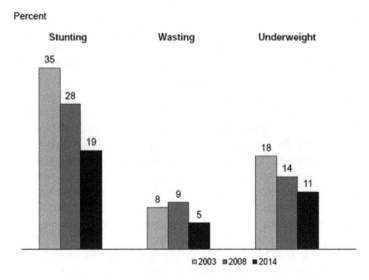

Fig. 4 Trends in nutritional status of children under Age 5, Ghana 2003-2014 (Ghana Statistical Service (GSS), Ghana Health Service (GHS), & ICF International, 2015)

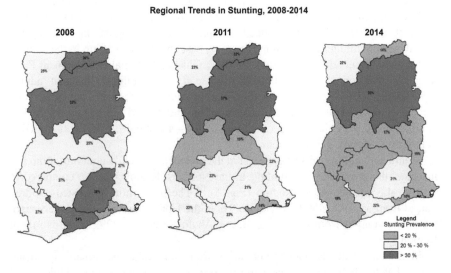

Fig. 5 Trends in stunting by region, 2008–2014 (Adapted from Amoaful, 2016)

women (GSS et al., 2015; United States Agency for International Development [USAID], 2014). The prevalence of child anemia decreased from 78% in 2008 to 66% in 2014 (GSS et al., 2015). Despite this marked decline, the prevalence of child anemia is still above the WHO's 40% threshold; child anemia prevalence above the 40% target is classified as a high public health concern (Pringle & Seal, 2013). Moreover, in the same year, the three northern regions had a significantly higher prevalence of child anemia—ranging from 73.8% to 82.1%—relative to other regions in the country (GSS et al., 2015).

Northern Ghana bears the greatest burden of food insecurity and consequent undernutrition in the country. These disparities point to critical determinants that will be discussed below and should be considered for appropriate targeting of programming and policy that can be most impactful for vulnerable populations.

Determinants of Malnutrition. The UNICEF conceptual framework on the determinants of malnutrition categorizes the causes of malnutrition into three levels: basic, underlying, and immediate (Fig. 6).[11] Basic causes represent broader contextual, structural, and societal determinants such as country-level policies and economic environment, culture, and gender norms. When these factors are not addressed, they undermine efforts taken to fight undernutrition. Underlying causes are household- and community-level factors that influence dietary intake and infectious disease, whereas immediate causes are related to inadequate dietary intake and infectious disease (UNICEF Evaluation Office, 2017).

Maternal factors. Undernutrition in Ghana is associated with a variety of maternal factors such as mother's BMI, age, education level, birth spacing/interval, marital status, and seeking prenatal or antenatal care during pregnancy.

Several studies have suggested that stunting in Ghanaian children was associated with lack of antenatal care during pregnancy, with stunting being more prevalent among children whose mothers did not receive prenatal care at least four times during pregnancy (Ali et al., 2017; Saaka & Galaa, 2016; Tette et al., 2015). Mother's age was also found to be positively associated with stunting and underweight, with younger mothers being more likely to have a malnourished child (Aheto et al., 2015; Darteh et al., 2014). Miah et al. (2016) found that marital status was a determinant of stunting; specifically, there was a positive association between stunting and households in which the husband had more than one wife.

There is evidence which suggests that Ghanaian women living in polygamous homes have lower dietary diversity because of competition with other wives for limited food and financial resources (Amugsi et al., 2016). Moreover, Ghanaian mothers living in polygamous households often have limited autonomy, and this significantly impacts their ability to make decisions on their own dietary needs as well as that of their children (Amugsi et al., 2016). Studies from Ghana have revealed that mothers with higher dietary diversity have children with better nutritional status (Amugsi et al., 2015; Saaka, 2012). The relationship between polygamous households and consequent child malnutrition should therefore be viewed in the vein of limited resources and mediating impact of maternal dietary diversity. In Northern Ghana, polygamous households are highly prevalent (Van Bodegom et al., 2012); this might explain the disproportionate burden of stunting in the region. Moreover, studies have indicated the presence of high child mortality rates—an established consequence of child undernutrition—in Northern polygamous households (Kanmiki et al., 2014; Van Bodegom et al., 2012).

---

[11] Black et al. (2008)

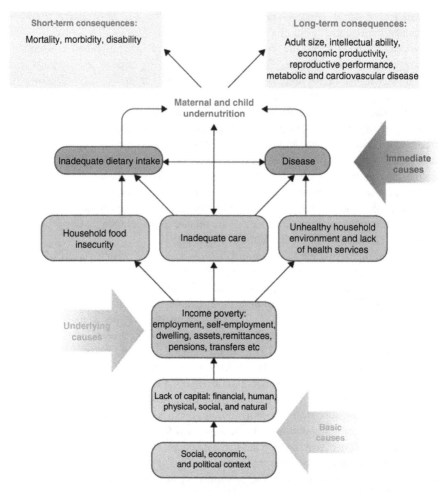

Fig. 6 UNICEF Conceptual Framework of the Determinants of Child Malnutrition (Black et al., 2008) (Reprinted from *The Lancet*, 371(9608), Robert E. Black, et al., Maternal and child undernutrition: global and regional exposures and health consequences, p. 243–260, Copyright 2008, with permission from Elsevier)

Shorter maternal height is also an established risk factor for child stunting and underweight; this relationship has been observed across low- and middle-income countries (Özaltin et al., 2010), in Northern Ghana (Ali et al., 2017), and in the rest of Ghana (Miah et al., 2016). Experts theorize that this relationship may be a result of an intergenerational cycle of malnutrition or growth failure—mothers who are stunted or underweight from childhood give birth to stunted or underweight children. Low maternal weight and inadequate dietary intake before and during pregnancy also affect the intergenerational vicious cycle (Ali et al., 2017; Miah et al., 2016; Özaltin et al., 2010). The probabilities of stunting, wasting, and underweight have also been found to be higher among Ghanaian children with low birthweight, compared to those born average or large in size (Aheto et al., 2015).

A mother's level of educational attainment is a predictor of child undernutrition, because education levels affect income generation and one's ability to purchase nutritious food, awareness of healthy behaviors, and good sanitation practices (Van De Poel et al., 2007). Studies in Ghana have found that mothers with lower levels of literacy and education were more likely to have stunted, wasted, or underweight children (Miah et al., 2016; Van De Poel et al., 2007). Generally, literacy rates, as well as rates of enrollment at the secondary and tertiary education levels, are lower for Ghanaian females relative to males (UNESCO Institute of Statistics, n.d.). With the established associations between maternal education and stunting, there is a strong imperative for equitable education as part of efforts aimed at reducing child undernutrition in Ghana.

Another maternal factor that affects child undernutrition in Ghana is birth spacing. When mothers give birth successively within short intervals, there is an increased risk for child undernutrition outcomes because it places a burden on the mother's nutritional and reproductive resources (Aheto et al., 2015; GSS et al., 2015; Van De Poel et al., 2007). Short birth spacing among Ghanaian women could be linked to Ghanaian cultural norms, which emphasize the importance of large families and therefore influence shorter birth intervals (Gyimah, 2005).

Feeding Practices. Different studies in Ghana have associated long duration of breastfeeding with higher rates of child undernutrition (Brakohiapa et al., 1988; Ross et al., 2014; Van De Poel et al., 2007); generally, these studies do not indicate whether the type of breastfeeding is exclusive or complementary. Beyond the recommended 6 months of exclusive breastfeeding, the WHO (2018a) recommends continued breastfeeding, along with complementary foods, for up to 24 months. About 50% of Ghanaian infants continue to breastfeed until they are 24 months, and the average duration of any breastfeeding in Ghana is about 21 months (GSS et al., 2015). Although these numbers align closely with the WHO's recommendations, Van De Poel et al. (2007) suggest that complementary foods may be lacking in most Ghanaian households where infants are breastfed for long periods of time; this may be a result of food insecurity or lack of resources to provide the infant with adequate nutrition. Moreover, longer duration of breastfeeding may signify infants' reluctance to eat other foods, as demonstrated in Brakohiapa et al.'s (1988) cohort of Ghanaian infants. It has been shown that prolonged breastfeeding predisposes a child to malnutrition, because the nutritional needs of the growing child may not be met solely with breastmilk (Brakohiapa et al., 1988).

For Northern Ghana, the median duration of any breastfeeding across the three regions in 2014 was high, ranging from 23 months to 25 months (GSS et al., 2015). Yet, there is evidence suggesting that delayed initiation of complementary feeding, inappropriate complementary feeding, and lack of dietary diversity remain as challenges and significant contributors to child undernutrition in Northern Ghana (Saaka et al., 2016).

Household Factors. Household factors that underlie child undernutrition in Ghana include large household size, food insecurity, inappropriate intrahousehold food distribution, and inadequate water, sanitation, and hygiene (WASH) practices and facilities.

Studies have shown that Ghanaian children who lived in large households with three or more other children under age 5 had higher prevalence of undernutrition outcomes (Glover-Amengor et al., 2016; Miah et al., 2016; Van De Poel et al., 2007). A study by Darteh et al. (2014) found that Ghanaian children in households with 5–8 children were 1.3 times more likely to be stunted compared to children in households with 1–4 children. When there are many young children in a household, there is competition for scarce resources, as well as decreased maternal attention and care for the children (Gyimah, 2005). Overcrowding in large households potentially leads to easier spread of infections, thereby increasing the risk of undernutrition among children (Miah et al., 2016; Van De Poel et al., 2007).

In Northern Ghana, the allocation of resources in the household is not dependent on who needs it the most, but on status within the household. For example, nutrient-rich foods, especially animal source foods (ASFs), are served to the male head of the household and not the children (Leroy et al., 2008; Malapit & Quisumbing, 2015). Therefore, when there are many children in the household, the status of the child matters and the unequal sharing of food is related to the intra-household inequality in growth (Leroy et al., 2008).

Poor household hygiene and inadequate access to sanitation increase a child's risk for diarrheal and other infectious diseases (Ngure et al., 2014; Schmidt, 2014). In their 2013–2017 nutrition policy, Ghana's Ministry of Health (2013) reported that potable water is accessible to less than half of the Ghanaian population. Moreover, about 17% of Ghanaian households lack toilet facilities and practice open defecation (GSS et al., 2015). The state of WASH in Ghana contributes to child malnutrition. For instance, Aheto et al. (2015) found that Ghanaian children living in homes without toilet facilities had significantly higher odds of wasting. Diarrhea and infections stemming from inadequate WASH influence child malnutrition through different pathways such as reduced appetite and decreased ability to absorb critical micronutrients via the small intestine (Bentley et al., 1995; Prendergast & Kelly, 2016). Efforts towards reducing child undernutrition should therefore work to improve the WASH infrastructure in order to reduce the impact of diarrheal and infectious diseases.

Different studies have identified poverty as a household-level risk factor for child undernutrition in Ghana (Anderson et al., 2010; Miah et al., 2016; Saaka & Galaa, 2016; Van De Poel et al., 2007). The link between poverty and child undernutrition may be due to factors such as inaccessibility to improved health, water and sanitation, and continued accumulative effects of food insecurity that characterize households living in poverty (Miah et al., 2016).

Community and societal determinants: Focus on Northern Ghana. There are several community- and societal-level factors—or basic causes—in Northern Ghana that may be linked to the disproportionate burden of food insecurity and malnutrition in the region. However, we explore the following factors that affect agricultural performance in the region: poverty and politics, as well as geography and climate.

These factors provide a deeper contextual overview of the situation in Northern Ghana.

Poverty and politics. Previous research has suggested that levels of poverty and economic development at the population level influence child malnutrition outcomes in a country (Moradi, 2010; Roth et al., 2017; Vollmer et al., 2014). Over the past decade, Ghana's poverty rate has decreased from 52% to 28%, but regional disparities remain—the poverty rate of Northern Ghana is nearly twice that of the South (USAID, 2014). Historically, this economic inequality has always been present. Experts posit that the origins of this inequality can be attributed to the colonial policies that encouraged labor migration of Northerners to the south and prevented the government from investing in the Northern economy (Shepherd et al., 2006). These circumstances constantly affirm the subordinate position of the north to the south in terms of economy and politics (Plange, 1979; Shepherd et al., 2006). Northern Ghana has also been plagued with conflict in the past. Past conflicts resulted in the destruction of families' properties and grave losses of cattle and other agricultural inputs and implements. This affected overall food security and farmers' ability to restart their livelihoods in agricultural production and trade (Van der Linde & Naylor, 1999). Rampant civil unrests, together with historic economic and political policies in Northern Ghana, have had significant impacts on economic growth in the region. These factors have also led to inequitable access to basic infrastructure in the northern region, compared to other regions in the south (Reinhardt & Fanzo, 2016). These political and economic factors have an effect on the underlying causes of malnutrition that are discussed earlier in this chapter.

Geography and climate. Northern Ghana is remote and often perceived as inaccessible. The area also comprises predominantly savanna vegetation and experiences erratic rainfall patterns, wildfires, flooding, droughts, and desertification (Armah et al., 2011; Plange, 1979; Shepherd et al., 2006). Moreover, the opportune time window for growing crops in Northern Ghana is limited because the region has one rainy season followed by a long dry season (Hjelm & Dasori, 2012).

Additional factors like land size, lack of crop diversity, limited agricultural inputs, and low soil fertility play a major role in the low agricultural output observed in Northern Ghana (Hjelm & Dasori, 2012; Quaye, 2008). For a region where agriculture is the dominant source of livelihood—an estimated 88% rely on cultivation for sustenance (Hjelm & Dasori, 2012)—this presents a considerable challenge. Past literature has also shown that climate and ecosystem changes influence the prevalence of stunting, not only through impacts on food security and local food systems; climate change affects infectious diseases and their transmission patterns and, therefore, increases malnutrition-related morbidity (Reinhardt & Fanzo, 2016; WHO, n.d.).

Consequences of Food Insecurity and Malnutrition

Undernutrition contributes to high mortality and global disease burden (Black et al., 2008), increases risk of infection, weakens the immune system (Tette et al., 2015; World Food Programme (WFP) & United Nations Children's Fund (UNICEF), 2006), and can also result in shorter adult height, which has implications for the birthweight of offspring. Below, we further detail evidence on child developmental and behavioral outcomes that stem from food insecurity and malnutrition.

Malnutrition and Child Developmental Outcomes. Undernutrition affects brain and nervous system development, leading to impaired cognitive functioning and delays in socio-emotional, language, and motor development (Hobbs & King, 2018; Victora et al., 2008). Research has proposed a number of mechanisms to explain relationships between undernutrition and these developmental delays. Grantham-McGregor and Ani (2001) suggest that small-sized, undernourished children are treated as younger children; this may contribute to impaired development. They also hypothesize that undernourished children "functionally isolate" themselves from their environment and, therefore, do not engage in as many activities as their well-nourished counterparts. Undernourished children are also more likely to be lethargic; hence, they acquire fewer skills, thereby worsening their development (Grantham-McGregor & Ani, 2001).

The brain develops rapidly in the first 1000 days of life—during gestation and children's first 2 years of life. Insults occurring early during brain development can have long-term effects on the brain's structure and function (Grantham-McGregor et al., 2007). Environmental quality—factors like stress; poor stimulation; early undernutrition; and deficiencies in critical micronutrient deficiencies like iron, zinc, iodine, choline, and vitamin B12—affects child brain development, structure, and function. Poor environmental factors result in insults to long-term cognitive, socio-emotional, and motor development (Bourre, 2006; Chattopadhyay & Saumitra, 2016; Grantham-McGregor et al., 2007).

Malnutrition and Child Behavioral Outcomes. Early delays in cognitive, socio-emotional, language, and motor development contribute to behavioral outcomes such as lower academic performance, increased risk for emotional and behavioral problems, mental distress, anxiety, and depression among children and youths (Grantham-McGregor et al., 2007; Masa et al., 2018). These behavioral outcomes can affect future income and earnings, leading to poverty, which has been shown to be "both a cause and outcome of poor human development" (Victora et al., 2008). Currently, there is limited evidence on long-term outcomes that result from food insecurity and malnutrition during childhood. There is therefore a need for more population-based cohort studies to fill this research gap.

Despite the limited availability of evidence on food insecurity among children and consequent long-term outcomes, many researchers have studied the impact of food insecurity on behavioral outcomes during childhood and adolescence. A systematic review that explored the association between food insecurity and child behavioral, emotional, and academic outcomes in Western industrialized countries (the United States, the United Kingdom, Canada, and Australia) found that food insecurity was associated with outcomes like increased aggressive behavior, limited self-control, impaired academic performance, and depression, among others in pre-schoolers, school-aged, and adolescents (Shankar et al., 2017).

Similar findings have been observed in the Ghanaian context. Appoh (2005) conducted a study that explored the effect of early malnutrition on children's social and emotional status among Ghanaian children between the ages of 8 and 16 years. The researcher found that children who were malnourished at an earlier age were more depressed, sad, withdrawn, and anxious; had poorer social relationships; and experienced more thought and attention problems relative to non-malnourished children. Another study by Masa et al. (2018) examined the role that food insecurity plays on the future orientation of Ghanaian youth. They define future orientation as "people's tendency to engage in future thinking and create images of their future possible selves." According to the researchers, future orientation is important because it influences the cultivation of desirable and healthy behaviors. They found that food insecurity was consistently associated with low future orientation among youth; youth from food-insecure households focus more on present circumstances and, therefore, lose sight of the future. This may be detrimental to how children and youth set present and future goals related to aspects of their life such as education and occupation.

Empirical evidence on behavioral outcomes and their associations with food insecurity and malnutrition is limited for Northern Ghana, where food insecurity and malnutrition rates are relatively high. For food insecurity, specifically, most of the existing evidence is from high-resource countries. Therefore, although the results from these contexts parallel findings from Ghana, measurement factors (e.g., different scales used to quantify food insecurity as well as different types of behavioral outcomes) may affect the generalizability of research findings to the Ghanaian context. Furthermore, differences in social safety nets such as government assistance programs in low- and high-resource countries may affect the construct validity of food security measures (Hobbs & King, 2018).

There is a wealth of evidence on the association between malnutrition and behavioral outcomes in sub-Saharan African countries and other middle- to low-income countries like Ghana. Inferences can be made regarding these findings and their applications to Northern Ghana and the rest of the country. Table 3 summarizes findings from research conducted in sub-Saharan Africa and other low- and high-resource countries.

Policy, Programming, and Research Solutions

Policy
On the national front, the government has shown considerable commitment to improving nutrition in Ghana, as evidenced by the many nutrition-related policies and initiatives headed by policy makers (Brantuo et al., 2009). Nutrition policies

Table 3 Food insecurity, malnutrition, and behavioral outcomes

Preschoolers	• Impaired social behavior (measured as exploratory behavior, extent of verbalization, friendliness, and active play) was observed among 3-year-old children who showed signs of malnourishment and the impairment increased with increased malnutrition[a]
	• Food insecurity was associated with internalizing and externalizing behavior such as increased aggressive behavior and limited self-control and interpersonal skills[b,c,d,e]
	• Preschoolers from food-insecure households were at an increased risk of mental health symptoms such as anxious or depressed moods[e]
School-aged children	• Food insecurity and malnutrition are associated with internalizing and externalizing behavior such as increased aggressiveness, increased hyperactivity, and inattention, among others[b,d,f,g,h,i]
	• Children from food-insecure households experience academic problems such as missing school (absenteeism) and impaired academic performance[j,k,l,m]
	• Food insecurity among school-aged children was found to be associated with depression and anxiety[d]
	• Food insecurity was also associated with less optimal self-control and interpersonal skills[h]
	• Bullying and being physically attacked were found to be significantly associated with hunger[x,**]
Adolescents	• Higher levels of depression, and anxiety, and lower self-esteem in adolescents who were stunted at age 2 years[n]
	• Higher depression levels in adolescents who experienced severe wasting during infancy[o]
	• Increased prevalence of executive function impairments and aggressive behaviors in adolescents between the ages of 9 and 15 who experience early childhood malnutrition[p]
	• Increased risk of suicide ideation and attempted suicide associated with adolescents from food-insecure households as well as those who were stunted at 24 months[q,r,s,*]
	• Adolescents who were malnourished in early childhood are more likely to be hyperactive in late adolescents and have attention deficits in adulthood[g,m,t]
	• Adolescents who were malnourished in early childhood are more likely to have conduct disorders[g]
	• Adolescents from food-insecure households are at an increased risk for mental and emotional problems such as anxiety, depression, dysthymia, and substance-abuse disorders[q,r,*,u,v]
	• Adolescents are more likely to have conduct and peer problems, and have worse psychosocial outcomes such as having fewer friends and having difficulty getting along with others[i,u]
	• Food insecurity was found to be independently associated with common mental problems that are characterized by symptoms of irritability, exhaustion, sleeplessness, concentration difficulties, somatic problems, poor memory, etc.[w,**]
	• Adolescents with lower levels of hunger had lower odds of depression, anxiety, loneliness, suicidal ideation, and suicide attempts[x,**,y,**].
	• Bullying and being physically attacked were found to be significantly associated with hunger[x,**]
	• Symptoms of depression and suicidal ideation with planning increased with increasing persistency and frequency of the hunger among adolescents aged 11–16[z]

(continued)

Table 3 (continued)

	• Among teenage girls, food insecurity has a strong association with depression, anxiety, behavioral control, and psychological distress[aa],* • Increased frequency of hunger was found to be associated with substance abuse (alcohol and tobacco use), psychological distress (anxiety, loneliness, suicidal ideation), and behavioral problems (physical fighting, bully victimization, and truancy) among adolescents from different countries in Southeast Asia[ab],*

**represents findings from sub-Saharan Africa, *represents findings from other low-resource settings

[a]Liu and Raine (2016).
[b]Slack and Yoo (2005).
[c]Kimbro and Denney (2015).
[d]Weinreb et al. (2002).
[e]Whitaker et al. (2006).
[f]Slopen et al. (2011).
[g]Liu et al. (2004).
[h]Howard (2011).
[i]Weigel and Armijos (2018).
[j]Alaimo et al. (2001).
[k]Jyoti et al. (2005).
[l]Ramsey et al. (2011).
[m]Winicki and Jemison (2003).
[n]Walker et al. (2007).
[o]Galler et al. (2010).
[p]Galler et al. (2011).
[q]Cheung and Ashorn (2009)
[r]Alaimo et al. (2002)
[s]McIntyre et al. (2013).
[t]Galler et al. (2012).
[u]McLaughlin et al. (2012).
[v]Poole-Di Salvo et al. (2016).
[w]Jebena et al. (2016).
[x]Arat (2016).
[y]Mwambene et al. (2013).
[z]Romo et al. (2016).
[aa]Rani et al. (2018).
[ab]Peltzer and Pengpid (2017).

dating back to Ghana's independence in 1957 primarily focused on implementing *nutrition-specific* interventions including food demonstration and nutrition education with strategies emphasizing behavior change and tackling micronutrient deficiencies (Ghartey, 2010). Nutrition efforts in the country only began to center on child malnutrition during the mid-1970s, when weaning and supplementary foods were first incorporated into nutrition policy (Ghartey, 2010). Moreover, micronutrient deficiencies had not been prioritized in Ghana's nutrition policy until the late 1980s (Ghartey, 2010).

Historically, nutrition policy efforts in Ghana had been fragmented, lacking coordination across multiple sectors and ministries (Ghartey, 2010). In 2013, the

Ministry of Health (MOH), the Ghana Health Service (GHS), and other key stakeholders from multiple disciplines joined forces to draft a national nutrition policy (Ministry of Health, 2013). The purpose of the 2013–2017 National Nutrition Policy (NNP) was to provide a framework for nutrition interventions and services in the country. This framework would guide implementation and effective delivery of these interventions while including nutrition in all mainstream national development efforts (Ministry of Health, 2013). The strengths of having an overarching policy is that it guides the organization and management of all nutrition programs in the country, spells out strategic objectives and measures of these objectives, and encourages stakeholders to collaborate and streamline their efforts (Brantuo et al., 2009). Northern Ghana, therefore, relies on the national policy to guide its work against food insecurity and malnutrition in the region.

While the NNP has designed several interventions to curb malnutrition in the country, it cites inadequate funding as a major barrier to program implementation (Ministry of Health, 2013). In the Ministry of Health's budgetary plans, nutrition has consistently remained a low priority (Ghartey, 2010). Given malnutrition's impact on children, the Ghanaian population at large, and the economy, it is imperative that advocacy efforts are directed towards increased investment in the prevention of malnutrition.

In addition to implementing the 2013–2017 NNP, Ghana signed on to the Scaling Up Nutrition (SUN) Movement[12] in 2011. The purpose of SUN in Ghana is to build a base of nutrition evidence to influence policy advocacy and program implementation in Ghana (Laar et al., 2015). Currently, although most of the research from SUN is at the national level, the researchers aspire to move into local research. Their research could be expanded to include food security in Northern Ghana, given that those areas have the highest burden of malnutrition in the country.

Programs

There are a number of programs that have been implemented to address food insecurity and malnutrition in Northern Ghana. Most of these interventions are based on global standards and policies, since funding comes from global agencies. For example, USAID has introduced a number of projects in the region including Systems for Health; Resiliency in Northern Ghana (RING); and Strengthening Partnerships, Results, and Innovations in Nutrition Globally (SPRING) (SPRING, 2017). RING aims to improve the livelihoods and nutritional status of vulnerable households in Northern Ghana, and SPRING's goal is to scale up high-impact nutrition practices and policies (SPRING, 2017). Components of these programs

[12] Scaling Up Nutrition (SUN) Movement is a global movement aimed at uniting national leaders, bilateral and multilateral organizations, private businesses, donors, civil society, and researchers in a collaborative effort to improve nutrition. Ghana joined the SUN Movement in 2011 and has USAID as its donor convener. As a donor convener, USAID's role is to work with other donor agencies to coordinate and increase financial support for the nation's nutrition interventions and to prioritize interventions based on identified gaps (Scaling Up Nutrition [SUN] 2014; U.S. Agency for International Development [USAID], 2016)

have the larger aim of reducing stunting in the region; thus they focus on addressing key determinants of stunting, including food insecurity. These interventions also aim to increase access to and consumption of diverse quality food; partner with regional and local governments to strengthen local support networks; link agriculture, nutrition, and income growth; increase competitiveness of major food value chains; and provide extension training or capacity building (SPRING, 2017).

Although these globally funded programs and projects perform well during the period when they are active, they are usually limited in their coverage, have minimal long-term impact, and are often unsustainable. This emphasizes the need for the government to have a certain level of ownership of the interventions to ensure their sustainability (Steiner-Asiedu et al., 2017).

A major program directly targeting child undernutrition and educational outcomes is the Ghana School Feeding Program (GSFP). Initiated in 2005, the program provides one hot and adequately nutritious meal to school pupils on school days. GSFP is modeled after school feeding programs from other countries which seek to improve children's nutritional status and their educational issues while offering livelihood avenues for local communities (Ghana School Feeding Program [GSFP], & Ministry of Gender, Children and Social Protection, 2016). Although the program has been largely successful in increasing school enrollment and improving nutrition for children, the Ghanaian Government is working to ensure that it delivers the optimum benefits for the children.

Current international guidelines recommend that school feeding programs provide at least 30% of school children's daily energy and micronutrient needs (Bhatia, 2013; Food and Agriculture Organization (FAO), 2018a). However, few studies assessing the GSFP have suggested that the program is found wanting in its ability to meet this need in Ghanaian school children (Danquah et al., 2012; Owusu et al., 2017). Despite this issue, some studies have suggested that the program increases dietary diversity among children participating in the program (Martens, 2007; Owusu et al., 2017).

In Ghana, as well as in many low- and middle-income countries where national school feeding programs are implemented, national nutrition guidelines and standards—which should ultimately inform nutrition quality in school feeding programs—have not been established (Buhl, 2010; Food and Agriculture Organization (FAO), 2018a). In 2016, the Ghanaian Government launched a national school feeding policy aimed at giving more structure to GSFP, streamlining the implementation of the program, and fostering its sustainability (GSFP, & Ministry of Gender, Children and Social Protection, 2016). The government is also currently in the process of establishing school meal and nutrition guidelines to address nutrition gaps in the GSFP (Food and Agriculture Organization (FAO), 2018a).

Research

There is a wealth of research in Ghana aimed at addressing malnutrition and food insecurity. We briefly highlight three landmark studies which were part of broader cross-national research initiatives and collaborations and yielded findings with the potential to influence practice and policy: 1. the International Lipid-Based Nutrient

Supplements (iLiNS) Project; 2. the Research to Improve Infant Nutrition and Growth (RIING) project; and 3. Enhancing Child Nutrition through Animal Source Food Management (ENAM) Project.

iLiNS project. The iLiNS project exemplifies a *nutrition-specific* approach, which addresses proximal and immediate factors of malnutrition (United Nations Children's Fund, 2015). The project used a randomized trial approach in Ghana, Burkina Faso, and Malawi to assess the efficacy of small-quantity lipid-based nutrient supplements (SQ-LNS) in pregnant and lactating women and infants and young children. Beyond efficacy, the project also explored possible product delivery systems and economic dimensions such as the cost-effectiveness and willingness of populations to pay for the products. Findings to date indicate that mothers who were given prenatal SQ-LNS had heavier and longer infants, with larger head circumference at birth compared to the control group. Additionally, SQ-LNS provided during the first 1000 days had a positive impact on the weight and length of the infant at 18 months compared to the control group (International Lipid-Based Nutrient Supplements (iLiNS) Project, 2015).

Over the past few years, the iLiNS project has expanded its efforts to assess the impact of nutrient supplementation on behavioral and cognitive development. Recent findings from the project have suggested that the intervention had limited impacts on children's cognition at the preschool stage (Ocansey et al., 2019). However, children of mothers who received the SQ-LNS during pregnancy presented signs of improved socio-emotional development at 4–6 years, despite evidence that most of these children were from households where the home environment was not sufficiently stimulating and nurturing (Ocansey et al., 2019). Current efforts are underway to follow up on the iLiNS cohort at the ages of 8–12 years to assess the impact of SQ-LNS on nervous system development (UC Davis Institute for Global Nutrition, 2020).

Researchers involved in the iLiNS project have suggested that scaling up interventions that incorporate SQ-LNS with programming addressesing broader social determinants of malnutrition may significantly reduce the public health and economic burden of child undernutrition. They therefore call on policy makers to consider potential returns on investment that may result from large-scale adoption of SQ-LNS (International Lipid-Based Nutrient Supplements (iLiNS) Project, 2015).

RIING study. The second project, RIING, did not have a direct interventional component. However, it sought to identify barriers and facilitators to optimal infant feeding practices and to improve the state of child nutrition among Ghanaian populations affected by HIV. Thus, mothers with HIV who were enrolled in the study were educated on infant feeding and were encouraged to exclusively breastfeed their babies (Lartey, 2015; Otoo et al., 2009).

The RIING study provided insights into food insecurity and its impacts on maternal nutrition in Ghana. After following a sample of women for 12 months postpartum, the investigators found that the prevalence of food insecurity increased over the course of follow-up for mothers with HIV (Garcia et al., 2013). Persistent food insecurity was also found to be associated with lower energy intake among lactating mothers and increased risk of maternal stress (Addo et al., 2011; Garcia et al., 2013). Additionally, women who were both HIV positive and food insecure were about 15 times more likely to report maternal stress (Garcia et al., 2013). These negative outcomes that characterize mothers with HIV in the study translate into child nutritional outcomes; the RIING project found that maternal HIV was a significant risk factor for reduced infant weight and length in the first 12 months of life (Lartey et al., 2014).

Ghana's 2013–2017 National Food Policy indicates that nutrition interventions specific to persons living with HIV/AIDS exist in select antiretroviral centers. These interventions provide assessment, counselling, and livelihood support. Nutrition services also provide antiretroviral therapy for pregnant women and lactating mothers who are HIV positive. An intervention that specifically targets pregnant women, mothers, and their children aged 0–59 months—the Essential Nutrition Actions (ENA) for integrated maternal and childcare—also promotes infant feeding and maternal nutrition in families affected by HIV (MOH, 2013). Currently, there is limited evidence demonstrating the impact of these interventions on maternal and child nutrition outcomes. Moreover, despite the potential that these interventions carry, there is no explicit mention of measures to directly tackle food insecurity, especially since findings from the RIING project highlight its rampancy and ramifications among mothers and families affected by HIV.

ENAM project. This project adopted a more *nutrition-sensitive* approach to curbing food insecurity and other basic, upstream contributors to malnutrition in Ghana. The project built on the success of the Global Livestock Collaborative Research Support Program's (GL-CRSP) Child Nutrition Project, a trial that demonstrated the effect of Animal Source Food (ASF) consumption on increased micronutrient intake and cognitive development among children in rural Kenya. The investigators sought to increase access to and use of ASF in the diets of Ghanaian children. The intervention, adopting a quasi-experimental approach, entailed a microcredit scheme and entrepreneurship training to drive caregivers' businesses as well as nutrition education to encourage consumption of ASF among children. For health, nutrition, and agricultural stakeholders at the regional and national levels, the intervention provided agriculture and nutrition extension education (Colecraft et al., 2012; Marquis & Colecraft, 2014).

Compared to the control groups, a majority of caregiver participants who received microcredit loans reported increased business earnings (Marquis & Colecraft, 2014). Moreover, findings revealed that there was a significant increase in children's consumption of livestock meat, organ meat, eggs, and dairy products (Marquis & Colecraft, 2014). This increase in ASF consumption and diversity was attributed to significant increases in nutrition knowledge among households receiving the intervention (Christian et al., 2016; Sakyi-Dawson et al., 2009). The ENAM project also reported that caregivers who received the intervention had 50% lower risk of food insecurity, be it moderate or severe, at the end of the intervention (Colecraft et al., n. d.; Harding et al., 2009). An essential finding regarding child growth from the study was the marked increase, in comparison to the control group, in height-for-age and weight-for-age z-scores of children living in households that received microcredit loans (Marquis & Colecraft, 2014). Mothers who were involved in the program also reported that acting on lessons from the nutrition education component of the intervention may have been associated with decreased events of illnesses among their children (Anyidoho et al., 2009).

The ENAM project demonstrates how nutrition education, combined with financial empowerment, enables households to obtain nutritious foods, thereby increasing their dietary diversity and food security (Christian et al., 2016; Marquis & Colecraft, 2014). Scholars have asserted that nutrition interventions and programming adopt a nutrition-sensitive approach, which includes providing social safety nets and empowering caregivers through the provision of adequate resources (Ruel & Alderman, 2013; United Nations Children's Fund, 2015). The ENAM project exemplifies a nutrition-sensitive approach and, therefore, highlights the importance of addressing underlying social determinants of malnutrition such as poverty and inadequate education in Ghana in order to tackle food insecurity and child malnutrition more holistically. Findings from the ENAM project were a key influence in USAID's 2011–2015 Multi-year Strategy for the Feed the Future Initiative[13] in Ghana, thereby creating an avenue for translation of this vital research into food and agricultural programming and policy in the country (Lartey et al., 2014; USAID, 2011).

In Northern Ghana, there is minimal evidence for interventions that can significantly reduce food insecurity in the region. With the high number of interventions implemented in Northern Ghana, there is the need for efficacy studies to determine the impact of these interventions in reducing food insecurity and malnutrition in the region. A recent systematic review by Adu et al. (2018) examined the effects of agricultural interventions on food security in Northern Ghana. They found some evidence for the contributions of these interventions to food security, but the overall impact on reducing food insecurity was weak because of the lack of counterfactuals. This has implications for monitoring and evaluation of policies, programming, and interventions.

Conclusions

Although the prevalence of food-insecure and malnourished households has decreased in Ghana over the years, the rates remain high, especially in Northern Ghana. Food insecurity and malnutrition, particularly during the first 1000 days of a child's life, can lead to impaired neurocognitive development. These insults also contribute to behavioral outcomes such as lower academic performance, increased

---

[13] Feed the Future (FTF) is a US Government initiative that aims at improving food security and reducing global hunger through partnerships with countries to improve agricultural sectors. The initiative also seeks to address root causes of poverty, hunger, and malnutrition (Feed the Future (FTF), n.d.; United States Agency for International Development (USAID), 2011).

risk of emotional and behavioral problems, mental distress, anxiety, and depression, among others in children and youths. Given the adverse developmental and behavioral outcomes that are associated with food insecurity and malnutrition, Ghana needs concerted efforts to confront the range of factors that lead to food insecurity and malnutrition. A multi-sectoral approach should be taken. Explicit nutrition objectives should be linked to programs and policies addressing poverty alleviation, agriculture development, and education interventions. At the household and individual levels, programs and policies to support optimal infant and young child feeding practices (e.g., breastfeeding and complementary feeding), parental education, maternal nutrition, and infection mitigation could all be supported. Ultimately, addressing food insecurity and malnutrition in Ghana contributes to achieving the second Sustainable Development Goal, which seeks to "end hunger, achieve food security and improved nutrition and promote sustainable agriculture" by 2030 (United Nations Statistics Division [UNSD], n.d.).

References

Addo, A. A., Marquis, G. S., Lartey, A. A., Pérez-Escamilla, R., Mazur, R. E., & Harding, K. B. (2011). Food insecurity and perceived stress but not HIV infection are independently associated with lower energy intakes among lactating Ghanaian women. *Maternal and Child Nutrition, 7* (1), 80–91. https://doi.org/10.1111/j.1740-8709.2009.00229.x

Adu, M. O., Yawson, D. O., Armah, F. A., Abano, E. E., & Quansah, R. (2018). Systematic review of the effects of agricultural interventions on food security in northern Ghana. *PLoS One, 13*(9). https://doi.org/10.1371/journal.pone.0203605

Aheto, J. M. K., Keegan, T. J., Taylor, B. M., & Diggle, P. J. (2015). Childhood malnutrition and its determinants among under-five children in Ghana. *Paediatric and Perinatal Epidemiology, 29* (6), 552–561. https://doi.org/10.1111/ppe.12222

Ali, Z., Saaka, M., Adams, A.-G., Kamwininaang, S. K., & Abizari, A.-R. (2017). The effect of maternal and child factors on stunting, wasting and underweight among preschool children in Northern Ghana. *BMC Nutrition, 3*(1). https://doi.org/10.1186/s40795-017-0154-2

Amoaful, E. F. (2016). Overview of nutrition situation in Ghana.

Amugsi, D. A., Lartey, A., Kimani-Murage, E., & Mberu, B. U. (2016). Women's participation in household decision-making and higher dietary diversity: findings from nationally representative data from Ghana. *Journal of Health, Population and Nutrition, 35*(1), 16. https://doi.org/10.1186/s41043-016-0053-1

Amugsi, D. A., Mittelmark, M. B., & Oduro, A. (2015). Association between maternal and child dietary diversity: An analysis of the Ghana demographic and health survey. *PLoS One, 10*(8), 136748. https://doi.org/10.1371/journal.pone.0136748

Anderson, A. K., Bignell, W., Winful, S., Soyiri, I., & Steiner-Asiedu, M. (2010). Risk factors for malnutrition among children 5-years and younger in the Akuapim-North District in the eastern region of Ghana. *Current Research Journal of Biological Sciences, 2*(3), 183–188.

Anyidoho, N. A., Kobati, G. Y., Butler, L. M., Marquis, G. S., Colecraft, E. K., Sakyi-Dawson, O., . . . Ahunu, B. K. (2009). Using case studies to understand successful entrepreneurship among Ghanaian women.

Appoh, L. Y. (2005). Consequences of early malnutrition for subsequent social and emotional behaviour of children in Ghana. *Journal of Psychology in Africa, 14*(2), 87–94. https://doi.org/10.4314/jpa.v14i2.30616

Armah, F. A., Odoi, J. O., Yengoh, G. T., Obiri, S., Yawson, D. O., & Afrifa, E. K. A. (2011). Food security and climate change in drought-sensitive savanna zones of Ghana. *Mitigation and Adaptation Strategies for Global Change, 16*(3), 291–306. https://doi.org/10.1007/s11027-010-9263-9

Bentley, M. E., Black, M. M., & Hurtado, E. (1995). Child-feeding and appetite: What can programmes do? *Food and Nutrition Bulletin, 16*(4), 340–349.

Bhatia, R. (2013). *Operational guidance on menu planning guide.* Retrieved from http://hgsf-global.org/en/bank/downloads/doc_download/347-operational-guidance-on-menu-planning

Bilinsky, P., & Swindale, A. (2010). *Months of Adequate Household Food Provisioning (MAHFP) for measurement of household food access: Indicator guide* (*Version 4*). Retrieved from www.fantaproject.org

Black, R. E., Allen, L. H., Bhutta, Z. A., Caulfield, L. E., de Onis, M., Ezzati, M., … Rivera, J. (2008). Maternal and child undernutrition: Global and regional exposures and health consequences. *The Lancet, 371*(9608), 243–260. https://doi.org/10.1016/S0140-6736(07)61690-0

Bourre, J. M. (2006). Effects of nutrients (in food) on the structure and function of the nervous system: Update on dietary requirements for brain. Part 1: Micronutrients. *Journal of Nutrition Health and Aging, 10*(5), 377.

Brakohiapa, L. A., Yartey, J., Bille, A., Harrison, E., Quansah, E., Armar, M. A., … Yamamoto, S. (1988). Does prolonged breastfeeding adversely affect a child's nutritional status? *Lancet, 2* (8608), 416–418. https://doi.org/10.1016/s0140-6736(88)90411-4

Brantuo, M. N. ., Okwabi, W., Adu-Afuawuah, S., Agyepong, E., Attafuah, N. T., Brew, G., … Ashong, J. (2009). *Landscape analysis of readiness to accelerate the reduction of maternal and child undernutrition in Ghana* (Vol. 252). Retrieved from http://apps.who.int/nutrition/landscape_analysis/SCNNews37_extract_Ghana.pdf?ua=1

Buhl, A. (2010). *Meeting nutritional needs through school feeding: A snapshot of four African nations.* Global Child Nutrition Foundation.

Chattopadhyay, N., & Saumitra, M. (2016). Developmental outcome in children with malnutrition. *Journal of Nepal Paediatric Society, 36*(2), 170–177. https://doi.org/10.3126/jnps.v36i2.14619

Christian, A. K., Marquis, G. S., Colecraft, E. K., Lartey, A., Sakyi-Dawson, O., Ahunu, B. K., & Butler, L. M. (2016). Caregivers' nutrition knowledge and attitudes are associated with household food diversity and children's animal source food intake across different agro-ecological zones in Ghana. *British Journal of Nutrition, 115*(2), 351–360. https://doi.org/10.1017/S0007114515004468

Clay, E. (2002). *Food security: Concepts and measurement* (pp. 25–33). FAO.

Colecraft, E K, Marquis, G. S., Sakyi-Dawson, O., Lartey, A., Ahunu, B., Butler, L. M., … Lonergan, E. (n.d.). *The Enhancing Child Nutrition through Animal Source Food Management (ENAM) Project.* Retrieved from http://www.fao.org/ag/humannutrition/34273-09cbd308d8aa06bda7edbba1ee173c961.pdf

Colecraft, E. K., Marquis, G. S., Sakyi-Dawson, O., Lartey, A., Butler, L. M., Ahunu, B., … Canacoo, E. (2012). Planning, design and implementation of the enhancing child nutrition through animal source food management (ENAM) project. *African Journal of Food, Agriculture, Nutrition and Development, 12*(1), 5687–5708.

Danquah, A. O., Amoah, A. N., Steiner-Asiedu, M., & Opare-Obisaw, & C. (2012). Nutritional status of participating and non-participating pupils in the Ghana school feeding programme. *Journal of Food Research, 1*(3), 264–271. https://doi.org/10.5539/jfr.v1n3p263

Darteh, E. K. M., Acquah, E., & Kumi-Kyereme, A. (2014). Correlates of stunting among children in Ghana. *BMC Public Health, 14*(1). https://doi.org/10.1186/1471-2458-14-504

Feed the Future (FTF). (n.d.). *Guidance and tools for global food security programs.* Retrieved October 28, 2019, from https://www.feedthefuture.gov/guidance-and-tools-for-global-food-security-programs/

Food and Agriculture Organization (FAO). (2008). *An introduction to the basic concepts of food security.* Retrieved from http://www.fao.org/3/al936e/al936e.pdf

Food and Agriculture Organization (FAO). (2017). *The state of food security and nutrition in the world: Building resilience for peace and food security.* Retrieved from http://www.fao.org/3/a-i7695e.pdf

Food and Agriculture Organization (FAO). (2018a). *Nutrition guidelines and standards for school meals.* Retrieved from http://www.fao.org/policy-support/resources/resources-details/en/c/1177795/

Food and Agriculture Organization (FAO). (2018b). *The state of food security and nutrition in the world: Building climate resilience for food security and nutrition.* Retrieved from www.fao.org/publications

Garcia, J., Hromi-Fiedler, A., Mazur, R. E., Marquis, G., Sellen, D., Lartey, A., & Perez-Escamilla, R. (2013). Persistent household food insecurity, HIV, and maternal stress in peri-urban Ghana. *BMC Public Health, 13,* 215. https://doi.org/10.1186/1471-2458-13-215

Ghana School Feeding Program (GSFP), & Ministry of Gender, C. and S. P (2016). *National School Feeding Policy.*

Ghana Statistical Service (GSS), Ghana Health Service (GHS), & ICF International. (2015). *Ghana demographic and health survey 2014.* Ghana Statistical Service (GSS), Ghana Health Service (GHS), & ICF International.

Ghartey, A. B. (2010). *Nutrition policy and programs in Ghana: The limitation of a single sector approach.* Washington, DC. Retrieved from www.worldbank.org/hnppublications

Glover-Amengor, M., Agbemafle, I., Hagan, L. L., Mboom, F. P., Gamor, G., Larbi, A., & Hoeschle-Zeledon, I. (2016). Nutritional status of children 0-59 months in selected intervention communities in northern Ghana from the Africa RISING project in 2012. *Archives of Public Health, 74*(1), 12. https://doi.org/10.1186/s13690-016-0124-1

Grantham-McGregor, S., Cheung, Y. B., Cueto, S., Glewwe, P., Richter, L., & Strupp, B. (2007). Developmental potential in the first 5 years for children in developing countries. *Lancet, 369* (9555), 60–70. https://doi.org/10.1016/S0140-6736(07)60032-4

Grantham-McGregor, S. M., & Ani, C. C. (2001). Undernutrition and mental development. Nestlé Nutrition Workshop Series. Clinical & Performance Programme. https://doi.org/10.1159/000061844.

Gyimah, S. O. (2005). The dynamics of timing and spacing of births in Ghana. *Journal of Comparative Family Studies, 36*(1), 41–60.

Harding, K. B., Marquis, G. S., Colecraft, E. K., Lartey, A., Sakyi-Dawson, O., Ahunu, B. K., ... Lonergan, E. (2009). An integrated economic and education intervention (the ENAM project) decreased household food insecurity in rural Ghana. *The FASEB Journal, 23*(S1), 336–331.

Hjelm, L., & Dasori, W. (2012). *Comprehensive food security and vulnerability analysis: Focus on Northern Ghana.* Retrieved from https://documents.wfp.org/stellent/groups/public/documents/ena/wfp257009.pdf?_ga=2.145224112.503299078.1544512191-1869174646.1544512191

Hobbs, S., & King, C. (2018). The unequal impact of food insecurity on cognitive and behavioral outcomes among 5-year-old urban children. *Journal of Nutrition Education and Behavior, 50* (7), 687–694. https://doi.org/10.1016/j.jneb.2018.04.003

International Lipid-Based Nutrient Supplements (iLiNS) Project. (2015). *Key results to date: iLiNS project, March 2015.* Retrieved from https://ilins.ucdavis.edu/sites/g/files/dgvnsk1776/files/inline-files/resultsToDate_0.pdf

Kanmiki, E. W., Bawah, A. A., Agorinya, I., Achana, F. S., Awoonor-Williams, J. K., Oduro, A. R., ... Akazili, J. (2014). Socio-economic and demographic determinants of under-five mortality in rural northern Ghana. *BMC International Health and Human Rights, 14*(1), 24.

Laar, A., Aryeetey, R. N. O., Akparibo, R., Zotor, F., & Ghana SUN Academic Platform. (2015). Nutrition sensitivity of the 2014 budget statement of Republic of Ghana. *The Proceedings of the Nutrition Society, 74*(4), 526–532.

Lartey, A. (2015). What would it take to prevent stunted growth in children in sub-Saharan Africa? In *Proceedings of the nutrition society* (Vol. 74, pp. 449–453). Cambridge University Press.

Lartey, A., Marquis, G. S., & Marquis CINE Bldg, G. S. (2014). *Nutrition for health and socioeconomic development in sub-Saharan Africa*. Retrieved from https://idl-bnc-idrc. dspacedirect.org/bitstream/handle/10625/53854/IDL-53854.pdf?sequence=1&isAllowed=y

Leroy, J. L., Razak, A. A., & Habicht, J.-P. (2008). Only children of the head of household benefit from increased household food diversity in Northern Ghana. *The Journal of Nutrition, 138*(11), 2258–2263.

Malapit, H. J. L., & Quisumbing, A. R. (2015). What dimensions of women's empowerment in agriculture matter for nutrition in Ghana? *Food Policy, 52*, 54–63. https://doi.org/10.1016/j.foodpol.2015.02.003

Marquis, G. S., & Colecraft, E. K. (2014). Community interventions for dietary improvement in Ghana. *Food and Nutrition Bulletin, 35*(4), S193–S197. https://doi.org/10.1177/15648265140354S305

Martens, T. (2007). *Impact of the Ghana school feeding Programme in 4 districts in central region, Ghana*. Wageningen University, Division of Human Nutrition.

Masa, R., Chowa, G., & Bates, C. (2018). Household food insecurity and future orientation of Ghanaian youth and their parents. *Vulnerable Children and Youth Studies, 13*(2), 170–182. https://doi.org/10.1080/17450128.2017.1392054

Miah, R., Apanga, P. A., & Abdul-Haq, Z. (2016). Risk factors for undernutrition in children under five years old: Evidence from the 2011 Ghana multiple Indicator cluster survey predictors of caesarean section in northern Ghana: A case-control study view project. *Journal of AIDS & Clinical Research, 7*, 585. https://doi.org/10.4172/2155-6113.1000585

Ministry of Health. (2013). *National Nutrition Policy for Ghana*.

Moradi, A. (2010). Nutritional status and economic development in sub-Saharan Africa, 1950-1980. *Economics and Human Biology, 8*, 16–21. https://doi.org/10.1016/j.ehb.2009.12.002

Napoli, M., De Muro, P., & Mazziotta, M. (2011). *Towards a food insecurity multidimensional index (FIMI)*. Retrieved from https://pdfs.semanticscholar.org/e37d/ad6f2c3e6d3f159ab68e6c7867b3ea3034ad.pdf

National Development Planning Commission (NDPC). (2016). *Social and economic impact of child undernutrition on Ghana's long-term development National Development Planning Commission (NDPC)*. Retrieved from https://reliefweb.int/sites/reliefweb.int/files/resources/GHANA.pdf

Ngure, F. M., Reid, B. M., Humphrey, J. H., Mbuya, M. N., Pelto, G., & Stoltzfus, R. J. (2014). Water, sanitation, and hygiene (WASH), environmental enteropathy, nutrition, and early child development: Making the links. *Annals of the New York Academy of Sciences, 1308*(1), 118–128. https://doi.org/10.1111/nyas.12330

Ocansey, M. E., Adu-Afarwuah, S., Kumordzie, S. M., Okronipa, H., Young, R. R., Tamakloe, S. M., ... Prado, E. L. (2019). Prenatal and postnatal lipid-based nutrient supplementation and cognitive, social-emotional, and motor function in preschool-aged children in Ghana: A follow-up of a randomized controlled trial. *The American Journal of Clinical Nutrition, 109*(2), 322–334.

Otoo, G. E., Lartey, A. A., & Pérez-Escamilla, R. (2009). Perceived incentives and barriers to exclusive breastfeeding among periurban Ghanaian women. *Journal of Human Lactation, 25*(1), 34–41. https://doi.org/10.1177/0890334408325072

Owusu, J. S., Colecraft, E. K., Aryeetey, R. N., Vaccaro, J. A., & Huffman, F. G. (2017). Nutrition intakes and nutritional status of school age children in Ghana. *Journal of Food Research, 6*(2), 11. https://doi.org/10.5539/jfr.v6n2p11

Özaltin, E., Hill, K., & Subramanian, S. V. (2010). Association of maternal stature with offspring mortality, underweight, and stunting in low- to middle-income countries. *JAMA - Journal of the American Medical Association, 303*(15), 1507–1516. https://doi.org/10.1001/jama.2010.450

Plange, N.-K. (1979). Underdevelopment in Northern Ghana: Natural causes or colonial capitalism? *Review of African Political Economy, 15*, 4–14.

Prendergast, A. J., & Kelly, P. (2016, June 1). Interactions between intestinal pathogens, enteropathy and malnutrition in developing countries. *Current Opinion in Infectious Diseases, 29*(3), 229–236. https://doi.org/10.1097/QCO.0000000000000261

Pringle, J., & Seal, A. (2013). *UNHCR Anaemia strategy review*. Retrieved from https://www.unhcr.org/5669540d9.pdf

Quaye, W. (2008). Food security situation in northern Ghana, coping strategies and related constraints. *African Journal of Agricultural Research, 3*(5), 334–342.

Reinhardt, K., & Fanzo, J. (2016). Addressing chronic malnutrition through multi-sectoral, sustainable approaches: A review of causes and consequences. *World Review of Nutrition and Dietetics. S. Karger AG*. https://doi.org/10.1159/000441823

Ross, K., Shanoyan, A., & Zereyesus, Y. (2014). Longitudinal analysis of child malnutrition trends in Ghana. In *Agricultural & Applied Economics Association's 2014* AAEA Annual Meeting

Roth, D. E., Krishna, A., Leung, M., Shi, J., Bassani, D. G., & Barros, A. J. D. (2017). Early childhood linear growth faltering in low-income and middle-income countries as a whole-population condition: Analysis of 179 demographic and health surveys from 64 countries (1993–2015). *The Lancet Global Health, 5*(12), E1249–E1257. https://doi.org/10.1016/S2214-109X(17)30418-7

Ruel, M. T., & Alderman, H. (2013). Nutrition-sensitive interventions and programmes: How can they help to accelerate progress in improving maternal and child nutrition? *The Lancet, 382* (9891), 536–551. https://doi.org/10.1016/S0140-6736(13)60843-0

Saaka, M. (2012). Maternal dietary diversity and infant outcome of pregnant women in Northern Ghana. *International Journal of Child Health and Nutrition, 1*, 148.

Saaka, M., & Galaa, S. Z. (2016). Relationships between wasting and stunting and their concurrent occurrence in Ghanaian preschool children. *Journal of Nutrition and Metabolism, 2016*, 4654920. https://doi.org/10.1155/2016/4654920

Saaka, M., Larbi, A., Mutaru, S., & Hoeschle-Zeledon, I. (2016). Magnitude and factors associated with appropriate complementary feeding among children 6–23 months in Northern Ghana. *BMC Nutrition, 2*(1), 1–8. https://doi.org/10.1186/s40795-015-0037-3

Sakyi-Dawson, O., Marquis, G. S., Lartey, A., Colecraft, E. K., Ahunu, B. K., Butler, L. M., ... Quarmime, W. (2009). *Impact of interventions on caregivers' nutrition knowledge and animal source food intake in young children in Ghana*. Davis.

Schmidt, C. W. (2014). Beyond malnutrition: The role of sanitation in stunted growth. *Environmental Health Perspectives, 122*(11), A298–A303. https://doi.org/10.1289/ehp.122-A298

Shankar, P., Chung, R., & Frank, D. A. (2017). Association of food insecurity with Children's behavioral, emotional, and academic outcomes: A systematic review. *Journal of Developmental and Behavioral Pediatrics, 38*(2), 135–150. https://doi.org/10.1097/DBP.0000000000000383

Shepherd, A., Gyimah-Boadi, E., Gariba, S., Plagerson, S., & Musa, W. A. (2006). *Bridging the north south divide in Ghana* (World Development Report 2006 No. 477383–1118673432908.).

SPRING. (2017). Opportunities for integrating nutrition into agricultural information Systems in Northern Ghana. Retrieved from https://www.spring-nutrition.org/sites/default/files/publications/reports/spring_integrating_nutrition_northern_ghana.pdf

Steiner-Asiedu, M., Dittoh, S., Newton, S. K., & Akotia, C. (2017). *Addressing sustainable development goal 2: The Ghana zero hunger strategic review*. Retrieved from https://docs.wfp.org/api/documents/WFP-0000071730/download/?_ga=2.47054116.2038938788.1535558371-1957203229.1486643929

Tette, E. M. A., Sifah, E. K., & Nartey, E. T. (2015). Factors affecting malnutrition in children and the uptake of interventions to prevent the condition. *BMC Pediatrics, 15*(1). https://doi.org/10.1186/s12887-015-0496-3

The DHS Program (2017). *Spatial data repository - Ghana 2017 MHS* [*Shapefile*]. Retrieved from http://spatialdata.dhsprogram.com/boundaries/#view=table&countryId=GH

UC Davis Institute for Global Nutrition. (2020). *Beth Prado and Seth Adu-Afarwuah launch new project examining long-term neural effects of early nutrition in Ghana*. Retrieved from https://globalnutrition.ucdavis.edu/news/prado-and-adu-afarwuah-launch-new-project-examining-long-term-neural-effects-early-nutrition

UNESCO Institute of Statistics. (n.d.). *Ghana, education and literacy*. Retrieved October 31, 2019, from http://uis.unesco.org/en/country/gh

UNICEF Evaluation Office. (2017). *Reducing stunting in children under 5 years of age: A comprehensive evaluation of UNICEF'S strategies and programme performance global synthesis report evaluation report evaluation office.*

United Nations Children's Fund. (2015). *UNICEF's approach to scaling up nutrition for mothers and their children.* Retrieved from https://www.unicef.org/nutrition/files/Unicef_Nutrition_Strategy.pdf

United Nations Children's Fund (UNICEF), World Health Organization (WHO), & World Bank Group. (2018). *UNICEF/ WHO/ World Bank Group - Joint Child Malnutrition Estimates 2018th edition. Levels and Trends in Child Malnutrition.* Retrieved from https://www.who.int/nutgrowthdb/2018-jme-brochure.pdf?ua=1

United Nations Statistics Division (UNSD). (n.d.). *Goal 2: End hunger, achieve food security and improved nutrition and promote sustainable agriculture — SDG Indicators.* Retrieved November 2, 2019, from https://unstats.un.org/sdgs/report/2016/goal-02/

United States Agency for International Development (USAID). (2011). *Feed the future Ghana FY 2011–2015 multi-year strategy.* Retrieved from http://mofa.gov.gh/site/wp-content/uploads/2014/09/USAID-FtF-Ghana-Strategy-2011-2015.pdf

United States Agency for International Development (USAID). (2014). *Ghana: nutrition profile.* Retrieved from https://www.usaid.gov/sites/default/files/documents/1864/USAID-Ghana_NCP.pdf

Van Bodegom, D., Eriksson, U. K., Houwing-Duistermaat, J. J., & Westendorp, R. G. J. (2012). Clustering of child mortality in a contemporary polygamous population in Africap. *Biodemography and Social Biology, 58*(2), 162–172. https://doi.org/10.1080/19485565.2012.720445

Van De Poel, E., Hosseinpoor, A. R., Jehu-Appiah, C., Vega, J., & Speybroeck, N. (2007). Malnutrition and the disproportional burden on the poor: The case of Ghana. *International Journal for Equity in Health, 6*, 21. https://doi.org/10.1186/1475-9276-6-21

Van der Linde, A., & Naylor, R. (1999). *Building sustainable peace: Conflict, conciliation, and civil society in northern Ghana.* Oxfam Working Papers.

Victora, C. G., Adair, L., Fall, C., Hallal, P. C., Martorell, R., Richter, L., & Sachdev, H. S. (2008). Maternal and child undernutrition: Consequences for adult health and human capital. *The Lancet, 371*(9609), 340–357. https://doi.org/10.1016/S0140-6736(07)61692-4

Vollmer, S., Harttgen, K., Subramanyam, M. A., Finlay, J., Klasen, S., & Subramanian, S. V. (2014). Association between economic growth and early childhood undernutrition: Evidence from 121 demographic and health surveys from 36 low-income and middle-income countries. *The Lancet Global Health, 2*(4), E225–E234. https://doi.org/10.1016/S2214-109X(14)70025-7

World Bank. (2018). *Ghana.* Retrieved November 20, 2018, from https://data.worldbank.org/country/ghana

World Food Programme, & United Nations Children's Fund. (2006). *Global framework for action.* Retrieved from https://www.unicef.org/about/execboard/files/Global_Framework_for_Action1.0%2D%2DDec2006.pdf

World Food Summit (WFS). (1996). *Rome Declaration on World Food Security.* Retrieved November 2, 2019, from http://www.fao.org/3/w3613e/w3613e00.htm

World Health Organization (WHO). (2010). *Nutrition landscape information system (NLIS) country profile indicators.* Retrieved from https://www.who.int/nutrition/nlis_interpretation_guide.pdf

World Health Organization (WHO). (2018a). *Breastfeeding.*

World Health Organization (WHO). (2018b). *Malnutrition.* Retrieved January 5, 2018, from https://www.who.int/news-room/fact-sheets/detail/malnutrition

World Health Organization (WHO). (2018c). *Obesity and overweight.* Retrieved November 2, 2019, from https://www.who.int/news-room/fact-sheets/detail/obesity-and-overweight

World Health Organization (WHO). (n.d.). Nutrition: Food Insecurity. Retrieved November 2, 2019, from http://www.emro.who.int/nutrition/food-security/

Child Labor in Ghana: Current Policy, Research, and Practice Efforts

Alice Boateng and Mavis Dako-Gyeke

Introduction

The Constitution and the Children's Act of Ghana define a child as any person of either sex who is below age 18 years, same as the definition provided by the UN Convention on the Rights of the Child. Children engaging in productive economic activities often are engaged in work that deprives them of their childhood, their potential, and their dignity, and that is harmful to their physical and mental development, defined as child labor (ILO, 2002). Child labor has emerged as an increasingly compelling and controversial issue in international policy debates. This is because what may constitute as child labor in one sociocultural context may not be seen as child labor in another. In Ghana, and many African countries, for example, it is normal for a child who is attending school to simultaneously be engaged in economic activities, such as petty trading, fishing, and farming, to support his/her family. These activities could be considered child labor in many Western industrialized countries.

The ambiguity surrounding what constitutes as unacceptable or exploitative work makes identifying cases of child labor a challenging task. Generally, although child labor may be defined differently in different sociocultural contexts, the International Labour Organization (ILO) defines child labor as work that deprives children of their childhood, their potential, and their dignity, and that is harmful to physical and mental development, work that is mentally, physically, socially, or morally dangerous and harmful to children, and interferes with their schooling, requiring them to attempt to combine school attendance with excessively long and heavy work (ILO, 2002).

A. Boateng (✉) · M. Dako-Gyeke
Department of Social Work, University of Ghana, Accra, Ghana
e-mail: aboateng@ug.edu.gh; mdako-gyeke@ug.edu.gh

© Springer Nature Switzerland AG 2022
F. M. Ssewamala et al. (eds.), *Child Behavioral Health in Sub-Saharan Africa*,
https://doi.org/10.1007/978-3-030-83707-5_13

Article 3 of ILO Convention 182[1] classifies the worst forms of child labor as: "(a) all forms of slavery or practices similar to slavery, such as the sale and trafficking of children, debt bondage and serfdom and forced or compulsory labour, including forced or compulsory recruitment of children for use in armed conflict; (b) the use, procuring or offering of a child for prostitution, for the production of pornography or for pornographic performances; (c) the use, procuring or offering of a child for illegal activities, in particular for the production and trafficking of drugs as defined in the relevant international treaties; and (d) work which, by its nature or the circumstances in which it is carried out, is likely to harm the health, safety or morals of children."

The ILO Convention 138[2] defines light work as work which is:

- "not likely to be harmful to [children's] health or development; and
- not such as to prejudice [children's] attendance at school, their participation in vocational orientation or training programmes approved by the competent authority or their capacity to benefit from the instruction received."

The Ghana Statistical Service (GSS) defines child labor as work that deprives children of their childhood, education, potential, and dignity, and that is harmful to their physical and mental development (GSS, 2014). The Children's Act of Ghana (1998) defines exploitative labor as work that deprives the child of his/her education, health, or development. It sets the minimum age for entering employment at 15 years for general employment, 13 years for light work, and 18 years for hazardous work. The Act defines hazardous work as work posing a danger to the health, safety, or morals of a person, and provides a long list, including mining, quarrying, fishing, porterage, or carrying of heavy loads; work involving the production or use of chemicals; and work in places where there is a risk of exposure to immoral behavior, also known as the worst forms of child labor. The ILO, GSS, and the Children's Act of Ghana's definitions agree that child labor is work that deprives children of their childhood, their potential, and their dignity, and that is harmful to their physical and mental development.

In addition, Article 32(1) of the Convention on the Rights of the Child (1989) defines child labor as any work that is likely to be hazardous or to interfere with children's education, or to be harmful to their health, physical, spiritual, mental, moral, or social development. What is common across all the definitions is the fact that the term child labor does not cover all economic activities carried out by children. Instead, it refers to work or employment undertaken by children that conforms neither to the provisions of national legislation, such as the Children's Act, 1998 (Act 560), nor to the provisions of international instruments, such as the ILO's Conventions 138 and 182, which clearly define the boundaries of work undertaken by children that must be abolished.

---

[1] Copyright © International Labour Organization 1999

[2] Copyright © International Labour Organization 1973

National laws and regulations may permit the engagement of persons 13–15 years to do light work, yet international law prohibits these activities. African laws for instance permit children to engage in light work, because children in Africa are socialized into work, right from early childhood. According to the Ghana Statistical Service (2014) whether or not particular forms of work can be called child labor depends on the child's age, the type and hours of work performed, and the conditions under which the activity is undertaken. In Ghana, children are considered to be in child labor if they are (a) doing hazardous work, (b) less than 12 years and involved in economic activity, or (c) aged 12–14 years and involved in economic activities that are not defined as light work. Economic activity is defined as any work or activity performed during a specified reference period for pay (in cash or in kind), for profit, or for family gain (GSS, 2014). It is clear from the Ghana Children's Act 1998 and the GSS (2014) documents that light work differs from hazardous work, depending upon age, type, length of work, and work conditions. However, these definitions have some things in common, such as work, and economic activity for cash or for family support.

Child Labor in Africa

The 2016 Global Estimates of Child Labor, according to the ILO (2017) report, show that one-fifth of all African children engage in child labor, a proportion more than twice as high as in other regions, and that the highest number of child laborers, 72.1 million African children, are estimated to be in child labor, with 31.5 million African children in hazardous work. Africa is thus falling further behind the rest of the world in fighting child labor, despite the number of targeted policies implemented by African governments.

Africa is also noted to be among the regions affected by state of crisis and fragility, such as civil wars and disasters, which turn to increase the risk of child labor. For instance, in conflict regions, where children often comprise more than half of the 65 million people displaced by war, children's labor is often used as a coping mechanism in situations of heightened vulnerability. Many displaced families lose their income, especially if the main breadwinner is killed or is separated from the rest of the family (UNICEF, 2016).

Additionally, child labor in Africa occurs largely in family agriculture. Child labor in agriculture relates primarily to subsistence, livestock, and commercial farming, and it is often hazardous in its nature and in the circumstances it is carried out. Of the remaining children in child labor in Africa, 8.1 million (11%) are found in the services sector and 2.7 million (4%) are found in industry. Most child labor is unpaid, and most children in child labor are not in an employment relationship with a third-party employer, but rather work on family farms and family businesses. Most of these children are kept out of school, and thus robbed of their childhood and guaranteed a life in poverty, which may perpetuate itself throughout generations.

The Concept of Childhood in the African and Ghanaian Contexts

Researchers, such as Boakye-Boaten (2010) and Jenks (1996), have argued that the concept of childhood needs to be understood through people's sociocultural backgrounds. To these researchers, a child is a social being whose world is constructed within a cultural and historical frame of reference. Changes in any society have a significant impact on its children, and any effort to universalize the concept of the child may lead to interpretational fallacies, as well as a misunderstanding of the world of children (Boakye-Boaten, 2010; Jenks, 1996; Mead & Wolfenstein, 1954). As custodians of the future, the continuous survival of any society depends on the ability of its members to socialize its children to thrive through imparting its culture onto its young ones. In many traditional African societies, socialization of children is done through the various institutional structures, including religious rituals and traditional tales/myths, to help children acquire the values, beliefs, customs, norms, and cultural behaviors of the society.

Most often, Africans managed to maintain and perpetuate their culture through stringent socialization techniques that embraced the inputs of all community members. Their community organization techniques and communal nature that sought to protect its members enabled their survival against the invasion of social, economic, and political exploitation by other cultures. Also, in many traditional African societies, including Ghana, children were considered economic assets for their families. This leads to an economic incentive to have many children and a man's wealth comprised his many children (Boakye-Boaten, 2010; Clerk, 2011). Usually, children are perceived as biologically vulnerable persons in need of nurturing and protection and childhood is also perceived as a social construction with prescribed functions.

In Ghana and other African countries, clear responsibilities and roles exist between male and female members' domestic work. While females perform household chores (sweeping, cleaning, cooking), males perform heavy chores, such as farming, fishing, and hunting (Adu-Gyamfi, 2014; Clerk, 2011. Children also have a long history of domestic work, and normally they work as part of household production. For instance, children in Tallensi in Northern Ghana were noted to start engaging in economic activities at age 5 or 6, in order to be fully responsible for some tasks at age 12 (Bass, 2004; Clerk, 2011). Some children performed tasks such as bird-scaring on farms and baby-tending to allow their parents to engage in other tasks (Bass, 2004). It would therefore be useful to emphasize that from the cultural point of view, children working is not the same as child labor.

According to ILO/IPEC (2004), child domestic labor is not the ordinary tasks children perform at home; rather, it is the domestic tasks children perform in the homes of third parties under exploitative conditions. Examples include children/ grandchildren of elderly relatives engaging in tasks like washing clothes, fetching and carrying water to the bathroom, running errands, and sweeping rooms for elderly relatives (Clerk, 2011; Van Der Geeest, 2002). These tasks have historically and culturally been backed by intergenerational obligation of reciprocity and support to parents and the elderly, as they are entitled to this support. In a way, this makes the concept of child labor controversial, because the tasks Van Der Geeest (2002) has listed as child labor may not be perceived as such in Ghana.

Even with the tasks that are classified as child labor under laws or conventions, there is a general perception among adults and children in Ghana "that children are simply engaging in work, which is essential for their socialization" (Clerk, 2011, p. 10). Of course, reciprocity and respect for elders are among the values inculcated into children in the course of the socialization process. Different cultures have diverse ways of classifying childhood and child labor. In this regard, there is the need for society to understand the nature of current global developments in child labor laws and child rights policies accordingly. Also, while globalization and urbanization are altering the concept of childhood in urban areas in Ghana, the concept still exists in rural communities where children reside within the extended family system with community solidarity as the norm.

Child Labor in Ghana

Child labor is a social problem, especially in developing countries, Ghana inclusive. Statistics released by the ILO (2017) report indicates that about one million children globally between the ages of 5 and 17 years work in mining and quarrying alone. The ILO estimates tell a story both of real progress and of an unfinished job. The estimates indicate a dramatic decline in child labor under the age of 16 years, since the ILO began monitoring child labor in 2000. But the estimates also indicate that the pace of decline has slowed considerably in the last 4 years. The report estimates a total of 152 million children (64 million girls and 88 million boys) to be engaged in child labor globally. This accounts for nearly one in ten of all children across the globe. In addition, ILO (2017) reports that nearly half of all children engaged in child labor, 73 million, are in hazardous work that directly endangers their safety, health, and moral development. Children in employment, many of them comprising both child labor and permitted forms of employment involving children of legal working age, number 218 million. Additionally, the report indicates that Africa ranks highest both in the percentage of children in labor (one-fifth) and the absolute number (72 million) of children engaged in child labor. Almost half of all those in child labor in absolute terms are in hazardous work that directly endangers their safety, health, and moral development.

The Ghana Statistical Service (2014) noted that the proportion of Ghanaian children who participated in economic activities among the age group of 15–17 years was 43.7%, while that of the 5- to 7-year-old age group was 10%. According to the Ghana Statistical Service, 21.2% of the population of children 5–14 years old were engaged in child labor, with 11% engaged in hazardous labor. Higher proportions of children within the age groups 12–14 and 15–17 years who were attending school participated in economic activities, compared to the other age groups. Another 2014 Report by the Ghana NGOs Coalition on the Rights of the Child (GNCRC) noted that half of rural children and one-fifth of urban children in Ghana were economically active.

According to a UNICEF (2016) report, child labor in Ghana continues to affect an estimated 1.9 million children aged 5–17 years, about 22% of this age group. These numbers indicate clearly that the battle against child labor in Ghana has not yet been won, and that efforts in this regard need to be accelerated and intensified, in order that the goal of eliminating child labor is reached in the nearest future. The report further notes that the difference in child labor involvement between rural and urban children is striking. For the 5- to 17-year-old age range as a whole, the rate of child labor in rural areas (30%) is more than twice that in urban areas (12%). Child labor varies by region from a high of 33% in the Brong Ahafo and Upper West Regions to a low 5% in Greater Accra, per the report.

In Ghana, children engaged in activities, such as fishing, illegal artisanal mining, cattle herding, quarrying, selling, carrying heavy loads on the streets, farming activities, and tobacco production, meet the definition of child laborers (Appiah, 2018; GNCRC, 2014). Child labor according to these reports is still a major problem. Increase in the number of children in economic activities in the homes and on some city streets of Ghana has been attributed to the breakdown of the traditional family system. By this system, childcare by extended family members is prevalent, and the lack of, or ineffective, social protection mechanisms to safeguard needy and vulnerable families is attributed to the African concept of socialization of children through work (Appiah, 2018).

Factors Contributing to Child Labor in Ghana

Generally, child labor is a complex phenomenon caused by myriad factors given that the phenomenon is found in many sectors of the Ghanaian economy (UNICEF, 2016; Ghana Statistical Service, 2014). This section discusses the following factors: poverty, income shocks on households and urbanization, lack of formal education and educational opportunities for children, conflict situations, and gender roles.

Poverty

Poverty is noted to be a major cause of child labor in both rural and urban areas of sub-Saharan Africa (Basu et al., 2010). According to the poverty hypothesis, child labor is an unavoidable effect of hardship as children's participation in the workforce contributes positively to household income, alleviates economic stress, and satisfies the consumption requirements of many families (Basu et al., 2010; Togunde & Carter, 2006). With more than 50% of sub-Saharan Africa's population living below the poverty line and its countries ranking among the poorest in the world, it has been argued that poverty is driving children to paid economic activities to provide income to support themselves and their families (ILO, 2017).

In many rural areas in the subregion of Ghana, these economic activities are linked to subsistence farming, fishing, and mining among others (Boateng, 2017; Ghana NGOs Coalition on the Rights of the Child (GNCRC, 2014)). The GNCRC's report further indicated that 2.7 million Ghanaian children aged 5–7 years were engaged in economic activities. Per the same report, children were engaged in small-scale mining, which is among the worst forms of child labor, since the children are exposed to chemicals, such as mercury, cyanide, and crude machines that could be injurious to their health. Approximately, one million children globally between the ages of 5 and 17 are working in mining and quarrying alone (ILO, 2004).

Poverty compels children to engage in child labor in both rural and urban areas in Ghana. For instance, children in villages alongside the banks of the Volta River in Ghana also engage in child labor in the fishing industry (Appiah, 2018). Also, in urban areas, poverty compels children to indulge in activities, such as petty trading, truck pushing, quarrying, prostitution, and carrying heavy loads on the streets of urban/city markets for a fee (Basu et al., 2010; Boateng & Korang-Okrah, 2013). It is observed from these studies that many girls migrate from the three northern regions of Ghana to southern cities to carry loads for money and endure many hardships to earn income. In the same northern regions, some children who do not migrate, but reside in their home regions, engage in herding cattle or driving away birds from farms, at the expense of their education.

In a study of 40 children, aged 8–15 years at Gbefi in the Volta Region, Appiah (2018) found that children walked through thorny bushes with their bare feet, were exposed to snake bites, and ate and drank with animals regularly, all because of poverty. It was further observed that the children were encouraged and forced into cultivating tobacco farms to support family incomes (Appiah, 2018). This suggests that children from poor households are more likely to be engaged in labor than their counterparts from wealthy families.

Income Shocks on Households and Urbanization

One of the means by which families are sustained is through a meaningful income. Some households find dealing with income shocks comparable to the effects of natural disasters, agricultural crises, HIV/AIDS, and deaths, and may resort to child labor as a coping mechanism (ILO/IPEC, 2008). For example, in war-torn countries of sub-Saharan Africa, some children now have to live with HIV/AIDS, while others have been orphaned. Such children may not have caregivers, or may have grand-mother caregivers, who are unable to work. Some of these children may have to drop out of school to engage in commercial activities in order to support their families. There have been cases where orphaned children were compelled to work to care for younger siblings (ILO, 2004). Also, there were instances where adults were unable to find jobs to support their families because industrialists and factory owners preferred hiring children as a form of cheap labor, since it was more profitable to employ children who worked more, but earned less income (Agarwal, 1997).

The most densely populated parts of Ghana are the southern industrial cities, comprising Accra, Tema, Kumasi, and Takoradi. Research posits that majority of porters who migrate from the three northern regions of Ghana, or rural parts of the country to the industrial cities, have very little or no education, are of very poor economic backgrounds, and therefore engage in domestic labor and petty trading (Bermudez et al., 2018). These workers include children who have migrated to work and engage with city life. Some of these children are used as load carriers to offset the difficulty of vehicles accessing the center of markets to load or discharge goods. In other words, the few roads constructed for trucks to drive through to the markets have been taken over by market women selling their wares, making the roads inaccessible by cars/trucks. Others who migrate from rural communities to the cities indulge in street hawking or selling along the streets (Boateng & Korang-Okrah, 2013; Hamenoo et al., 2018; Opare, 2003). The rapid growth of these menial jobs, among other things, attributes to the fact that rural poverty alleviation programs are not attractive enough to incentivize the youth to participate in rural community enterprises (Bangirigah & Hilson, 2010) with implications for rural-urban migration, such as overcrowding, unemployment, and limited access to social amenities.

Lack of Formal Education and Educational Opportunities for Children

Most often, parents who do not have formal education do not find it necessary for their children to attend school. Children in families where high levels of illiteracy exist are more likely to be candidates of domestic work (ILO, 2004). There are instances where children have dropped out of school to help with farmwork or household chores. Normally, there is a perception that in developing countries, the decision to enroll children in school is influenced by the educational levels of their parents. For example, findings from a study by Fetuga et al. (2000) conducted in Ogun State, Nigeria, concluded that the prevalence of child labor increased with decreasing parental education and socioeconomic status. Similar conclusions were made by Khanam (2008) in a study conducted in rural Bangladesh that parents' educational level significantly increases the probability that school-aged children would further their education to a higher level. However, there may be instances where parents without formal education support and encourage their children to pursue higher education. Hilson (2010) for instance noted that despite the acute shortage of jobs in Tallensi-Nabdam and surrounding townships, parents continued to value their children's education.

Lack of educational opportunities could also drive children into various kinds of child labor. This is stipulated in the ILO report on eliminating child labor in mining and quarrying (ILO, 2005), which posits that lack of access to quality education,

particularly secondary education, is common and children with no access to education have little or no alternative than to enter the labor market. Many of the ILO's
studies have drawn conclusions to reinforce this claim. For example, almost 70% of
child laborers interviewed as part of an ILO study carried out in mining camps in the
Chunya, Geita, and Tunduru districts of Tanzania reported that children were forced
to end their studies because they lacked the finances to attend school (Mwami et al.,
2002). Similarly, another ILO study conducted in Burkinabe artisanal mining sites
and communities found that several child laborers had dropped out of school because
of lack of funds (Groves, 2004). These findings notwithstanding, it was suggested
that while endemic poverty is fueling child labor in artisanal mining sites, its
impoverished educational facilities have not diminished children's ambitions to
attend school (Groves, 2004).

Conflicts and Gender Roles

There is a link between child labor and situations of conflict and disaster. According
to the ILO (2017) report, the African region has been among those most affected by
conflicts and disasters, which in turn heighten the risk of child labor. The incidence
of child labor in countries affected by armed conflict is noted to be 77% higher than
the global average, while the incidence of hazardous work is 50% higher. This
situation calls for prioritization of child labor within humanitarian responses and
during reconstruction and recovery. In addition, governments, employers' organizations, and humanitarian actors, including social workers and public health professionals, have a critical role to play in this context. For instance, the Government of
Ghana partners, UNICEF and USAID, aim to strengthen the social protection programs, such as the Livelihood Empowerment Against Poverty and the National
Health Insurance. The International Organization for Migration supports the government's efforts in rescuing children from forced labor at fishing villages along the
Volta Lake.

Traditional and cultural roles could have detrimental impacts on childhood and
children in Ghana. Debates on gender issues are currently central in discussions on
child domestic labor, as gender plays a role in determining the nature and patterns of
labor that children are engaged in at home. Child domestic work is generally
considered as a female role in Ghana. Doubtless to say that girls in many Ghanaian
localities face social, economic, and cultural barriers, which may further impede
their ability to fully enjoy their childhood, and as well impact their ability to access
formal education (Hilson, 2010).

Consequences of Child Labor in Ghana

Child labor has adverse effects on children's development and well-being, especially their education and health (Hamenoo et al., 2018). Children who engage in child labor may suffer from many ill effects, such as risks and dangers at work, poor school attendance, and health complications.

Risks and Dangers at Work

Children engaged in child labor and other kinds of hazardous work are exposed to various kinds of abuses at their workplaces. Findings from the Ghana Statistical Service (2014) indicated that about nine in every ten (91%) children engaged in child labor reported experiencing some form of abuse, with another 87.4% of those exposed to hazardous forms of work reporting abuses at the workplace. Abuses in child labor include rape, customers yelling at the child laborers, receiving lower wages, employers not paying the children their wages at all, and constant exposure to poor working conditions. Certainly, these experiences can physically damage a child's health (Boateng & Korang-Okrah, 2013). Children often suffer psychological and emotional damage from working and living in an environment where they are exposed to harassment, violence, and physical and sexual abuse. These may result in serious emotional effects, such as depression, low self-esteem, hopelessness, guilt, shame, and loss of confidence that could lead to a higher risk of mental illness and antisocial behaviors.

In a study on children fishing on the Volta Lake of Ghana, it was noted that the children faced double jeopardy of death due to diseases such as bilharzia, guinea worm, or even drowning, as they dive to release fishing nets stuck to tree stumps in the water (Clerk, 2011). Since these are children under 18 years of age, this is a violation of Sect. 91 of the 1998 Children's Act of Ghana. Also, illegal artisanal gold mining is noted to be one of the worst forms of child labor, since the children are exposed to chemicals and machines that could be harmful, together with potential drowning in the mining pits (Hilson, 2010). Consequences of work-related hazards may lead to permanent disabilities and premature death in children.

Poor School Attendance

The Ghana Statistical Service Survey (2014) sought to find out whether children engaged in child labor were also attending school and the findings showed that 20.1% of children who were attending school were engaged in child labor. Nearly two-fifths of the males (39.9%) and 31.2% of the females who were engaged in child labor were not attending school. The distribution by locality indicated that the proportion of children in rural areas (28.8%) who were attending school and engaged in child labor was higher, compared to those in urban areas (11.2%). Ghana's rural savannah had the highest proportion of children (32.2%) attending school and at the same time engaged in child labor, while the rural forest had the highest proportion of children (20.4%) engaged in hazardous forms of child labor. The ILO (2004) asserts that if a child combines school with work, it might be difficult for him/her to attend school because the long hours of work could interfere with class or homework.

Another study observed that child labor negatively affects children's education with regard to school attendance, enrollment, and performance (Odonkor, 2007). In many rural areas of developing countries where more than 70% of the world's child labor occurs (ILO, 2017), it becomes an activity that makes children part-time pupils, rather than full-time students (Beegle et al., 2009). It was noted by Anumaka (2012) that child labor has an adverse impact on children's academic performance. Also, Bezerra et al. (2009) found that children who worked 7 h or more per day had a 10% decrease in their test scores, in comparison to their counterparts who did not engage in any kind of work. Furthermore, Heady (2003) conducted a household study in Ghana and reported a negative relationship between child labor and measures of reading and mathematics competence.

Health Complications

There are several risks involved in the kind of work children do, which can have a negative impact on their health. Porter et al. (2011) asserted that many of the trades children engaged in required them to carry loads and this adversely affected their health. Among the negative health effects of child labor are energy cost of head-loading, long-term biomechanical impacts, risk of acute injury, and physical deficiencies (Porter et al., 2013). Additionally, working as a child could lead to ill health and road traffic accidents (Hamenoo et al., 2018; Omokhodion et al., 2005). Many children who are engaged in child labor, especially the worst forms of child labor, are likely to experience health complications because they may not have enough time to rest.

Findings from the Ghana Living Standards Survey conducted by the Ghana Statistical Service (2014) indicated that 11.1% of females were exposed to gas, fire, or fumes, compared to 6.4% of males, and 21.3% and 18.3% of males and females, respectively, were exposed to chemicals at their workplaces. More than 58.9% of male and 55.5% of female children engaged in economic activities were exposed to dangerous tools (knives). Additionally, 43.1% of males and 42.1% of females were exposed to dust and fumes, while 27.4% of males and 28.2% of females (more than one-quarter in each case) were exposed to extreme heat and cold. The findings also indicated that almost two out of every five (38.1%) working children had insect bites at work, while 33.6% experienced fatigue. Nearly equal proportions of males and females experienced skin problems, extreme fatigue, and fever in the course of their work.

Legal Framework and Policies in Place for Tackling Child Labor

Given the adverse effects of child labor on children's well-being and development, various laws and policy measures have been put in place at the international, regional, and national levels, to lessen its intensity and ultimately prevent its occurrence. As noted by Awadey (2011), since 1990, key conventions that are relevant to the rights of children, as well as their protection from labor, have been ratified in Ghana. These include:

- United Nations Convention on the Rights of the Child in 1990
- ILO Convention on the Worst Forms of Child Labor in 2000
- African Charter on the Rights and Welfare of the Child of the African Union, which states that children should be protected from all forms of economic exploitation and from performing work that is likely to be hazardous or to interfere with the child's physical, mental, spiritual, moral, or social development (Organization of African Unity, 1999)

Ghana also joined other nations in 1999 on a 3-year ILO/IPEC, International Programme on the Elimination of Child Labour, a regional project to eliminate the trafficking of children for labor purposes within the African subregion. In 2000, a Memorandum of Understanding (MoU) was signed by the government with ILO/IPEC to formulate a national policy and plan of action to combat child labor (Hamenoo et al., 2018; Kukwa, 2013). In addition, at the national level, the Government of Ghana has strengthened the legal protection of children as stipulated in the provisions for fundamental human rights and freedoms in Chap. 5 of the 1992 Constitution for all Ghanaians, children inclusive. In addition, the entire Sect. 28 of Chap. 5 of the Constitution relates to children's rights, while Sect. 28(2) specifies that every child has the right to be protected from engaging in work that constitutes a threat to their health, education, or development. Moreover, Section 16 of the Constitution prohibits slavery and forced labor by any person; Section 24 states that it is the right of every person to work in satisfactory, safe, and healthy conditions; and Sect. 28 guarantees children the right to be protected from engaging in work that comprises a threat to their health, education, or development (Awadey, 2011).

Further, in 1998, the Parliament of the Republic of Ghana passed the Children's Act (Act 560) that combined all previous child-related laws for protecting children to reflect the standards of the United Nations and the ILO. The Act made a provision for the creation of child panels in all metropolitan, municipal, and district assemblies (MMDAs). A child panel is established in each district of Ghana to mediate in any civil matter concerning the rights of the child and parental duties. The Legal Aid Scheme Act, 1997 (Act 542), also made provision for legal aid services. These laws sought to establish institutions for welfare and access to justice for previously excluded segments of the society like children engaged in worst forms of child labor. Additionally, other laws have been passed to further strengthen the legal framework and ensure favorable treatment of children with regard to their protection from exploitation, growth, and development. These laws included the Human Trafficking Act, 2006, (Act 694); the Domestic Violence Act, 2007 (Act 732); the Criminal Code Amendment Act, 1998 (Act 554), that abolished all forms of customary servitude, including those involving children; the Juvenile Justice Administration Act, 2003 (Act 653); and the Whistle Blower's Act, 2006 (Act 720) (Awadey, 2011).

Since the program on the elimination of child labor was introduced in Ghana in 2000, many steps have been initiated to withdraw or prevent children from engaging in child labor (Ghana Statistical Service, 2014). In support of these efforts, a legal framework and a National Plan of Action (NPA) were developed to guide the prevention or fight against child labor. The action plan involved the establishment of systems and development of different instruments and guidelines, which aimed to assist in combating the phenomenon and included:

- The Ghana Child Labor Monitoring System (GCLMS), which is an active process to regularly check workplaces in order to ensure that children are not working there, and that young workers are adequately protected.
- The Hazardous Activity Framework for the Cocoa Sectors of Ghana (HAF), which provides guidelines for identifying hazards associated with the occupation and specifies economic activities that are hazardous and must not be done by children. It also provides the list of work that is permissible and those that are not permissible for children in each sector where child labor is found.
- The Standard Operating Procedures and Guidelines (SOPs) for Child Labor Elimination in Ghana, which provides procedures for dealing with the worst forms of child labor and specific guidelines for dealing with children engaged in child labor in each sector.

Notwithstanding the existence of various laws and programs to prevent or withdraw children from child labor, the phenomenon is still in existence. Children engage in economic activities in different sectors of the Ghanaian economy, including agriculture, which has the largest proportion (80%) of children engaged in child labor (UNICEF, 2016). This is disturbing because as argued by Holgado et al. (2014), child labor is a disinvestment in social and human capital as it adversely affects the development of children, as well as hinders the development of their skills, abilities, and knowledge necessary to make a significant contribution to society.

Implications for Social Work, Social Policy, and Public Health in Ghana

In order to prevent or reduce children's engagement in exploitative economic activities, which has negative effects on their development and well-being, there is the need to enforce the implementation of laws, policies, and programs that have been developed to protect children and guarantee their development. It would be useful, therefore, to create more awareness about the dangers of child labor as some people in Ghana perceive it as essential since it is part of children's socialization. This suggests the need for social workers and public health professionals to collaborate with community members, especially traditional and religious leaders, to draw society's attention on how child labor is abusive and injurious and deprives children of their rights.

In view of the fact that high levels of poverty and unemployment are major factors that contribute to child labor, many poor and impoverished children and their families depend on children's work to meet their basic daily needs. Thus, children are pulled by the prospect of getting instant money for survival as it has become the bait, luring them into labor. In the absence of adequate viable economic opportunities for adults, jobs like artisanal mining, tobacco production, and load carrying where children are involved in could then be described as income generation avenues to support the livelihoods of households. Children are therefore expected to work, whether unpaid or paid, to assist their families/households. In such a situation, work is regarded as an opportunity to fulfill filial and other socioeconomic obligations in families and communities. Consequently, the intricate relationship between push and pull factors for child labor in Ghana cannot be overemphasized.

Furthermore, poverty reduction in Ghana needs to be addressed by both governmental and nongovernmental organizations through the strengthening of social protection programs (social insurance, social assistance, and child protection) in order to alleviate the plight of vulnerable children and their families. For instance, the introduction of the Livelihood Empowerment Against Poverty (LEAP), a cash transfer program that benefits the most vulnerable in Ghana, is a step in the right direction. Another effort of the Government of Ghana is the replacement of school fees with the capitation grant where schools receive a grant per student to cover their fees. This grant is also complemented by a school feeding program, which fosters improved nutrition and has a positive impact on education through improved attendance and performance. However, these programs do not cover all schools in Ghana, mainly due to financial constraints, and should therefore be expanded to benefit all eligible children and families.

In addition, given that child labor constitutes a major social and public health problem, it is important to prioritize it in social policy discussions. It is negatively associated with the physical and psychological health of children involved as it exposes children to health and safety risks, such as exposure to chemicals, injuries, vehicular accidents, and neck and bodily pains. The harm experienced by children manifests itself in many guises with acute, latent, and chronic effects on the children themselves, their families and communities, and the nation as a whole. Thus, it is essential for social workers and community health nurses to collaborate with relevant stakeholders to identify exploitative and hazardous economic activities that children are engaged in and design interventions that would eliminate, mitigate, or halt such activities. Social workers could introduce and create linkages between communities and cooperatives/microfinance schemes to engage families in sustainable development projects to generate income to support their households.

Adopting a multidisciplinary and multi-sectoral approach would help understand, prevent, and address the issue.

Also, it would be useful for child protection agencies to collaborate and ensure the removal, recovery, and reintegration of children who are engaged in child labor, particularly the worst forms of child labor. In addition, the provision of psychosocial support for children engaged in child labor and their families would be a step in the right direction, as child labor could be difficult, hazardous, and exploitative. Furthermore, given that child labor is a complex, multidimensional phenomenon associated with many risk factors, it is essential to conduct more research on the psychosocial and health impacts of the phenomenon. This is necessary because child labor is a wound that is visible, but seems invisible and far from being addressed. Future research could consider implications for measurement, definitions, and concepts.

References

Adu-Gyamfi, J. (2014). Childhood construction and its implications for children's participation in Ghana. *African Journal of Social Sciences, 4*(2), 1–11.

Agarwal, B. (1997). Bargaining and gender relations: Within and beyond the household. *Feminist Economics, 3*(1), 1–51.

Anumaka, I. B. (2012). Child labour: impact on academic performance and social implication: A case of Northeast Uganda. *Journal of Educational Science and Research, 2*(2).

Appiah, S. O. (2018). Child labor or child work? Children and tobacco production in Gbefi, Volta region. *Ghana Social Science Journal, 15*(1), 147–176.

Awadey, C. (2011). *National social mobilization strategy for the elimination of the worst forms of child labour in Ghana: A call to action.* Child Labour Unit of the Labour Department, Ministry of Employment and Social Welfare.

Bangirigah, S. M., & Hilson, G. (2010). Re-orienting livelihoods in African artisanal mining. *Policy Sciences, 43*, 157–180.

Bass, L. E. (2004). Child labor in sub-Saharan Africa. In R. K. Ame, D. L. Agbenyiga, & N. A. Apt (Eds.), *Children's rights in Ghana: Reality or rhetoric?* (p. 102). Lexington Books.

Basu, K., Das, S., & Dutta, B. (2010). Child labor and household wealth: Theory and empirical evidence of an inverted-U. *Journal of Development Economics, 91*(1), 8–14.

Beegle, K., Dehejia, R., & Gatti, R. (2009). Why should we care about child labor? The education, labor market, and health consequences of child labor. Journal of Human Resources, 44(4), 871–889. https://doi.org/10.3368/jhr.44.4.871

Bermudez, L. G., Bahar, O. S., Dako-Gyeke, M., Boateng, A., Ibrahim, A., Ssewamala, F. M., & McKay, M. (2018). Understanding female migrant child labor within a cumulative risk framework: The case for combined interventions in Ghana. *International Social Work, 63*(2), 147–163.

Bezerra, M. G., Kassouf, A. L., & Arends-Kuenning, M. (2009). The impact of child labour and school quality on academic achievement in Brazil. IZA Discussion Paper No. 4062.

Boakye-Boaten, A. (2010). Changes in the concept of childhood: Implications on children in Ghana. *The Journal of International Social Research, 3*(10), 104–115.

Boateng, A. (2017). Rethinking alternative livelihood projects for women of the pits: The case of Atiwa. *Academic Journal of Interdisciplinary Studies, 6*(2), 17–25.

Boateng, A., & Korang-Okrah, R. (2013). The predicament of rural urban migration in Ghana: The case of visible, but voiceless Kayayei girls. *Journal of Social Sciences, 3*(4), 46–61.

Clerk, G. (2011). Child labor in Ghana: Global concern and local reality. In Ame, R.K., Agbenyiga, D.L., & Apt, N.A.. *Children's rights in Ghana: Reality or rhetoric?*. Lexington Books.

Fetuga, B., Njokama, F. O., & Olowu, A. D. (2000). Prevalence, types and demographic features of child labour among school children in Nigeria. *International Health and Human Rights, 5*(1), 2.

Ghana NGOs Coalition on the Rights of the Child. (2014). *Convention on the rights of children (CRC) report.* Retrieved on December 10, from https://tbinternet.ohchr.org/Treaties/CRC/Shared%20Documents/GHA/INT_CRC_NGO_GHA_17939_E.pdf

Ghana Statistical Service. (2014). *Ghana living standards survey.* Retrieved on 03/26/2020, from http://www.statsghana.gov.gh/nada/index.php/catalog/72/data-dictionary

Government of Ghana. (1998). Children's Act (560). Government Printer.

Groves, L. (2004). Implementing ILO Child labour convention 182: Lessons from the gold mining sector in Burkina Faso. *Development in Practice, 15*(1), 49–59.

Hamenoo, E. S., Dwomoh, E. A., & Dako-Gyeke, M. (2018). Child labour in Ghana: Implications for children's education and health. *Children and Youth Services Review, 93*, 248–254.

Heady, C. (2003). The effects of child labour on learning achievement. *World Development, 31*, 385–398.

Hilson, G. (2010). Child labor in African artisanal mining communities: Experiences from Northern Ghana. *Development and Change, 41*(3), 445–473.

Holgado, D., Maya-Jaiego, I., Ramos, I., Palacio, J., Oviedo-Trespalacios, O., Romero-Mendoza, V., & Amar, J. (2014). Impact of child labor on academic performance: Evidence from the program Educame Primero Colombia. *International Journal of Educational Development, 34*, 58–66.

ILO. (1999). *C182 – Worst Forms of Child Labour Convention*, 1999 (No. 182). Retrieved from: https://www.ilo.org/dyn/normlex/en/f?p=NORMLEXPUB:12100:0::NO::P12100_ILO_CODE:C182

ILO. (2002). *The International Labour Organization's fundamental conventions.* Retrieved on December, 01, 2018 from http://www.ilo.org/legacy/english/inwork/cb-policy-guide/ilodeclarationonfundamentalprinciplesandrightsatwork

ILO. (2004). *Global child labour developments: Measuring trends* from 2004-2008. Retrieved on November 19, 2018 from www.ilo.org/ipecinfo/product/download.do?type=document&id=13313

ILO. (2005). *Eliminating child labour in mining and quarrying.* Retrieved on October 16, 2018 from http://www.ilo.org/public/portugue/region/eurpro/lisbon/pdf/minas.pdf

ILO. (2017). *Global estimates of child labour: Results and trends*, 2012–2016. Retrieved on October 30, 2018 from https://www.ilo.org/wcmsp5/groups/public/@dgreports/@dcomm/documents/publication/wcms_575499.pdf

ILO/IPEC. (2008). *Children in hazardous work: What we know, what we need to do.* Retrieved on October 23, 2018 from https://www.ilo.org/wcmsp5/groups/public/@dgreports/@dcomm/@publ/documents/publication/wcms_155428.pdf.

Jenks, C. (1996). Changes in the concept of childhood: Implications on children in Ghana. *The Journal of International Social Research, 3*(10), 104–115.

Khanam, R. (2008). Child labour and school attendance: Evidence from Bangladesh. *International Journal of Social Economics, 35*(1/2), 77–98.

Kukwa, P. A. (2013). *Analytical study on child labour in Lake Volta fishing in Ghana.* ILO/IPEC.

Mead, M., & Wolfenstein, M. (1954). *Childhood in contemporary cultures*. Chicago University Press.

Mwami, J. A., Sanga, A. J., & Nyoni, J. (2002). *Child labour in mining: A rapid assessment*. ILO.

Odonkor, M. (2007). *Addressing child labour through education: A study of alternative complementary initiatives in quality education delivery and their suitability for cocoa-farming communities*. Retrieved on 09 December 2018, from http://citeseerx.ist.psu.edu/viewdoc/download?doi=10.1.1.732.5631&rep=rep1&type=pdf.

Omokhodion, F. O., Omokhodion, S. I., & Odusote, T. O. (2005). Perceptions of child labour among working children in Ibadan, Nigeria. *Child: Care, Health & Development, 32*(3), 281–286.

Opare, J. A. (2003). Kayayei: The women head porters of southern Ghana. *Journal of Social Development in Africa, 18*(2), 33–48.

Porter, G., Blaufuss, K., & Acheampong, F. (2011). Filling the family transport gap in sub-Saharan Africa: Young people and load carrying in Ghana. In L. Holt (Ed.), *Geographies of children, youth and families: An international perspective*. Routledge.

Porter, G., Hampshire, K., Dunn, C., Hall, R., Levesley, M., Burton, K., ... Panther, J. (2013). Health impacts of pedestrian head-loading: A review of the evidence with particular reference to women and children in sub-Saharan Africa. *Social Science & Medicine, 80*, 90–97.

Togunde, D., & Carter, A. (2006). In their own words: Consequences of child labour in urban Nigeria. *Journal of Social Sciences, 16*(2), 173–181.

UNICEF. (2016). *Child labour and the youth decent work deficit in Ghana: Inter-agency country report* http://www.ucw-project.org/attachment/13052016890Ghan_child_labour_youth_employment_report.pdf

Van Der Geest, S. (2002). Respect and reciprocity: Care of the elderly people in rural Ghana. In R. K. Ame, D. L. Agbenyiga, & N. A. Apt (Eds.), Children's rights in Ghana: Reality or rhetoric? (p. 102). Lexington Books.

Children Living on the Street: Current Efforts in Policy Research and Practice in Ghana

Ernestina Korleki Dankyi

Introduction

The situation of children and youth growing up on the streets is a global phenomenon that has attracted considerable interest both in academic and policy research and in debates. The concern about children living on the street becomes even more crucial with the adoption of the Sustainable Development Goals (SDGs). In September 2015, the United Nations General Assembly adopted the 2030 Agenda for Sustainable Development that includes 17 SDGs with a firm pledge of "leaving no one behind". Street children represent a vulnerable group that is furthest behind in terms of development—as they lack shelter, access to education and healthcare, and general social support and if the goal to leave no one behind is to be achieved, the needs of these vulnerable social groups must be deliberately targeted.

According to the United Nations, there are more than 150 million street children in the world today. The lack of national level data on street children globally makes it challenging to ascertain an accurate number of children living in vulnerable conditions on the streets (Dabir & Athale, 2011). The large numbers of children living on the streets are due to global challenges such as poverty, rapid urbanisation, overcrowded cities, uneven distribution of wealth, privatisation, high rates of migration and breakdown of family structures (Amantana, 2012; Boakye-Boaten, 2008; Conticini & Hulme, 2006; Patel, 1990; van Blerk, 2012; Young, 2003)—a challenge confronting both developed and developing countries.

The growing incidence of children living on the streets of Ghana and factors driving this trend mirror the global picture. It is uncertain how many children live and work on the streets of Ghana; however, the last census of children living and working on the streets of Accra revealed that about 61,492 children live and work on

E. K. Dankyi (✉)
Centre for Social Policy Studies, College of Humanities, University of Ghana, Legon, Ghana
e-mail: ekdankyi@ug.edu.gh

© Springer Nature Switzerland AG 2022
F. M. Ssewamala et al. (eds.), *Child Behavioral Health in Sub-Saharan Africa*,
https://doi.org/10.1007/978-3-030-83707-5_14

the streets (Department of Social Welfare, 2011). The majority (65%) of these children are categorised as "children of the street" (Ennew, 1994) for whom a street is a place of residence and work. The situation of children living and working on the street is assuming more problematic dimensions as the numbers soar and their living conditions get worse (Amantana, 2012; Awumbila & Ardayfio-Schandorf, 2008; Boakye-Boaten, 2008; Oppong, 2015). The trend of increasing numbers of children living on the streets may continue in the foreseeable future, considering the rapid rate of urbanisation across Africa and the lack of mechanisms to reduce urban poverty.

Whereas the subject has received a lot of attention in research (Mizen & Ofosu-Kusi, 2013; Mizen & Ofosu-Kusi, 2010; Oppong, 2015; Oppong Asante & Meyer-Weitz, 2015; Ungruhe, 2019) the same cannot be said for policy efforts and actual actions towards addressing the situation. The Government of Ghana, like many other African governments, has not attached the needed aggression and urgency to match the rising concern of children living in unsafe conditions on the street. Ghana was the first country in the world to ratify the UN Convention on the rights of a child in 1990 which was followed by the passing of the Children's Act (Act 560) in 1998, a clear commitment to promote and protect the rights of all children including those living on the street. However, these policies have not translated into any concrete actions as far as children living on the streets are concerned. Other efforts made by the government in this regard can be best described as ad hoc, reactive and not sustainable.

One important group that has shouldered the problem of street children in Ghana has been non-governmental organisations (NGOs). In Ghana, NGOs have been at the forefront with or without government support in addressing the problem of children living and working on the street for almost three decades now. NGOs have proven to be a critical party in working to address the problem of children living on the streets in several countries (Desai & Potter, 2014; Kassa, 2018; Niboye, 2013). With a focus on international conventions and the Sustainable Development Goals, this chapter examines the efforts that have been made to address the situation of children living on the streets in Ghana. Specifically, I assess the activities of 15 NGOs that work with street children and the alignment of their activities with the international and local conventions and the SDGs. Attention is paid to the SDGs 1 (ending poverty), 2 (no hunger), 3 (quality health and well-being for all), 4 (education), 8 (employment and decent income), 10 (reducing inequality) and 17 (partnerships). These goals were selected based on their direct relevance to the day-to-day experiences of children living on the street.

Street Children in Ghana

In Ghana, the situation of street children has been an important focus of research for almost three decades now. Research areas covered include reasons for moving to the streets, livelihood strategies and violence that characterises the daily lives of children living on the streets (Agarwal et al., 1997; Awumbila & Ardayfio-Schandorf, 2008;

Boakye-Boaten, 2008). There is also growing interest in the mental health experiences of children living on the street with common themes such as resilience and coping mechanisms for navigating the harsh conditions of the street as they seek food, shelter and safe spaces receiving the most attention (Mizen & Ofosu-Kusi, 2013; Oppong Asante & Meyer-Weitz, 2017; Ungruhe, 2019).

A census taken in the Greater Accra region of Ghana in 2011 revealed that about 61,492 persons below the age of 18 are working on the streets (Department of Social Welfare, 2011). A significant proportion (65%) of these children live and work on the streets, the majority of whom have migrated from rural areas into the big cities. Some of them migrate to the cities in the company of friends and adults, while others migrate alone. These children, often of ages 4 and above, are found in the largest cities of Ghana, also known as Ghana's golden triangle cities (Kwankye and Addoquaye-Tagoe, 2009). The golden triangle entails Accra and Tema in south-eastern Ghana in the Greater Accra region, where Accra is Ghana's capital and also serves as the commercial, industrial and cultural nerve centre of Ghana. Tema, located to the east of Accra, has Ghana's largest port and serves as the industrial centre of Ghana, making it attractive to various categories of migrants including children. Kumasi is the capital city of the Ashanti region and is the second largest city in Ghana almost centrally located; the city is attractive to many migrants in pursuit of various livelihood activities. In south-western Ghana is the oil city of Sekondi-Takoradi which also hosts Ghana's main export port. As an industrial city, Sekondi-Takoradi has always attracted migrants in search of jobs at the port and the various industries there. The commercial discovery of oil and gas in 2007 and the subsequent surge in business activities also boosted the attractiveness of Sekondi-Takoradi to migrants (Ablo, 2018). The population of migrants in these cities comprises both girls and boys in almost equal proportion, the majority of whom have migrated from mostly rural parts of less endowed regions of Ghana.

Once on the street, the children engage in various forms of income-generating activities. Whereas the girls from the northern parts of Ghana are noted for engaging in head porterage and are usually referred to as "Kayeyei", other girls engage in petty trading, hawking in the street and selling different kinds of "fast-moving commodities" on the streets of these cities (Awumbila & Ardayfio-Schandorf, 2008; Boakye-Boaten, 2008; Kwankye et al., 2009). The boys, on the other hand, work as errand boys in large markets where they stay in front of large shops and assist customers who come to buy products in bulk; others serve as shoeshine boys, some beg for alms and others hawk fast-moving commodities like their female counterparts. After a hard day's work, majority of the 65% for whom the street is home too sleep on the pavements of lorry stations, in front of shops and in marketplaces and the few who can afford may rent wooden structures in a slum (Department of Social Welfare, 2011; Mizen & Ofosu-Kusi, 2013; Mizen & Ofosu-Kusi, 2010). In most cases, they sleep in the open and manage to get some covering to protect themselves against mosquitoes.

Street children in Ghana, according to Anarfi (Anarfi, 1997), have had to pay for almost every essential service including toilet, shower in public bathrooms, their food and drinking water and places that they keep their valuable belongings (if any).

Thus, life on the street is particularly expensive for these children. There is also a growing number of what has become known as the "second generation" of street children, referring to children born on the streets to street children. Some children live on the streets with their mothers, sleep in open places and are mostly carried on their mothers' backs during the day as the mothers try to work to earn a living. Sometimes, to allow them room to work without distractions, some of these second-generation children are sent back to their relatives to whom the mothers remit money regularly for their upkeep.

Successive governments have tried to address the situation of children living on the streets. Several social protection programmes, aimed at promoting the rights of all children, including the vulnerable ones, have been rolled out in the last 10 years. The Ministry of Gender, Children and Social Protection and other relevant ministries have rolled out 44 social intervention programmes aimed at reducing the burden of unemployment, poverty and other related socioeconomic challenges. Notably, 5 out of the 44 programmes directly target child and family welfare. These are the National Health Insurance Scheme (NHIS), Livelihood Empowerment Against Poverty (LEAP), School Feeding Programme, Capitation Grant and Free School Uniform Programme. In 2015, the Government of Ghana launched the Child and Family Welfare Policy. The overall goal of the Child and Family Welfare Policy was to help formulate child and family welfare programmes and activities to more effectively prevent and protect children from all forms of violence, abuse, neglect and exploitation (Ministry of Gender, Children and Social Protection, 2015). The policy stressed on the collaboration of key actors in the area of child protection to set standards for addressing harm to children in a comprehensive way. It also emphasised the empowerment of children and families to understand abusive situations better and make choices to prevent and respond to cases of risk. However, street children have barely benefitted from these interventions because they are primarily family and household based, thereby resulting in increasing numbers and worsening condition of street children. Thomas de Benitez (Thomas de Benitez, 2011) noted that social welfare and development policies aimed at protecting vulnerable children are inadequate for street children, whose multiple deprivations and street-connectedness overwhelm service capacity.

Non-governmental and faith-based organisations have augmented these efforts working with street children for about three decades now, and these have collaborated with government agencies on several issues and activities. Notable among these collaborations are attempts and policies that guide the work of NGOs and make provisions for street children to be catered for as stipulated in the many conventions that govern and promote the welfare of all children.

Study Framework

The study was analysed using a policy framework comprising the international and national level policies, namely the UN Convention on the Rights of the Child, Ghana's 1998 Children's Act (Act 560), the Child and Family Welfare Policy

(2015) and the Sustainable Development Goals which are deemed to make adequate provision for the protection and promotion of the rights of all children including children living on the street. The UNCRC compels signatory states to regularly evaluate implementation and enforcement of laws and policies towards children, including street children (see, e.g., (Veeran, 2004)). It is anticipated that these local and international conventions will inform efforts to address the situation of street children.

Activities of NGOs assessed according to principles of the best interest of the child, protection of the child and participation of children in the matters that concern their lives as enshrined in the UNCRC and the Children's Act (Act 560) and the principle of leaving no one behind that guides the Agenda 2030 of the SDGs. Assessing the best interests of a child, according to the UNCRC, means to evaluate and balance all the elements necessary to decide in a specific situation for a particular individual child or group of children. Best interests of children in street situations must be a primary concern in all actions that concern them—by parents, carers, lawmakers, policymakers, welfare institutions and those who influence or control resource allocation, including decisions throughout government, judiciary and parliamentary (OHCHR, n.d.). Protection includes immediate protection from danger, abuse, and exploitation, but also covers more long-term proactive approaches designed to promote the development of children's skills and knowledge, build support structures for children and lower their vulnerability. This further implies the need to protect children and prevent experiences of multiple deprivations that push them to connect with the street (OHCHR, n.d.). Participation is a human right with particular significance for street children. It is essential to actively engage children living on the street in addressing their problems from the design stage to the implementation and evaluation stages of interventions. The opinion of street-connected children should inform policies, plans and interventions designed to address them (OHCHR, n.d.). The principle of participation aligns with the modern conception of childhood as put forward by James and Prout (James & Prout, 1997) in their seminal work of the reconstruction of childhood. They advocate for children to be seen as social agents capable of making meaning of their world and responding to the meanings they make of their lifeworld.

Leaving no one behind and reaching the furthest behind first is the mantra for Agenda 2030. Based on the five characteristics that indicate which populations are at risk of being left behind, namely discrimination, geography, governance, socio-economic status, and shocks and fragility, street children easily fall into the categories of the at-risk population. Including the principle of leaving no one behind in the framework was used to assess how the activities of these NGOs are targeted at reducing street children's risk of being left behind by 2030.

Methods and Materials

This project explored the range of services and interventions focused on street children in Ghana and the institutions that provided them. Fifteen NGOs that work exclusively with street children in Accra and Kumasi were purposively selected using a snowball sampling technique (Bryman, 2012). Their directors or founders were interviewed using a semi-structured interview guide. The study framework informed the interview guide. The interviews also explored how the institutions were regulated and financed and how they could be better positioned towards the achievement of the SDGs for street children. The interviews were audio-recorded with the consent of the participants and transcribed verbatim. Thematic analysis (Braun & Clarke, 2006) was conducted, and three main themes emerged: services provided, partnerships, and policy environment emerged from the data. Interpretation of the data was guided by the principles of the Convention on the Rights of the Child (1989), the 1998 Children's Act (Act 560) and the SDGs, namely best interest of the child, protection from harm, participation in decisions concerning their lives and leaving no one behind.

Findings

The data have been synthesised and presented under three main themes: (1) services rendered by the NGOs for street children, (2) partnerships for advancing the needs of street children and (3) policy environment.

Characteristics of NGOs and Services Provided for Street Children

The NGOs that have been working with street children have been operating for almost three decades now. Five out of the 15 were established in the 1990s with the oldest starting operations in 1993. Four of them began to operate between 2000 and 2010, and the remaining six started after the year 2010. Whereas most of them target both street boys and girls, two of them focus mainly on street girls and another uniquely targets the children of street mothers. Three out of the 15 were faith-based organisations (two Christian and one Islamic). Majority of the NGOs are based in Accra and Kumasi. Street children are also found in the other cities including Sekondi-Takoradi and Tamale; however, the scope of this study was limited to Accra and Kumasi primarily because of the pioneering role these cities play in issues of street children.

The institutions provided a similar range of critically needed services for these children. They provided employable skills (vocational skill training, scholarships for education, functional literacy), drop-in centre facilities, residential facilities, psycho-social services and reintegration/reunification with families. Almost all 15 NGOs provided some form of employable skills for the children. Children were usually assessed and based on their interest and availability of resources; they were then placed in their respective vocational skill training programmes, such as hairdressing and beauty care, dressmaking and tailoring, catering, bead making and soap making. In some organisations, the training took place in-house as they had their own training centres. Others paid for the children to undertake their apprenticeships with approved training centres.

"We are into scholarships; we have a curriculum that we have written with a three months' duration. It could be more, it could be less, but the average is three months, and within these three months 50% of our focus is on life skills" (Accra NGO 3, 2019).

The NGOs also supported the children to acquire formal education. The institutions provided in-house introductory lessons that included basic numeracy and literacy lessons for the children. The introductory lessons also assessed children's preparedness and their commitment to pursue formal education. Following this, the organisations placed them in schools and absorbed all their expenses. Depending on the children's progress and determination, they could be sponsored all the way to college or university. Other NGOs ran daily drop-in facilities from morning till 5: 00 pm. The drop-in centres offered a place where the children can take a break from their daily pursuit to rest, take a shower and play with other children. In some cases, the children are provided cooked meal and also join any of the literacy lessons organised in-house. Children who visited drop-in centres had to return to the streets or slums where they looked for shelter for the night.

In addition to the drop-in centres, five of the NGOs provided residential facilities for children living on the street. Their boarding and lodging were adequately catered for by the organisations. Further, children in residential facilities were mostly placed in either formal education or vocational skill training until the time of completion. According to Mokomane and Makaoaes (Mokomane & Makoae, 2015), shelters for homeless children offer some form of therapeutic, developmental and recreational programmes and seek to reach the street children at a preventive level.

Given the association between homelessness and mental health (Davou et al., 2019; De-Graft & Ofori-Atta, 2007; Oppong, 2015) the interviews also inquired into mental health intervention programmes that the institutions had in place for the children. All 15 NGOs had some form of support for the mental health challenges that children faced. They had counsellors who were either in-house or external who were invited when the need arose. However, all 15 NGOs admitted that they either did not follow any comprehensive mental health plan or intervention or were in the process of consulting an expert to develop one.

"Yes, mental health has been a big issue regarding when it comes to life skills. Like I mentioned before, what we are trying to do with life skill is trying to get into their minds, trying to get them to see things from a different perspective and when it comes to actual clinical mental health, we have not done clear programmes on that, but we have done referrals to situations like massive counselling that needs psychiatric help" (Accra NGO 2, 2019).

"Traumatised children are counselled and where necessary, taken to a psychologist. Giving them stability in a setting which puts them in groups of 'brothers and sisters' with a caregiver, and also having a social worker assigned to them for counselling helps them feel safe, and assists in the healing process" (Accra NGO 5, 2019).

Reintegration with families was another service that was provided by the NGOs. They highlighted the importance of collaborating with the families of these children to offer holistic interventions. One of the primary steps they took as part of engaging a child and providing for the needs of that child was to trace the families. The aim was to establish a relationship with them, ascertain the factors that pushed their children into the street and work with them to ensure that the factors that drove the children to the street are reduced considerably. Also, they obtained the financial (where possible) and emotional commitment of the families towards the future of the child. In some cases, once the negative family factors were deemed to have considerably reduced, children were placed back with families where they continued to receive support for their education or training. The Director of this NGO that works with street girls explained how they worked with families:

"Normally, what we do is that we get the family involved in the whole process. So when the girls deliver, maybe from the hospital, the parent will take her home or if the case is not yet settled, the girl comes in until we find a solution to that. So that is just another aspect of the . . . . And when they come in the house, you will teach them how to bath their babies, how to do baby food, weani-mix and all those kind of things" (Accra NGO 5, 2019).

One particular organisation had a different approach to working with families. Given the close relationship between poverty and children living on the street (Boakye-Boaten, 2008; Conticini & Hulme, 2006; Patel, 1990; Ofosu-Kusi 2017; van Blerk, 2012); 2009), this NGO sought to empower the primary caregivers or parents of the child by providing economic assistance to the families so that they could engage in income-generating activities. The idea was to wean the children off the organisation's sponsorship package after 5 years by which time the parents would be in the position to take over the care of their children. In addition to economic empowerment, they also provided social and emotional support to help the parents deal with their day-to-day challenges in taking care of their children. The Director describes the approach as follows:

". . . The other angle is where we do the protection itself, we have children that we give scholarships to, and we have the hand skills training for children who don't want to go to school. They go and learn that the child protection program of bringing them in and giving education, we have the parents program where we have the savings and loans, and they can take loans and start their little business little by little. That's what it has always been" (Accra NGO 3, 2019).

Challenges Encountered While Providing Services: Funding

Their primary sources of funding are benevolent individuals, families, friends, churches and in some cases development partners. It takes a lot of money to rescue, rehabilitate and get a child in the street situation on the "straight and narrow". The data analysis indicated that the activities of these institutions were and are still very donor dependent. The situation of street children attracted a lot of donor funding in the past, and donors supported various aspects of the lives of the children. Following Ghana's attainment of a middle-income-level status, the donor landscape in the country has been adversely affected as donor support to the institutions that work with street children has dwindled. The following illustrates some of the challenges with funding:

"Donors leave all the time. Sometimes, it is a matter of their in-house policy. Some stay longer, though. We have two donors that have been with us for the past ten years. Before that there were others . . . it is really terrible because you cannot get the money here and you cannot get it abroad because they recognised Ghana as a middle-income country so you look after your problems and that is all you can do" (Accra NGO 1, 2019).

The kind of support that NGOs can offer street children and the number of children who could benefit from these services were also adversely affected. The following concerns by some of the NGOs were expressed by the others as well:

"We have actually reduced the number of intakes because we used to take 100 at a time, but now we have only 30 we were even supposed to take 20, but we partnered with other organisations" (Accra NGO 6, 2019).

"For the legal aid for abused street children, we had to halt it till we found donors and partners that are willing to help or simply do referrals. For the referrals, Ghana legal aid has similar financial challenges, and so does FIDA also has similar challenges. So, the legal aids that could take some of these cases don't have the funding to do that. So we have kind of slow down on that" (Accra NGO 2, 2019).

Other sources of finance for the help of NGO work included philanthropists, family and friends, and for the FBOs contribution from their mother organisations. However, these supports are mainly ad hoc and not long-term planned support for the NGOs. This negatively affected the extent to which these institutions can plan and initiate medium- to long-term interventions for street children. The implication of the ad hoc funds' flow is that instance where these organisations attempt a medium-term response, and funds dry out in the middle of such initiatives which adversely affects beneficiaries. Others also relied on internally generated funds raised from the sale of products that the children produced as part of their training. When asked how they plan to mitigate the effect of the dwindling donor support, most of them said that they were going to rely more on the internally generated funds from their in-house activities.

Partnerships to Advance the Needs of Street Children

Partnerships were explored in the study because of goal 17 of the SDGs. It is for good reasons that the last of the 17 SDGs talks about partnerships. According to the Office of the High Commission on Human Rights, defending children from violence and other rights violations that push children into developing connections with the streets requires a coordinated and comprehensive approach. The approach must involve all government departments (from finance, through trade, employment, social sectors—such as recreation and sports, health, education and social well-being) and duty bearers at the family and community levels (OHCHR, n.d.). The United Nations has found multilevel partnerships (at macro, meso, micro levels) to be very useful in the pursuit of agendas like this one. Macro-level partnerships entailed relevant government institutions and agencies that lead to governmental recognition and action towards social inclusion of street children. Meso-level part-nerships involved a strong collaboration among different services and different NGOs working with street children whereas at the micro level lies the essence of care, which is the collaboration and relationship between practitioners and children/ youth and their guardians. The study revealed that the NGOs were doing well with micro-level partnerships with the children in their care and their families.

"If a child is found on the street we look for the extended family, and we make sure that the family agrees to give good shelter. When they give good shelter, then we give scholarship and start working with them (the family) to economically improve themselves to take over from us as families and sometimes their local communities" (Accra NGO 6, 2019).

The institutions endeavoured to know and understand the children they worked with. The interviews revealed a strong sense of wanting to understand these children; hence some of the NGOs invested in research and other activities such as street corner activities to achieve that objective. One Director intimated:

"We wanted to understand the situation of the children and know how to help them, so we conducted a lot of research that brought us closer to the children and their families" (Accra NGO 1, 2019).

Another Director shared this about when he started:

> Yes, so when I started, the goal was just to get to know them, understand why they were coming to the street and that was it. So, every Saturday I'll show up, go to different sections, sit on the floor with them, and I'll give them food and ask some questions, every Saturday evening (Accra NGO 2, 2019).

Consequently, they conducted many surveys and interviews to understand the factors and determinants of the children's situation before embarking on developing interventions. The concept of involving the children, their families and communities as part of their interventions illustrates the institutions' commitment to the micro-level partnerships and the principle of participation. In addition to research, all the NGOs boast of some qualified social workers who were always on the street engaging with street children, some of whom may not be direct beneficiaries of their organisations. They organised street corner education, mentoring sessions and other services on the street to, among other things, strengthen their relationship with the children.

"We send our social workers to the central market every day to interact with these children. We conduct street corner education for them and also give them tips on how to make good reproductive health choices. Sometimes, a few of them follow the social workers to the centre to get some help" (Kumasi NGO, 2019).

Partnerships at the meso level, which looks at the peer-to-peer partnerships among the various institutions and their critical services, were almost non-existent. To date, no alliance or network brought these institutions together to pursue a common policy goal and demand social justice from the government for these children. Interviews with the NGOs that started in the 1990s revealed that efforts in the past to establish this kind of partnerships had proved futile. At best, a number of institutions connected on ad hoc basis for different reasons. The absence of meso-level alliances had resulted in working in silos, and a duplication of efforts with very minimal results. During the interviews, I discovered that some of the NGOs that started after the year 2010 did not know about the existence of the older NGOs and vice versa.

"My expectations for attending that conference were really high because I had not heard of any organisation or group of people that actually deal with street children, I didn't know of any. So it was good news to know that there are other people that are actually involved in the same thing I do, they would understand and will be able to help me better" (Accra NGO 9, 2019).

This respondent was meeting other NGOs for the first time at a conference that had been organised by some NGOs to commemorate the world day for street children. She also learned about other organisations for the first time from my interview with her.

Partnerships at the macro level entail the active engagement between the government represented by relevant ministries and agencies and the NGOs. At the time of the study, the only active relationship that existed was that between the NGOs and the Department of Social Welfare (DSW) that had a regulatory role over these NGOs. So far, this partnership had also proven inadequate to advance and promote the needs of street children in Ghana. The DSW was expected to provide technical advice and expertise, such as social workers, to help these NGOs provide the needed service to the vulnerable groups in society. They were also tasked with monitoring and evaluating the activities of the NGOs, reviewing their annual reports and renewing their license to operate annually. The study reveals that the DSW had a cordial relationship with these NGOs; they attended programmes and also referred cases, particularly those involving residential placements to some of these NGOs. The DSW was unable to provide the full bouquet of support that these NGOs required. Some NGOs reported that the DSW had not visited the premises for the periodic inspection and monitoring of their activities. More critical was the annual reports that they submitted; they have received neither feedback and queries nor suggestions to improve their operations.

"They inspect your institution, they take your documents and check if you have the GRA certificate with the registrar general. If you have them, then in most cases they do not even go and see the site, then you keep waiting, and you pay a lot of money until you are registered" (Accra NGO 6, 2019).

"I met with social welfare, but I don't know. I honestly view it like anyone can get up and start something, and no one would know. So, on my part, I was having a chat with my board, and I told them I was going to do all these reports and send to them (social welfare). Whether someone shows up or not, for due diligence and for us to know that we are doing our part, I'll write the report on what is going on and send it to them and if they choose to do something then good but if they choose to do nothing then that's their problem" (Accra NGO 9, 2019).

Some of the NGOs that started operating in the 1990s and early 2000s indicated attempts that had been made in the past to partner with government to address some of the peculiar challenges they were facing, one of which was the absence of a policy on street children. This attempt and several others failed woefully, and the policy never saw the light of day after almost two decades since it was proposed. When I interrogated the reasons for the failed efforts, it emerged that they were inhibited by the interference of partisan politics. One of the Directors hinted that partisan politics interferences make the partnership with government challenging and often unproductive. He said:

"You meet politics ... politics mixed with reality, Yeah, so you think that in the case of government they just to be willing, you said you need a politician who is willing and who understands. All the other findings we have on children and all the solutions we think it could be implemented, they do not accept them at all" (Accra NGO 1, 2019).

He added:

"At one point you are working with a politician who is interested and is cooperating with you, but when they are replaced, you have to start all over again with the new person, and sometimes this new person is not interested at all" (Accra NGO 1, 2019).

The data further revealed that because of the lack of active macro-level partnerships, specifically a collaboration between the government and the NGOs, the government has often employed some inhumane approaches to dealing with issues of street children. This is because the government fails to consult the NGOs who have painstakingly studied and understood the situation. The NGOs bemoaned interventions such as children being arrested and rounded up by police and placed in some shelters that were not fit for the purpose. The children ran back to the street from that shelter because no concrete plans were accompanying the action.

"the former minister said that the children should be arrested and placed at the shelter in Madina by force though she promised us she would not use force and she was still using force. And I said you just pick a child from the street and put them there without knowing the child and she said we would put a psychologist there who can work on the child and then move on. I said madam, not all children need psychologist (psychologist yes). We work with the child on the street first to know them, and then finally we decide with the children what to do next, but you pick the child from the street just like that the state does not give you the right to do that ... After two days, they realised they could feed them" (Accra NGO 1, 2019).

A lack of macro-level partnerships with organisations that work with these children thus often led to inadequate interventions and poor results.

Policy Environments

Ghana is noted to have rich policies in every sector, including that which is responsible for children. Ghana's ratification of UNCRC (the first country to do so), followed by Ghana's Children's Act (Act 560) in 1998, a Child and Family Welfare Policy and Juvenile Justice Policy both launched in 2015 and the adoption of the SDGs in 2015, attests to Ghana's commitment to the promotion and protection of the rights of children. As part of the study, I sought to examine whether the services provided by the NGOs aligned with any of the existing policies and the SDGs. I first inquired about their knowledge of the polices and how they were incorporating this in their work. It is worth noting that almost 85% of the organisations were conversant with UNCRC, the various national level frameworks that guide working with children and the principles that drive them. A number of the organisations had developed their child protection policy based on these international and national level frameworks to guide their day-to-day engagement with the children.

"We wrote our child protection policy earlier before Ghana had its child protection policy, so we were part of the few NGOs that were consulted. I can say that in terms of policy we have formally used all of them" (Accra NGO 4, 2019).

Concerning the SDGs, although, not explicitly indicated or intended, the services they provided contributed to meeting certain critical SDGs, particularly 1 (no poverty), 2 (zero hunger), 3 (good health and well-being), 4 (quality education), 8 (decent work and economic growth) and 10 (reduced inequality). Another had this to say about the SDGs:

"We are actively pursuing the SDGs. I think goal eight, employment and decent work, is one of the things we incorporate into whatever we are doing and we are also looking at gender equality so as we said earlier on that the girls are more vulnerable so we want to create a platform where we can raise their standard to be able to know certain things and also do self-assessment and have a voice that they can ask for what is theirs instead of always just waiting for somebody to decide for him or her all the time should be able to upgrade themselves to the level that they can also have a voice and be mentors to their communities" (Accra NGO 6, 2019).

Another revelation from the data is that the institutions are operating within a poor policy environment. Although Ghana has several policies and action plans that work at promoting and protecting the rights of children, these policies and action plans have a visible gap of not catering to the specific needs of street children. These children, therefore, fall through the cracks even when the broader category of orphaned and vulnerable children have been catered for adequately making it a big challenge to sufficiently address the needs of street children. Another reason accounting for the poor policy engagement is the political interference and the frequent change of sector ministers that have varying levels of interest in the welfare of children.

Although the DSW has the mandate to execute interventions that support the interest of children, much of the funding from the government is locked up at ministry which is mandated to provide the policy guideline for children's welfare. Thus, changes in government and frequent change of ministers have stalled past interventions for the children. Another critical challenge they were confronted with revolved around regulation and provision of technical support to the NGOs. The Department of Social Welfare oversees the registration of NGOs and provides them with the requisite license to operate after they have met all requirements. Consequently, all 15 NGOs had registered with the DSW; however, the technical support required and feedback from monitoring are mostly lacking.

Discussion

In this chapter, I aimed to examine the efforts that have been made to address the situation of the children living on the street in Ghana. Specifically, I assessed the activities of 15 NGOs that work with street children and how these activities are aligned with the international and local conventions and the SDGs, particularly goals 1, 2, 3, 4, 8, 10 and 17. The study found that all 15 NGOs are providing critical services to the street children in their care albeit on a small scale considering the increasing spate of the phenomenon. The NGOs are aware of the legal provision made for all children, including street children at both international and national levels, and make efforts to align their activities by catering to these provisions.

NGOs form a critical force in the development agenda of many nations. In the area of upholding child rights and protection, they serve as a bridge and mediator between families and governments and that gives them central importance in the implementation of policies concerning children (Debrito, 2014). While they work downwards with families to strengthen their capacities to support their children, they work upwards with the government to, among other things, demand accountability for the care of children.

Knowledge of the children, context in which they are operating, and existing policies and framework guiding their work is key to the effective running of NGOs in any given sector. Other elements include a positive collaboration with governments of the jurisdiction in which they are operating, responsive policies and funding to carry out their activities. The NGOs in this study were knowledgeable about the situation of the children they worked with and also of existing policies that seek to protect them and to a large extent were doing their best to provide needed care for the children. However, as it happens in many jurisdictions, there is an extent to which NGOs can go in achieving their targets. There are realistic limitations, such as funding.

NGOs are heavily dependent on funding sources that are external to them and so are their services, the number of children they can support and for how long specific programmes could run. All 15 NGOs bemoaned the fact their activities and number of beneficiaries were dwindling by the years as donors' funding runs out mainly due to donors' in-house policies or a change of focus for the donors. It is safe to say that as long as funding for these NGOs is concerned, they are no longer thriving. Older

NGOs from the 1990s and early 2000s are no longer flourishing, and the newer ones (post-2010) are struggling to keep afloat with their core business. This also means that the efforts of these NGOs are currently not enough to reduce the risk of street children being left behind in the Agenda 2030.

Consequently, other critical roles such as holding governments accountable and getting the government to ensure that the policy environment and comprehensive policy to address the issues of street children are developed become secondary as they are saddled with their day-to-day operations. There is indeed a low level of collaborations among NGOs and between NGOs and the government. As powerful as these NGOs are in the protection and promotion of the rights of children including street children, their voices are not represented in the corridors of influence specifically among government, judiciary and parliament because of the lack of partnerships among themselves to provide a united front to demand the needed social justice for street children. Whereas some governments may not be too responsive and engage positively with NGOs and other partners due to their own challenges and sometimes low levels of commitment towards the course, the absence of meso-level partnerships plays a significant role in their omission. A strong partnership among the NGOs can fill this gap and attain more sustainable results for these children. There is also the clash between the rights-based approach and government actions. The actions of the latter, some of which have been mentioned earlier, seem to be inclined towards the repressive approach of addressing the situation of street children which sees children as deviants that need rehabilitation. This clash presents another lacuna that a strong meso-level partnership can address and demand the government to adopt and commit to a rights-based approach.

Conclusion

The study concludes that the identified challenges existed primarily because of the non-existence of effective multilevel partnership. Saddled with donor fatigue and weak regulations, the activities of these institutions are far from being sustainable. Multilevel and multifunctional partnerships are therefore needed to achieve the very ambitious goals that each of these NGOs sets for themselves and to ensure that these children are not left behind. Partnerships are critical to the work needed to build a sustainable world (the United Nations): multi-stakeholder partnerships (MSPs) between private enterprises, public agencies, academics and civil society groups. The last of the 17 SDGs focuses on partnerships, and the UN is explicit about the need for partnerships to achieve all the other goals. Partnerships are also key vehicles for mobilising and sharing knowledge, expertise, technologies and financial resources to support the achievement of SDGs in all countries. The same will go for these institutions that are working so hard for street children all over the country. It is concluded that there is a disconnect between policy and practice when it comes to the protection of the welfare of street children. While national level policies exist to protect street children in Ghana, it lacks the national level financial commitments and interventions. Government efforts have been ad hoc and piecemeal in many instances. The DSW has failed to provide the needed support for street children, and as this study has shown, the DSW relies on NGOs for long-term support for street children they rescue. For effective synergy between macro-level international policies, meso-level national policies and micro-level implementation, there is the need for a more inclusive approach that tackles the multidimensional nature of streetism among children that bridges the gap between policy and practice.

References

Ablo, A. D. (2018). Scale, local content and the challenges of Ghanaians employment in the oil and gas industry. *Geoforum, 96*, 181–189.

Agarwal, S., Attah, M., Apt, N., Grieco, M., Kwakye, E. A., & Turner, J. (1997). Bearing the weight: The kayayoo, Ghana's working girl child. *International Social Work, 40*(3), 245–263.

Amantana, V. (2012). *A sociological study of street children in Ghana: Victims of kinship breakdown and rural-urban migration.* Edwin Mellen Press.

Anarfi, J. (1997). Vulnerability to sexually transmitted disease: Street children in Accra. *Health Transition Review, 7*, 281–306.

Awumbila, M., & Ardayfio-Schandorf, E. (2008). Gendered poverty, migration and livelihood strategies of female porters in Accra, Ghana. *Norwegian Journal of Geography, 62*(3), 171–179.

Boakye-Boaten, A. (2008). Street children: Experiences from the streets of Accra. *Research Journal of International Studies, 8*, 76–84.

Braun, V., & Clarke, V. (2006). Using thematic analysis in psychology. *Qualitative Research in Psychology, 3*(2), 77–101. https://doi.org/10.1191/1478088706qp063oa

Bryman, A. (2012). *Social research methods* (4th ed.). Oxford University Press.

Conticini, A., & Hulme, D. (2006). Escaping violence, seeking freedom: Why children in Bangladesh migrate to the street. *Development and Change, 38*, 201–227. https://doi.org/10.1111/j.1467-7660.2007.00409.x

Dabir, N., & Athale, N. (2011). *From street to Hope: Faith based and secular programs in Los Angeles, Mumbai and Nairobi for street living children.* Sage Publication.

Davou, J., Yu-sha'u, A. A., Philip, T., & Taru, M. (2019). Street children: Implication on mental health and the future of West Africa. *Psychology, 10*, 667–681. https://doi.org/10.4236/psych.2019.105041

Debrito, A. (2014). *Street children and the implementation of child protection regulations: comparing Brazil and South Africa.* Master thesis, Linnaeus University, Faculty of Social Sciences. Retrieved 2016-01-07 from http://lnu.diva-portal.org/smash/get/diva2:748332/FULLTEXT01.pdf.

De-Graft, A. A., & Ofori-Atta, A. (2007). Homelessness and mental health in Ghana: Study everyday experiences of Accra's migrant squatters. *Journal of Health Psychology, 12*(5), 761–778.

Department of Social Welfare (2011). *Census on street children in the Greater Accra region, Ghana.* Accra.

Desai, V., & Potter, R. B. (2014). *Doing development research.* Sage Publications.

Ennew, J. (1994). *Street and working children: A guide to planning (development manual for save the children).* AbeBooks.

James, A., & Prout, A. (1997). *Constructing and reconstructing childhood* (2nd ed.). Routledge.

Kassa, S. (2018). The situation of street children in urban centers of Ethiopia and the role of NGO in addressing their socio-economic problems: The case of Hawassa City. *International Journal of*

Academic Research in Education and Review, 3(3), 45–57. https://doi.org/10.14662/ IJARER2015.012

Kwankye, S. O., & Addoquaye Tagoe, C. (2009). City life outside the home: the experiences of independent child migrants in Ghana. In J. K. Anarfi & S. O. Kwankye (Eds.), *Independent migration of children in Ghana* (pp. 132–170). Institute of Statistical Social and Economic Research.

Kwankye, S. O., Anarfi, J., Addoquaye, T., & C. Castaldo A. (2009). Independent north-south child migration in Ghana: The decision-making process among Accra's street children. *Childhood, 17*(4), 441–454.

Ministry of Gender, Children and Social Protection. (2015). *Child and Family Welfare Policy.* Accra.

Mizen, P., & Ofosu-Kusi, Y. (2010). Asking, giving, receiving: Friendship as survival strategy of trajectory and behavioural experiences of homelessness. *Global Social Welfare, 17*(4), 441–454. https://doi.org/10.1007/s40609-015-0039-8

Mizen, P., & Ofosu-Kusi, Y. (2013). Agency as vulnerability: Accounting for children's movement to the streets of Accra. *The Sociological Review, 61*, 363–382. https://doi.org/10.1111/ 1467-954X.12021

Mokomane, Z., & Makoae, M. (2015). An overview of programmes offered by shelters for street children in South Africa. *Child and Family Social Work, 22*(1), 378–387. https://doi.org/10. 1111/cfs.12251

Niboye, E. P. (2013). Effectiveness of non-governmental organizations in the rehabilitation of street children – experiences from selected NGOs in Dar es Salaam, Tanzania. *Journal of Education and Practice, 4*(1), 2013.

Ofosu-Kusi, Y. (2017). *Children's agency and development in African societies.* African Books Collective.

OHCHR. (n.d.) *Report of the United Nations High Commissioner for Human rights on the protection of the rights of children working and/or living on the street, OHCHR, Geneva* https://www.ohchr.org/Documents/Issues/Children/Study/OHCHRBrochureStreetChildren.pdf

Oppong, A. K. (2015). Street children and adolescents in Ghana: a qualitative study of trajectory and behavioural experiences of homelessness. *Global Social Welfare, 3*, 33–43. https://doi.org/ 10.1007/s40609-015-0039-8

Oppong Asante, K., & Meyer-Weitz, A. (2015). International note: Association between perceived resilience and health risk behaviours in homeless youth. *Journal of Adolescence, 39*, 36–39.

Oppong Asante, K., & Meyer-Weitz, A. (2017). Prevalence and predictors of suicide ideation and attempts among a sample of homeless children and adolescents in Ghana. *Journal of Child & Adolescent Mental Health, 29*(1), 111. https://doi.org/10.2989/17280583.2017.1287708

Patel, S. (1990). *Street children, hotel boys, children of pavement dwellers and construction workers in Bombay – How they meet their daily needs.* Society for the Promotion of Area Resource Centres (SPARC).

Thomas de Benitez, S. (2011). *State of the world's street children.* Consortium for street children Retrieved from https://www.streetchildren.org/wpcontent/uploads/2013/02/State_of_the_ Worlds_Street_Children_Research_final_PDF_online.pdf

Ungruhe, C. (2019). Beyond Agency's limits. "Street Children's" Mobilities in southern Ghana. *Cadernos de Estudos Africanos* 37.

van Blerk, L. (2012). Berg-en-see street boys: Merging street and family relations in Cape Town, South Africa. *Children's Geographies, 10*(3), 321–336. https://doi.org/10.1080/14733285. 2012.693381

Veeran, V. (2004). Working with street children: A child-centred approach. *Child Care in Practice, 10*(4), 359–366.

Young, L. (2003). Journeys to the street: The complex migration geographies of Ugandan street children. *Geoforum, 35*(4), 471–478.

Part V
Interventions Focused on Child Behavioral Health in Sub-Saharan Africa: Case Examples

Caregiver-Child Communication: The Case for Engaging South African Caregivers in Family-Based Interventions

Tyrone M. Parchment, Latoya Small, and Arvin Bhana

Introduction

South Africa has one of the highest HIV prevalence rates in the world with KwaZulu-Natal (KZN), a province in the city of Durban, having the highest density of people living with HIV. HIV infection is one of the direct threats to the health and well-being of young people worldwide (Mellins et al., 2007; Vreeman et al., 2017). According to UNAIDS (2019), 1.7 million children were living with HIV worldwide. Given the various efforts to stabilize the HIV epidemic both locally and internationally, there remains a high level of new HIV infections and AIDS death, particularly in sub-Saharan Africa (UNAIDS, 2019). While there has been a downward trend in provincial HIV prevalence for children in South Africa (SA), KwaZulu-Natal, a province of SA where the study was based, continues to have the highest national HIV infection rates (Shisana et al., 2014). Life expectancy in KZN is primarily driven by reductions in HIV-related mortality (Reniers et al., 2017). In light of this, SA's National Strategic Plan for 2017–2022 identified children as a key population requiring renewed focus as they face a chronic, stigmatizing, and transmittable illness at heightened risk of HIV infection.

T. M. Parchment (✉)
School of Social Work, Boston College, Boston, MA, USA
e-mail: parchmet@bc.edu

L. Small
Luskin School of Public Affairs, University of California Los Angeles, Los Angeles, CA, USA

A. Bhana
Department of Psychology, School of Applied Human Sciences, University of KwaZulu-Natal, Durban, South Africa

© Springer Nature Switzerland AG 2022
F. M. Ssewamala et al. (eds.), *Child Behavioral Health in Sub-Saharan Africa*,
https://doi.org/10.1007/978-3-030-83707-5_15

Background

Caregiver Well-Being in South Africa

Approximately one-third of South African adults experience some form of emotional challenges, with more than 17 million experiencing depression, anxiety, substance abuse, bipolar disorder, and schizophrenia (SAFMH, 2015). Additionally, the prevalence rate for psychiatric disorders is 5.9% among females and about 5% for males on the African continent (WHO, 2017). In South Africa, the prevalence of emotional disorders for individuals aged 15 years and up is 4.6% of the population (over two million cases), the fourth highest in the African Region (WHO, 2017). Many of these individuals are caregivers, adults who take on the responsibility of raising children. Caregivers are not only birth parents but also include extended family (e.g., grandparents, aunts, uncles), older siblings, and neighbors. In South Africa, there is limited research regarding the relationship between caregiver well-being and adolescent possible engagement in risky situations. Caregiver psychological distress is associated with adolescent health (including youth mental health; Meinck et al., 2017). However, caregivers can emit a positive, protective effect on their children's behaviors. Caregivers control much of youth's environment by acting as a buffer to contextual stressors (i.e., violence, poverty) since the bond between a child and their primary caregiver mediates their understanding and conceptualization of their world (De Bellis et al., 1999; McKay et al., 2010; Small et al., 2019; Spannring, 2012). This helps the child feel safe and secure and that improves their functional and normal development. When an adult caregiver has a strong support system, it also improves their capability to parent effectively (Casale et al., 2015; Lindsey et al., 2008; Lindsey et al., 2012; McKay et al., 1999; Ward et al., 2015). This improves their children's chances of experiencing better mental health outcomes and reduces the risk of engaging in sexual situations (Goodrum et al., 2017). This remains salient even if they reside in areas that are poverty (McKay et al., 2014; Morris et al., 2017) and HIV impacted in South Africa (Bhana et al., 2004; Casale et al., 2015; Paruk et al., 2005; Pedersen et al., 2019).

Early Adolescence

Early adolescence (9–14 years) is a time of inexperience and immaturity coupled with multiple new stressful situations as youth move in and out of the world of childhood and try to obtain guidelines to define their new status (Hamburg, 1990; Mellins et al., 2007; Paikoff, 1995; Whitbeck et al., 1999). It is also a developmental period marked by experimentation with adult behaviors and peer pressure to engage in risky sexual situations (Levitt et al., 1991; Mellins et al., 2007). Young people growing up in poverty-impacted communities are exposed to potential dangers (i.e., poverty, violence, and sexual situations) that impact their psychosocial development and are challenged to navigate these often-challenging circumstances (Hamburg, 1990; Holloway et al., 2012; Mellins et al., 2007; Tarantino et al., 2014).

Apartheid not only changed the Black South African family structure, but also contributed to challenges in parenting (Tarantino et al., 2014). During apartheid, families were weakened as many men were forced to work in distant areas away from their families under strenuous conditions, receiving insufficient wages. Some would be away for months or years at a time. Strain from these separations caused some men to break ties with their families, further exacerbating family hardship. Others might have experienced loneliness or associated psychological stressors due to these conditions (Knight, 2019). The land where many Black South Africans lived was often barren (Taitt, 1980). In 2015, approximately 51% of children in SA experienced poverty, with higher numbers among Black SA youth compared to their colored, Indian, and White counterparts (SSA, 2018). These disadvantages and their associated traumas can have long-term effects on Black South Africans (Adonis, 2018; Knight, 2019).

Youth in KwaZulu-Natal are at an increased risk of illicit drug use, early onset of alcohol use, and engaging in destructive internalizing behaviors (Reddy et al., 2013). Conversely, there is strong evidence that positive interaction among youth and adult caregivers can influence child mental health and reduce their engagement in risky sexual situations (Bell et al., 2008; Bhana et al., 2004; Eddy et al., 2013; Guilamo-Ramos et al., 2011; Hutchinson & Montgomery, 2007; Hutchinson, 2002; Li et al., 2000; Pequegant & Szapocznik, 2000; Whitaker & Miller, 2000). Caregiving that encompasses nurturing behaviors (Maccoby, 1992), communication around pro-social behaviors including sex (Namisi, 2004), and monitoring of supervised and unsupervised time (Dishion & McMahon, 1998) can reduce the incidence of risk-taking behaviors in children. Research on early adolescence is necessary to identify not only factors that contribute to the possible initiation of possible engagement in sexual situations, but also adaptive behaviors that can deflect such behaviors (Krauss, 1995; Krauss, 1997; Mellins et al., 2007; Paikoff, 1995). The longer an individual postpones sexual risk-taking behaviors, the less likely he or she is to initiate them (Botvin et al., 1990; Donovan et al., 1983; Kanfer & Goldstein, 1991; Mellins et al., 2007). Adult caregivers can provide an *adult protective shield*, where they serve as a buffer between children and external stressors (e.g., peer pressure, poverty, community violence). Parents as protective shields are a potentially important prevention strategy in protecting children and bolstering their well-being.

Caregiver-Child Communication

Children and youth residing in low- and middle-income countries (LMICs) tend to experience adverse circumstances such as poverty, neighborhood instability, and lack of mental health resources (Pedersen et al., 2019). Caregivers play an integral role in improving child well-being (e.g., reduced depression and anxiety symptoms) while promoting healthy sexual development that is achieved through dyadic communication. When there is mutual trust and confidence in each other, communication is said to be more effective (Botchway, 2004; Wang, 2009). Caregiver-child communication is known as the process through which expectations, beliefs, attitudes, values, and knowledge are transmitted between the caregiver and the child, often playing a critically formative role in child development (Coetzee et al., 2014; Jerman & Constantine, 2010). The development of healthy attitudes and beliefs is influenced by familial, communal, and contextual factors (Boyas et al., 2012). Thus, the comfort and frequency of the caregiver communicating to their child about alcohol, drugs, HIV/AIDS, having sex, sexually transmitted infections, negative peer influences, and puberty are essential.

Degree of communication between caregivers and children is contingent on empathy. Empathy necessitates both affective and cognitive elements that vary with the situation age and personality of a child (Feshbach, 1987). It often motivates caring and pro-social actions toward others (Zahn-Waxler & Van Hulle, 2011). This form of empathy is key in the development of a healthy relationship between caregiver and child. Caregiver empathy can be conceived as the sympathetic reaction to their child's distress that reflects social understanding and emotional identification (Feshbach, 1987). A caregiver who is empathic attends to the youth's point of view and feelings and can understand and share these feelings, which enhances the attachment they have with their child (Feshbach, 1987). This, in turn, directly influences the young person's emotional development and adjustment. A child's perceived empathy of their caregiver is correlated with higher levels of self-esteem and lower levels of depression (Trumpeter, Watson, O'Leary, Weathington, 2008). A longitudinal analysis in understanding the link between empathy and child development found that increased empathy predicted lower stress reactivity and emotional dysregulation (Abraham et al., 2018). The affective relationship between the South African adult caregiver and child that incorporates empathy in monitoring can lead to improved child well-being and behavior.

The focus on early adolescence (9–13 years) can contribute to the literature of preventing risk behavior and the potential development of mental health disorders in later adolescence. Indeed, earlier intervention has been proven to increase pro-social behavioral development in youth (Baptiste et al., 2006; Bell et al., 2008; Bhana et al., 2010; McKay et al., 2004; Mellins et al., 2007). Identifying preventive mechanisms that will bolster the well-being of young people also improves family functioning. There are a few researches in South Africa that empirically investigate how caregiver might influence early-adolescent outcomes and whether these protective factors have a familial effect (Casale et al., 2015).

Overall, as detailed above, caregiver-child relationship is critical in influencing youth mental and well-being more so in poverty-impacted communities heavily impacted by HIV/AIDS—such as KwaZulu-Natal. Caregivers enable children and adolescents to navigate social, environmental, and sexual risks (Pedersen et al., 2019). This has implications for child and adolescent mental health. In the proceeding section, we use data from a program, called Collaborative HIV Prevention Adolescent Mental Health Program, implemented in South Africa—in the KwaZulu-Natal region—to examine this further. Specifically, we examine the relationship between neighborhood disadvantages, caregiver mental health, and early adolescent report on caregiver communication around various developmental issues.

Collaborative HIV Prevention Adolescent Mental Health Program in South Africa

Collaborative HIV Prevention Adolescent Mental Health Program (CHAMP) was originally launched as a researcher–community-based partnership in the United States to address increasing rates of adolescent HIV/AIDS exposure in urban neighborhoods. CHAMP is a ten-session, manualized, family-focused, group-format intervention that is developmentally grounded, targeting pre- and early adolescence (9–13 years), providing a model of primary and secondary HIV prevention (Baptiste et al., 2006; Bhana et al., 2010). The program sessions run 90 min and involve delivery of content via multiple family groups (children and their caregivers). It includes education and skill-building activities to strengthen parental monitoring, discipline effectiveness, conflict resolution, support, and caregiver and youth frequency and comfort in communication about sensitive topics (Baptiste et al., 2006; Bhana et al., 2010). The intervention also targets youth social problem-solving abilities, such as recognition of risk and refusal and assertiveness in handling sexual pressure from peers and adults (Baptiste et al., 2006). CHAMP was tested and demonstrated effectiveness in studies in the United States (McKay et al., 2004; Madison et al., 2000) and in the Caribbean (Baptiste et al., 2006).

The first phase of adapting CHAMP for the South African context involved the ethnographic process of working with community members on the design, delivery, and evaluation of the first manual, which was theoretically informed by the Theory of Triadic Influence (Bell et al., 2008; Paruk et al., 2002; Paruk et al., 2005). The Theory of Triadic Influence is an ecological theory that focuses on the explanation and prediction of health behavior change, and the development of health-promoting interventions (Bhana et al., 2010). The final stage involved piloting the adapted manual using formative evaluation from each session to inform the final CHAMPSA, a cartoon-based, illustrated prevention manual (Bell et al., 2008; Bhana et al., 2004; Pedersen et al., 2019). A steering committee comprised of researchers, as well as traditional and political leaders from the community, oversaw the implementation of CHAMPSA within the township of Kwadedangendlale in the KwaZulu-Natal province of South Africa. Further information regarding the adaptation process can be found elsewhere (Paruk et al., 2005).

Trained facilitators, many of whom were South African caregivers, delivered the intervention, mostly on weekends. The sessions were designed for Black South African families to increase knowledge about HIV, authoritative parenting, caregiver decision-making, and caregiver monitoring of children; increase family frequency and comfort discussing hard-to-discuss subjects (i.e., alcohol, drugs,

HIV/AIDS, having sex, sexually transmitted infections, peer relationship, and puberty); and increase connectedness to caregiver social networks. The sessions also intended to decrease HIV-related stigma and increase social control and cohesion while helping families identify protective aspects to combat against neighborhood disorganization (Bell et al., 2008). How to apply these skills was introduced to group members through dramatic depiction in a cartoon-based storyline (Bell et al., 2008). CHAMPSA also provided necessary group context for caregivers to collectively renegotiate their parenting norms and practices toward healthier and more productive alternatives (Bell et al., 2008; McKay et al., 2002). The CHAMPSA study was a collaborative effort between four institutes: the Community Mental Health Council, Inc. and the Mount Sinai School of Medicine in the United States, and the Human Sciences Research Council and University of KwaZulu-Natal in South Africa. Considerable attention was paid to cultural and language differences in the wording of measures. This required facilitators to help adult caregivers by reading the items and responses aloud (just under 50% had a fifth-grade-level education; Bell et al., 2008).

Methods

To further support the case of engaging caregivers/families in HIV prevention, baseline data was used from 290 Black adult caregivers in the Collaborative HIV Prevention Adolescent Mental Health Program in South Africa (CHAMPSA; R01 MH55701). CHAMPSA is a family-based, HIV prevention intervention to reduce risk behaviors among uninfected SA youth. Structural equation modeling (SEM) was employed to explore the relationship between neighborhood disorganization and caregiver-child frequency of communication (i.e., having sex, HIV, puberty, peer pressure, alcohol use) and whether the relationship is mediated by caregiver socio-emotional well-being. Socio-emotional well-being was created as a latent variable using 12 items from the General Health Questionnaire (Goldberg & Hillier, 1979) and the Global Indicator of Well-Being (Bell et al., 2007).

Results

Mediation effects were analyzed, indicated by the joint significance test (MacKinnon et al., 2002). The results pointed toward good model fit ($\chi2 = 0.047$, df $= 1$, p-value <0.8281; CFI $= 1.00$, RMSEA $= 0.000$, p-value for close fit $= 0.880$, standardized RMR $= 0.001$). Findings indicated that South African caregiver socio-emotional well-being does not significantly mediate the relationship between neighborhood disorganization and frequency of communication with their child regarding sex, HIV, puberty, drugs, sexually transmitted infections, alcohol, and negative influences of peers. There was a significant direct effect for neighborhood disorganization and frequency of communication. For every unit increase in neighborhood disorganization, on average, there is an associated 0.991 unit (MOE $\pm$ 0.02, CR $= -0.027$, p < 0.001) increase in the frequency of the SA caregiver communication with their child. It also accounted for 97.3% of the variance for adult-to-child communication. In short, the more problems that exist in their neighborhoods, caregivers increase the frequency of discussing with children about alcohol, drug use, HIV/AIDS, having sex, sexually transmitted infections, negative peer influences, and puberty.

Implications for Policy

The comfortability and frequency of an adult caregiver communicating to children about alcohol, drugs, HIV/AIDS, having sex, sexually transmitted infections, negative influences of friends, and puberty are necessary for improved well-being in youth. The more comfortable and frequent South African caregivers are in discussing these developmental topics, the less likely children are to engage in harmful behaviors (Adjei & Saewyc, 2017; Bastien et al., 2011; Tarantino et al., 2014). The policy of apartheid grievously impaired Black families in South Africa through the deliberate splitting apart of families as a consequence of the implementation of the migrant labor system (Pillay, 2010). Following the end of apartheid, which brought about the establishment of a new democratic dispensation in 1994, the post-apartheid government instituted various policy and legislative reforms aimed at realigning the country's institutions in order to transform South African society (Department of Social Development Republic of South Africa, 2012). While government-sanctioned racial discrimination might have been formally abolished, attempts to reform the country's welfare system were doomed under the direction of the same leadership that previously implemented the policies that played a major role in strengthening white families, while undermining the capacities of Black South African families (Bozalek, 1999). The detrimental effects of policies during colonial apartheid on the Black South African family (i.e., land dispossessions, migrant labor) are connected to the multiplicity of social ills that continue to plague contemporary South Africa (Department of Social Development Republic of South Africa, 2012).

The family was not explicitly addressed in policy and legislative reforms; rather, it was inferred. As a consequence, the majority of government-delivered socioeconomic benefits filtered down to the family indirectly. The country's five major social assistance policies were focused on children (the Child Support Grant, the Foster Care Grant, and the Care Dependency Grant), individuals with disabilities (the Disability Grant), and the elderly (the State Old Age Pension). As important and pivotal as these policies are, the needs of such individuals may not be congruent with those of the family unit (Department of Social Development Republic of South Africa, 2012).

Findings from this study support the notion that the family, in particular Black South African adult caregivers, is integral in potentially preventing the youth from engaging in risky situations. It also reinforces the need for policies to strengthen family stability and relationships (Groenewald & Bhana, 2018). According to the 1994 International Conference on Population and Development (ICPD) Plan of Action, the family is the basic unit of society and as such should be strengthened (Department of Social Development Republic of South Africa, 2012). Despite well-documented evidence, including findings from this study, the family has not been a high priority in the political sphere and in social sciences research in South Africa (Department of Social Development Republic of South Africa, 2012; Zeihl, 2001). The family was not explicitly addressed in policy and legislative reforms; rather, it was inferred. As a consequence, the majority of government-delivered socioeconomic benefits filtered down to the family indirectly.

In South Africa, communication around sex and sexuality occurs in youth-centered programs and in the education system (Coetzee et al., 2014). Projects such as loveLife (loveLife, 2018) and Soul City (Soul City, 2018) focus on preventing HIV and reducing teenage pregnancy. In addition, sexual education is addressed in Life Orientation classes in the South African school system (Coetzee et al., 2014). Recently, the South African Government made a commitment to implement the Comprehensive Sexuality Education (CSE) programs in public schools (Badenhorst, 2018). The intent of the CSE is to provide comprehensive sexuality education which enables young people to protect their health and well-being. However, the rate of new HIV infections for adolescents has not decreased (Coetzee et al., 2014; Shisana et al., 2014). Given that adult caregivers are influential in reducing early sexual debut for adolescents, it is important to identify ways in which parents can also provide education around sex and sexuality. Bridging the gap of intergenerational differences between adults and children as it relates to viewpoints on sex can reduce misunderstandings and improve communication around it (Wang, 2009).

The White Paper on Families in 2012 was a landmark document in South African policy history where the diversity of family structures was acknowledged but implementation of addressing family needs is still underway (Department of Social Development Republic of South Africa, 2012). The importance of understanding the diversity of families in South Africa is a necessary step in implementing specific family policies. The white paper addressed three strategic priorities related to family stability: (1) promoting healthy family life, (2) family strengthening, and (3) family preservation. Chapter Eight of the Children's Amendment Act (Act No. 41 of 2007) mandates interventions in South Africa to support and develop positive parenting (Gould & Ward, 2015). It deals with prevention and early intervention that focuses on developing the capacity of parents to operate in the best interests of their children by (1) strengthening healthy relationships in families, (2) improving caregiver capacities of parents, and (3) assisting caregivers in using nonviolent forms of discipline (Gould & Ward, 2015). This mandate provides the legal basis for the provision of parenting programming in South Africa. Given its focus on improving caregiving capacities among families, it can be an optimal place to implement and roll out family-based treatment modalities such as CHAMPSA, where it has been documented to have great promise when embedded within community-based clinics

(Bhana et al., 2004). The Children's Act also has implications for preventive services for children and adolescents (Flisher et al., 2015). This would provide an opportunity to incorporate evidence-based practices that can improve caregiver's ability to effectively communicate with early adolescents about alcohol, drugs, HIV/AIDS, having sex, sexually transmitted infections, negative peer influences, and puberty. The mandate can also serve as an opportunity to magnify rather than minimize the opportunity to engage fathers/male caregivers in parenting programs.

References

Abraham, E., Raz, G., Zagoory-Sharon, O., & Feldman, R. (2018). Empathy networks in the parental brain and their long-term effects on children's stress reactivity and behavior adaptation. *Neuropsychologia, 116*, 75–85.

Adjei, J. K., & Saewyc, E. M. (2017). Boys are not exempt: Sexual exploitation of adolescents in sub-Saharan Africa. *Child Abuse & Neglect, 65*, 14–23. https://doi.org/10.1016/j.chiabu.2017.01.001

Adonis, C. K. (2018). Generational victimhood in post-apartheid South Africa: Perspectives of descendants of victims of apartheid era gross human rights violations. *International Review of Victimology, 24*(1), 47–65.

Badenhorst, A. N. (2018). *CSE in south African schools – Sexuality education, or sex education? ForSA.* Retrieved from https://forsa.org.

Baptiste, D. R., Bhana, A., Petersen, I., McKay, M., Voisin, D., Bell, C., & Martinez, D. D. (2006). Community collaborative youth-focused HIV/AIDS prevention in South Africa and Trinidad: Preliminary findings. *Journal of Pediatric Psychology, 31*(9), 905–916.

Bastien, S., Kajula, L. J., & Muhwezi, W. W. (2011). A review of studies of parent-child communication about sexuality and HIV/AIDS in sub-Saharan Africa. *Reproductive Health, 8* (1), 25.

Bell, C. C., Bhana, A., McKay, M. M., & Petersen, I. (2007). A commentary on the triadic theory of influence as a guide for adapting HIV prevention programs for new contexts and populations: The CHAMP-South Africa story. *Social Work in Mental Health, 5*(3–4), 243–267.

Bell, C. C., Bhana, A., Petersen, I., McKay, M. M., Gibbons, R., Bannon, W., & Amatya, A. (2008). Building protective factors to offset sexually risky behaviors among black youths: A randomized control trial. *Journal of the National Medical Association, 100*(8), 936.

Bhana, A., McKay, M. M., Mellins, C., Petersen, I., & Bell, C. (2010). Family-based HIV prevention and intervention services for youth living in poverty-affected contexts: The CHAMP model of collaborative, evidence-informed programme development. *Journal of the International AIDS Society, 13*(Suppl 2), S8.

Bhana, A., Petersen, I., Mason, A., Mahintsho, Z., Bell, C., & McKay, M. (2004). Children and youth at risk: Adaptation and pilot study of the CHAMP (Amaqhawe) programme in South Africa. *African Journal of AIDS Research, 3*(1), 33–41.

Botchway, A. T. (2004). Parent and adolescent males' communication about sexuality in the context of HIV/AIDS–A study in the eastern region of Ghana. Unpublished Master's thesis, University of Bergen, Bergen, Norway.

Botvin, G. J., Baker, E., Dusenbury, L., Tortu, S., & Botvin, E. M. (1990). Preventing adolescent drug abuse through a multimodal cognitive-behavioral approach: Results of a 3-year study. *Journal of Consulting and Clinical Psychology, 58*(4), 437.

Boyas, J. F., Stauss, K. A., & Murphy-Erby, Y. (2012). Predictors of frequency of sexual health communication: Perceptions from early adolescent youth in rural Arkansas. *Child and Adolescent Social Work Journal, 29*(4), 267–284.

Bozalek, V. (1999). Contextualizing caring in black South African families. *Social Politics: International Studies in Gender, State & Society, 6*(1), 85–99.

Casale, M., Cluver, L., Crankshaw, T., Kuo, C., Lachman, J. M., & Wild, L. G. (2015). Direct and indirect effects of caregiver social support on adolescent psychological outcomes in two South African AIDS-affected communities. *American Journal of Community Psychology, 55* (3–4), 336–346. https://doi.org/10.1007/s10464-015-9705-3

Coetzee, J., Dietrich, J., Otwombe, K., Nkala, B., Khunwane, M., van der Watt, M., Sikkema, K. J., & Gray, G. E. (2014). Predictors of parent-adolescent communication in post-apartheid South Africa: A protective factor in adolescent sexual and reproductive health. *Journal of Adolescence, 37*, 313–324.

De Bellis, M. D., Baum, A. S., Birmaher, B., Keshavan, M. S., Eccard, C. H., Boring, A. M., … Ryan, N. D. (1999). Developmental traumatology part I: Biological stress systems. *Biological Psychiatry, 45*(10), 1259–1270.

Department of Social Development. (2012). *White paper on families in South Africa*. Republic of South Africa.

Dishion, T. J., & McMahon, R. J. (1998). Parental monitoring and the prevention of child and adolescent problem behavior: A conceptual and empirical formulation. *Clinical Child and Family Psychology Review, 1*(1), 61–75.

Donovan, J. E., Jessor, R., & Jessor, L. (1983). Problem drinking in adolescence and young adulthood. A follow-up study. *Journal of Studies on Alcohol, 44*(1), 109–137.

Eddy, M. M., Thomson-de Boor, H., & Mphaka, K. (2013). *So we are ATM fathers. A study of absent fathers in Johannesburg, South Africa. Johannesburg, South Africa*. Centre for Social Development in Africa, University of Johannesburg.

Feshbach, N. D. (1987). Parental empathy and child adjustment/maladjustment. In N. Eisenberg & J. Strayer (Eds.), *Cambridge studies in social and emotional development. Empathy and its development* (pp. 271–291). Cambridge University Press.

Flisher, A. J., Dawes, A., Kafaar, Z., Lund, C., Sorsdahl, K., Myers, B., … & Seedat, S. (2012). Child and adolescent mental health in South Africa. *Journal of Child & Adolescent Mental Health, 24*(2), 149–161.

Goldberg, D. P., & Hillier, V. F. (1979). A scaled version of the general health questionnaire. *Psychological Medicine, 9*, 139–145.

Goodrum, N. M., Armistead, L. P., Tully, E. C., Cook, S. L., & Skinner, D. (2017). Parenting and youth sexual risk in context: The role of community factors. *Journal of Adolescence, 57*, 1–12.

Gould, C., & Ward, C. L. (2015). *Positive parenting in South Africa: Why supporting families is key to development and violence prevention (Policy brief 77)*. Retrieved from http://137.158.155.94/bitstream/handle/11427/12694/PolBrief77.pdf?sequence=1.

Groenewald, C., & Bhana, A. (2018). Substance abuse and the family: An examination of the south African policy context. *Drugs: Education, Prevention and Policy, 25*(2), 148–155. https://doi.org/10.1080/09687637.2016.1236072

Guilamo-Ramos, V., Bouris, A., Jaccard, J., Gonzalez, B., McCoy, W., & Aranda, D. (2011). A parent based intervention to reduce sexual risk behavior in early adolescence: Building alliances between physicians, social workers, and parents. *Journal of Adolescent Health, 48*, 159–163. https://doi.org/10.1016/j.jadohealth.2010.06.007

Hamburg, B. A. (1990). *Life skills training: Preventive interventions for young adolescents: Report of the life skills training working group (working paper no. ED323018)*. Retrieved from Carnegie council on adolescent development website: https://eric.ed.gov/?id=ED323018.

Holloway, I. W., Traube, D. E., Schrager, S. M., Levine, B., Alicea, S., Watson, J. L., … McKay, M. M. (2012). The effects of sexual expectancies on early sexualized behavior among urban minority youth. *Journal of the Society for Social Work and Research, 3*(1), 1–12.

Hutchinson, M. K. (2002). Sexual risk communication with mothers and fathers: Influence on the sexual risk behaviors of adolescent daughters. *Family Relations, 51*, 238–247.

Hutchinson, M. K., & Montgomery, A. J. (2007). Parent communication and sexual risk among African Americans. *Western Journal of Nursing Research, 29*(6), 691–707.

Jerman, P., & Constantine, N. A. (2010). Demographic and psychological predictors of parent–adolescent communication about sex: A representative statewide analysis. *Journal of Youth and Adolescence, 39*(10), 1164–1174.

Kanfer, F. H., & Goldstein, A. P. (1991). *Helping people change: A textbook of methods.* New York, NY: Pergamon Press.

Knight, Z. G. (2019). In the shadow of apartheid: Intergenerational transmission of black parental trauma as it emerges in the analytical space of inter-racial subjectivities. *Research in Psychotherapy: Psychopathology, Process and Outcome, 22*(1), 345.

Krauss, B. J. (1995). *Calm down, Mom, let's talk about sex, drugs and HIV: 10–13-year-old girls' prescriptions for HIV prevention conversations in their high HIV seroprevalence neighborhood.* Paper presented at the HIV Infection in Women Conference, Washington, DC.

Krauss, B. (1997). HIV education for teens and preteens in a high-seroprevalence inner-city neighborhood. Families in Society: *The Journal of Contemporary Social Services, 78*(6), 579–591.

Levitt, M. Z., Selman, R. L., & Richmond, J. B. (1991). The psychosocial foundations of early adolescents' high-risk behavior: Implications for research and practice. *Journal of Research on Adolescence, 1*(4), 349–378.

Li, X., Feigelman, S., & Stanton, B. (2000). Perceived parental monitoring and health risk behaviors among urban low-income African-American children and adolescents. *Journal of Adolescent Health, 27*(1), 43–48.

Lindsey, M. A., Browne, D. C., Thompson, R., Hawley, K. M., Graham, J. C., Weisbart, C., ... Kotch, J. B. (2008). Caregiver mental health, neighborhood, and social network influences on mental health needs among African American children. *Social Work Research, 32*(2), 79–88.

Lindsey, M. A., Gilreath, T. D., Thompson, R., Graham, J. C., Hawley, K. M., Weisbart, C., ... Kotch, J. B. (2012). Influence of caregiver network support and caregiver psychopathology on child mental health need and service use in the LONGSCAN study. *Children and Youth Services Review, 34*(5), 924–932.

LoveLife. (2018). *loveLife.* Retrieved July 20, 2018, from http://www.lovelife.org.za/

Maccoby, E. E. (1992). The role of parents in the socialization of children: An historical overview. *Developmental Psychology, 28*(6), 1006.

MacKinnon, D. P., Lockwood, C. M., Hoffman, J. M., West, S. G., & Sheets, V. (2002). A comparison of methods to test mediation and other intervening variable effects. *Psychological Methods, 7*(1), 83.

Madison, S. M., McKay, M. M., Paikoff, R., & Bell, C. C. (2000). Basic research and community collaboration: Necessary ingredients for the development of a family-based HIV prevention program. *AIDS Education and Prevention, 12*(4), 281.

McKay, M. M., Alicea, S., Elwyn, L., McClain, Z. R., Parker, G., Small, L. A., & Mellins, C. A. (2014). The development and implementation of theory-driven programs capable of addressing poverty-impacted children's health, mental health, and prevention needs: CHAMP and CHAMP+, evidence-informed, family-based interventions to address HIV risk and care. *Journal of Clinical Child & Adolescent Psychology, 43*(3), 428–441.

McKay, M. M., Chasse, K. T., Paikoff, R., McKinney, L. D., Baptiste, D., Coleman, D., ... Bell, C. C. (2004). Family-level impact of the CHAMP family program: A community collaborative effort to support urban families and reduce youth HIV risk exposure. *Family Process, 43*(1), 79–93.

McKay, M. M., Gonzales, J., Quintana, E., Kim, L., & Abdul-Adil, J. (1999). Multiple family groups: An alternative for reducing disruptive behavioral difficulties of urban children. *Research on Social Work Practice, 9*(5), 593–607.

McKay, M. M., Gopalan, G., Franco, L. M., Kalogerogiannis, K., Umpierre, M., Olshtain-Mann, O., ... Goldstein, L. (2010). It takes a village to deliver and test child and family-focused services. *Research on Social Work Practice, 20*(5), 476–482.

McKay, M. M., Harrison, M. E., Gonzales, J., Kim, L., & Quintana, E. (2002). Multiple-family groups for urban children with conduct difficulties and their families. *Psychiatric Services, 53* (11), 1467–1468.

Meinck, F., Cluver, L. D., Orkin, F. M., Kuo, C., Sharma, A. D., Hensels, I. S., & Sherr, L. (2017). Pathways from family disadvantage via abusive parenting and caregiver mental health to adolescent health risks in South Africa. *Journal of Adolescent Health, 60*(1), 57–64.

Mellins, C. A., Dolezal, C., Brackis-Cott, E., Nicholson, O., Warne, P., & Meyer-Bahlburg, H. F. (2007). Predicting the onset of sexual and drug risk behaviors in HIV-negative youths with HIV-positive mothers: The role of contextual, self-regulation, and social-interaction factors. *Journal of Youth and Adolescence, 36*(3), 265–278.

Morris, A. S., Robinson, L. R., Hays-Grudo, J., Claussen, A. H., Hartwig, S. A., & Treat, A. E. (2017). Targeting parenting in early childhood: A public health approach to improve outcomes for children living in poverty. *Child Development, 88*(2), 388–397.

Namisi, F. S. (2004). *Communicating on sexuality within the Kenya family setting in the context of HIV/AIDS: The perceptions of parents and 14–17 year old adolescents.* University of Bergen, Department of Health Promotion and Development.

Paikoff, R. L. (1995). Early heterosexual debut: Situations of sexual possibility during the transition to adolescence. *The American Journal of Orthopsychiatry, 65*(3), 389–401.

Paruk, Z., Petersen, I., Bhana, A., Bell, C., & McKay, M. (2002). A focused ethnographic study to inform the adaptation of the NIMH funded CHAMP project in South Africa. In *xIV international AIDS conference.* Bologna: Moduzzi Editore (pp. 295–298).

Paruk, Z., Petersen, I., Bhana, A., Bell, C., & McKay, M. (2005). Containment and contagion: How to strengthen families to support youth HIV prevention in South Africa. *African Journal of AIDS Research, 4*(1), 57–63.

Pedersen, G. A., Smallegange, E., Coetzee, A., Hartog, K., Turner, J., Jordans, M. J., & Brown, F. L. (2019). A systematic review of the evidence for family and parenting interventions in low- and middle-income countries: Child and youth mental health outcomes. *Journal of Child and Family Studies*, 1–20.

Pequegant, W. & Szapocznik, J. (2000). The role of families in preventing and adapting to HIV/ AIDS: Issues and answers. In W. Pequegant & J. Szapocznik (Eds.), *Working with families in the era of HIV/AIDS* (pp. 3–26). Thousand Oaks, CA: Sage.

Pillay, A. (2010). *The influence of household and family structure on children in the Chatsworth area with special reference to primary school learners* (Master's thesis). Retrieved from http://citeseerx.ist.psu.edu/viewdoc/download?doi=10.1.1.1024.1855&rep=rep1&type=pdf.

Reddy, S. P., James, S., Sewpaul, R., Sifunda, S., Ellahebokus, A., Kambaran, N. S., & Omardien, R. G. (2013). *Umthente Uhlaba Usamila: The 3rd south African National Youth Risk Behaviour Survey 2011.* Human Sciences Research Council.

Reniers, G., Blom, S., Calvert, C., Martin-Onraet, A., Herbst, A. J., Eaton, J. W., . . . Bärnighausen, T. (2017). Trends in the burden of HIV mortality after roll-out of antiretroviral therapy in KwaZulu-Natal, South Africa: An observational community cohort study. *The Lancet HIV, 4* (3), e113–e121.

Shisana, O., Rehle, T., Simbayi, L. C., Zurra, K., Jossle, S., Zungu, N., Labadarios, D., Onoya, D., et al. (2014). *South African national HIV prevalence, incidence and behavioral survey, 2012.* HSRC Press.

Small, L. A., Parchment, T. M., Bahar, O. S., Osuji, H. L., Chomanczuk, A. H., & Bhana, A. (2019). South African adult caregivers as "protective shields": Serving as a buffer between stressful neighborhood conditions and youth risk behaviors. *Journal of Community Psychology, 47*(8), 1850–1864.

Soul City. (2018). *About soul city.* Retrieved from http://www.soulcity.org.za.

South African Federation for Mental Health. (2015). *Annual report April 2014 – March 2015.* Retrieved from http://www.safmh.org.za/documents/annual-reports/2015/index.html#p=1.

Spannring, J. R. (2012). *The role of parental mental health issues in the development of child and adolescent psychological crisis symptoms* (doctoral dissertation), Palo Alto University

Statistics South Africa. (2018). *Men, women, and children: Findings of the living conditions survey 2008/2009*. Statistics South Africa.

Taitt, A. L. (1980). *The impact of apartheid on family life in South Africa*. United Nations, Centre Against Apartheid, Dept. of Political and Security Council Affairs.

Tarantino, N., Anthony, E. R., Zimmerman, L., Armistead, L. P., Cook, S. L., Skinner, D., & Toefy, Y. (2014). Talking to young people about sex in South Africa: Neighborhood and social influences. *Journal of Community Psychology, 42*(6), 656–672. https://doi.org/10.1002/jcop. 21644

Trumpeter, N. N., Watson, P. J., O'Leary, B. J., & Weathington, B. L. (2008). Self-functioning and perceived parenting: Relations of parental empathy and love inconsistency with narcissism, depression, and self-esteem. *The Journal of Genetic Psychology, 169*(1), 51–71.

UNAIDS. (2019). *Fact sheet world AIDS day*. Retrieved from https://www.unaids.org/sites/default/files/media_asset/UNAIDS_FactSheet_en.pdf

Vreeman, R. C., McCoy, B. M., & Lee, S. (2017). Mental health challenges among adolescents living with HIV. *Journal of the International AIDS Society, 20*, 21497.

Wang, Z. (2009). Parent-adolescent communication and sexual risk-taking behaviours of adolescents (Doctoral dissertation), University of Stellenbosch (Stellenbosch, South Africa).

Ward, C. L., Gould, C., Kelly, J., & Mauff, K. (2015). Spare the rod and save the child assessing the impact of parenting on child behaviour and mental health. *SA Crime Quarterly, 51*, 09–22.

Whitaker, D., & Miller, K. (2000). Parent-adolescent discussions about sex and condoms: Impact on peer influences of sexual risk behavior. *Journal of Adolescent Research, 15*, 251–273.

Whitbeck, L. B., Yoder, K. A., Hoyt, D. R., & Conger, R. D. (1999). Early adolescent sexual activity: A developmental study. *Journal of Marriage and Family, 61*(4), 934–946.

World Health Organization. (2017). *Depression and other common mental disorders: Global health estimates* (Report No. WHO/MSD/MER/2017.2). Retrieved from http://apps.who.int/iris/handle/10665/254610.

Zahn-Waxler, C., & Van Hulle, C. (2011). Empathy, guilt, and depression. In B. Oakley, A. Knafo, G. Madhavan, & D. Sloan Wilson (Eds.), *Pathological altruism* (pp. 321–344). Oxford University Press.

Ziehl, S. C. (2001). Documenting changing family patterns in South Africa: Are census data of any value? *African Sociological Review, 5*(2), 36–62.

Social Enterprises for Child and Adolescent Health in Sub-Saharan Africa: A Realist Evaluation

Juliet Iwelunmor, Sarah Blackstone, Ucheoma Nwaozuru, Chisom Obiezu-Umeh, Florida Uzoaru, Stacey Mason, Titilola Gbaja-Biamila, David Oladele, Oliver Ezechi, and Collins Airhihenbuwa

Introduction

Improving the health and well-being of children and adolescents in sub-Saharan Africa (SSA) has been the focus of significant attention for several decades. Yet global and regional progress in reducing morbidity and mortality rates has been limited (Kassebaum et al., 2017). The statistics are dire. While sub-Saharan Africa has the largest cohort of young people in history (Agyepong et al., 2017), 45% of deaths and 35% of disability-adjusted life years (DALYs) occur among Africa's adolescent population. Adolescent health in the region is influenced by childhood well-being, which in turn sets the trajectory for adult health (Berhane et al., 2020). Children living in sub-Saharan Africa currently have the highest rates of under-five mortality globally, with an under-five mortality rate of 76 deaths per 1000 live births in 2017, leading to 2.7 million deaths in the region (Nilsson et al., 2016; Van Malderen et al., 2019). The major causes of under-five mortality among children in sub-Saharan Africa are malaria, diarrhea, acute respiratory infection, anemia, and growth failure from malnutrition (Boah et al., 2019; Liu et al., 2016; McAllister et al., 2019). Likewise, childhood and adolescence malnutrition is a major public health concern in sub-Saharan Africa. The region has the world's highest rate of stunting (43%) and undernutrition (25%) among children, while also grabbling with overweight and obesity (Akombi et al., 2017; Osgood-Zimmerman et al., 2018). Currently, an estimated 15% of adolescents in sub-Saharan Africa are overweight or obese with increased risk for diabetes, and other noncommunicable diseases later in life (Berhane et al., 2020). However, goal 3 of the United Nations Sustainable

J. Iwelunmor (✉)
Saint Louis University, College for Public Health and Social Justice, Department of Behavioral Science and Health Education, Saint Louis, MO, USA
e-mail: julietiwelunmor@slu.edu

© Springer Nature Switzerland AG 2022
F. M. Ssewamala et al. (eds.), *Child Behavioral Health in Sub-Saharan Africa*,
https://doi.org/10.1007/978-3-030-83707-5_16

Development Goals (SDGs) seeks "to ensure healthy lives and promote well-being for all at all ages" (UN., 2015). Nowhere is this goal more significant than in sub-Saharan Africa where children and adolescents continue to experience significant unmet health and well-being needs (Berhane et al., 2020), highlighting the need for holistic research and action that embrace their needs across the life cycle (Bundy et al., 2018).

Social enterprises have emerged as potential cost-effective and scalable solutions to intractable health improvement challenges faced by children and adolescents in sub-Saharan Africa. In this chapter, we define social enterprises "as organizations that combine social missions with the pursuit of financial sustainability and self-sufficiency via trading activity" (Farmer et al., 2020). Social enterprises create models for efficiently catering to basic human needs that existing markets and institutions have failed to satisfy (Macaulay et al., 2018; McKague & Harrison, 2019). It is also typically designed and governed so that improvements to the business will deliver improvements in health outcomes (McKague & Harrison, 2019). Over the past several decades, social enterprises have emerged as a way to identify and bring about potentially transformative societal change that ultimately improves health and well-being (Gordon et al., 2018; Roy et al., 2013; Roy et al., 2014). It also aligns with the principle of the UN's SDG goal 8 that seeks to promote economic growth for all. However, the knowledge of how social enterprises influence child and adolescent health outcomes in sub-Saharan Africa remains limited.

Although social enterprises involve the use of market-based strategies to enact social change (Kerlin, 2010; Roy et al., 2014), the health impacts of social initiatives remain largely unknown (Farmer et al., 2020). Roy and colleagues argue that social enterprises may influence the unequal distribution of power, income, goods, services, and health outcomes (Marmot et al., 2008; Roy et al., 2014; Wilkinson & Marmot, 2003). They may also create solutions to social challenges, offering more cost-effective and sustainable strategies than those provided by other entities (Addicott, 2011; Smith et al., 2015). Social enterprises also differ from other market-generating entities in that the profits from the enterprises are reinvested into the community they serve or into the development of innovative services to serve the target population (Clancy & Mayo, 2009; Gordon et al., 2018).

Given the promise of social enterprises, in this chapter, we examine its potential in improving the health and well-being of children and adolescents in sub-Saharan Africa. We extend prior reviews on social enterprises, by using realist evaluation to explore how and why these enterprises are utilized to address child and adolescent health outcomes challenges in sub-Saharan Africa. Realist evaluation enables an understanding of how contextual factors influence health outcomes, by exploring how, why, for whom, and under which conditions interventions or social enterprises work (Pawson & Tilley, 1997). We begin by describing how realist evaluation was applied to understand social enterprises in sub-Saharan Africa. Next, we identify existing social enterprises and how and why they work to address child and adolescent health outcomes in sub-Saharan Africa. We conclude with implications on the potential of using social enterprises to improve the health and well-being of children and adolescents in sub-Saharan Africa.

Applying Realist Principles to Social Enterprises for Child and Adolescent Health Outcomes in Sub-Saharan Africa

Realist evaluation, a theory-driven approach developed by Pawson and Tilley (1997), builds an understanding of the underlying processes that explains what works for whom and in what circumstances it works (Pawson & Tilley, 1997). Through a realist evaluation, our findings are summarized and presented in context-mechanism-outcome (CMO) configurations to assess the impact of social enterprises on improving child and adolescent health and thus can support the production of future evidence. Context may refer to broad factors (i.e., cultural, social, or institutional features) in the backdrop environment of a program that may influence its outcomes (Jagosh, 2019). Mechanisms refer to the underlying program processes, entities, or structures that interact in a specific context to influence an outcome (Astbury & Leeuw, 2010). Outcomes are intended or unintended effects of a program (Jagosh, 2019). In our evaluation, the problem and target population make up the social enterprise context, then the mechanism is the approach or process in which the social enterprise is implemented to address the needs, and the program impacts are considered to be the outcome.

Identification of Social Enterprises for Child and Adolescent Health in Sub-Saharan Africa

To identify the social enterprises working in the child and adolescent health space, we searched for social enterprise interventions appraised by the Schwab Foundation for Social Entrepreneurship (Schwab Foundation, 2020). Schwab Foundation for Social Entrepreneurship is a global platform which identifies a select community of social enterprises that are engaged in global, national, and regional agendas to improve the quality of life internationally. It is one of the world's most influential social entrepreneurship organizations and repositories for social entrepreneurs working on making global social impacts. Inclusion criteria of social enterprises in the realist evaluation were as follows: (1) at least one region of target for the program was in sub-Saharan Africa; (2) the program utilized social enterprise mechanisms, such as skills training and capacity building to improve the health and well-being of children and adolescents; and (3) the long-term outcome of the program was related to child and adolescent health. To identify the organizations, the keyword filters used for the search on Schwab's website were the following: (1) Sector—Global Health; (2) Region of Impact—Africa; (3) Population—Children and Adolescents; and (4) Award—Social Entrepreneur. There was no restriction on the year of the award. Each enterprise was reviewed by two separate researchers to establish a consensus on the goal of each program, target audience, social program to be addressed, and potential solutions that each program offered to combat issues affecting children and adolescent health and well-being. A final list of nine social enterprise organizations met the inclusion criteria of social enterprises operating in sub-Saharan Africa and targeting child and adolescent health issues. The social enterprises included in this chapter are summarized in Table 1. These programs include mothers2mothers, Last Mile Health, Living Goods, Embrace Innovations, Zipline, GiftedMom, VisionSpring, Table for Two International, and BasicNeeds. We also provide an overview of a social enterprise led by the authors in Nigeria focused on promoting HIV self-testing among adolescents and young people in Nigeria.

Components of Social Enterprise for Adolescent and Child Health in Sub-Saharan Africa

All of the programs in some way incorporated workforce development and/or job creation for disadvantaged populations by providing a product or service needed by the respective communities (Schwab Foundation, 2020). To aid in the understanding of our synthesis of these enterprises, our results are presented in four categories: physical health, mental health, social determinants, and health systems. However, it is important to note that in practice, these categories are interrelated and continually impact each other.

Physical Health

Three of the social enterprises identified focused on physical health: Living Goods, M2M, and GiftedMom. *Living Goods* is a social enterprise, founded in 2007, that seeks to address preventable and treatable infectious diseases that account for high mortality rates, particularly among children under 5 years of age, including malaria, diarrhea, and pneumonia (Living Goods, 2020). This social enterprise also addresses family planning, immunization, nutrition, and clean air and water. Living Goods operates in Uganda and Kenya using an "Avon-like" system, in which local women serve as entrepreneurs, going door to door to provide health education and sell families essential products that are difficult to access (e.g., hard to reach, overpriced). The Living Goods program has reduced under-five mortality by nearly 27% and stunting by 7% in over 200 villages and 8000 families according to the organization's 2020 enterprise report (Children's Investment Fund Foundation, 2020). Furthermore, the products offered by Living Goods entrepreneurs are being sold for 17% less than other venues, making these services affordable to more families who otherwise might not have access to these products.

Another program *mothers2mothers (M2M)*, founded in 2001, focuses on preventing mother-to-child HIV transmission by engaging local mothers to educate and empower pregnant women to improve the health and well-being of women and

Table 1 Description of social enterprise programs

Social enterprise	Context (the problem)	Mechanism (the approach)	Outcomes (the impact)
Living Goods	Millions of children die each year from preventable and easily treated diseases including malaria, diarrhea, and pneumonia. There is a lack of scalable and sustainable cost-effective delivery systems of dependable medications.	Living Goods supports networks of "Avon-like" health entrepreneurs (in the form of community health workers) who go door to door to teach families how to improve their health and wealth and sell life-changing products such as simple treatments for malaria and diarrhea, safe delivery kits, fortified foods, clean cookstoves, water filters, and solar lights.	Reduction in under-five mortality by more than 27% and stunting by 7%, in over 200 villages and 8000 families.
mothers2mothers (M2M)	In the past two-and-a-half decades, 25 million people died from HIV/AIDS. Currently, 33 million people are living with HIV and more than two million people are newly infected each year. Of these, 1.5 million pregnant women with HIV give birth annually, 90% of whom live in sub-Saharan Africa.	M2M trains, employees, and empowers local mothers living with HIV, called mentor mothers, as frontline healthcare workers in understaffed health centers and within communities. In one-on-one and group sessions, mentor mothers provide essential health education and support to women on how they can protect their babies from HIV infection, and keep themselves and their families healthy.	The program has reached more than 11 million women and children <2 in SSA. The mother-to-child transmission rate was as low as 1.3% (which is less than the <5% UN benchmark for virtual elimination of HIV).
Embrace Innovations	Every year, 20 million premature and low-birth-weight babies are born. In developing countries, mortality for these infants is particularly high because incubators are extremely rare.	Embrace Innovations has developed a low-cost infant warmer for premature and low-birth-weight babies. It works without electricity and costs less than 1% of a traditional incubator.	Embrace Innovations has reached over 300,000 babies in 22 countries including Somalia.
Last Mile Health	There is little or no access to healthcare services in Monrovia, Liberia. Of the existing health facilities, 45% are without power and 13% do not have access to safe water.	Last Mile Health supports community healthcare workers (CHW) to bring life-saving services to the doorsteps of communities that live far from healthcare facilities.	Under the program, 60% of sick children in Rivercess County, Liberia, reporting fever, acute respiratory illness, or diarrhea (within the last 2 weeks of treatment time) have received treatment from a qualified health

(continued)

Table 1 (continued)

Social enterprise	Context (the problem)	Mechanism (the approach)	Outcomes (the impact)
			provider, more than the 45% of children that were recorded at the start of the national program. Additionally, there was a 40% increase in children under five who had received medical care from the start of the national program.
Zipline	Medical equipment/medication stockouts and expiry rates remain high in sub-Saharan African countries. These stockouts cause missed opportunities for preventive interventions, unnecessary emergency trips, urban hospital overcrowding, and preventable deaths.	Zipline, founded in 2011, uses drones known as Zips to deliver medical supplies, vaccines, and blood to health facilities.	Zipline has delivered medical products, such as blood and vaccines for infants and their mothers, to 20 hospitals and health centers in Rwanda since its inception in 2011.
GiftedMom	About 800 women worldwide die every day from pregnancy-related causes, but most of these deaths could be prevented with access to antenatal care and information, vaccinations, or timely health advice. Pregnant women and nursing mothers living in developing countries like Cameroon often delay decisions to seek healthcare. Less than 60% of women in Cameroon receive the recommended amount of care during pregnancy, and the country is among the world's top 20 countries with the highest maternal mortality rates.	GiftedMom, founded in 2015, provides pregnant women and nursing mothers access to health information and monitoring services provided by health specialists. The service is accessible to end users across multiple platforms, including USSD, SMS, web, and a mobile app. One of GiftedMom's key offerings is the "ask a doctor" service, which provides a two-way text-based communication service accessible via SMS and an in-app chat. The social enterprise also works closely with 42 hospitals across eight of Cameroon's ten regions to offer a mobile-based hospital appointment reminder solution.	By the end of 2018, 170,831 users had access to GiftedMom's services, with about 40,000 active users who are provided with health information and monitoring services from health specialists.

VisionSpring	In developing countries, an estimated 703 million people suffer from vision impairment that affects their ability to work and learn. Particularly among children and adolescents, it affects their ability to learn and continue with schooling which affects their life trajectory.	VisionSpring, founded in 2001, focuses on providing affordable eyeglasses and vision screenings to communities, including children and adolescents. By training local villagers to conduct outreach and vision screenings and to sell high-quality, low-cost eyeglasses, VisionSpring provides a cost-effective, high-impact intervention that instantly improves the productivity and quality of life for the underprivileged in the developing world.	By 2018, VisionSpring had provided 176,000 school students with glasses in participating countries. Overall, VisionSpring has sold eyeglasses to 6.9 M customers, with more than 50% acquiring their first ever pair, and is on track to provide a clear vision for 10 M people by 2021.
Table for Two International	In our world of 7 billion, 1 billion suffer from hunger while another 2 billion suffer from obesity and other health-related issues due to unhealthy eating.	Table for Two International, founded in 2007, focuses on eliminating global hunger and reducing health issues related to unhealthy eating among children and adolescents in resource-constrained settings. This is achieved through a unique meal-sharing program, where they partner with corporations and organizations to provide healthier options in cafeterias, restaurants, food trucks, and vending machines for an extra $0.25, which is donated to providing school meals in areas of need throughout the world. They support children and adolescents in East Africa (Malawi, Ethiopia, Uganda, Rwanda, Kenya, and Tanzania) and Southeast Asia as well as low-income communities in the United States.	Since 2007, Table for Two International has served meals to over 70 million children and adolescents globally, including the six sub-Saharan African countries in their network.
BasicNeeds	Mental illness has an enormous impact on individuals and families, yet many countries do not have adequate resources to address these conditions; 40% of countries have no	BasicNeeds, founded in 2000, uses community engagement to promote awareness of mental illness, trains medical and volunteer workers to treat affected community	As of December 2016, over 686,000 people had been reached through the BasicNeeds programs globally. This included providing treatment access and

(continued)

Table 1 (continued)

Social enterprise	Context (the problem)	Mechanism (the approach)	Outcomes (the impact)
	mental health policies and 25% have no mental health legislation. Furthermore, many individuals with mental health conditions have difficulty finding regular employment, which prohibits them from obtaining regular health services.	members to avoid institutionalization, creates peer support and advocacy networks for mentally ill people and caregivers, and provides opportunities for income generation or participation in productive work to enable sustainable recoveries and reintegration into society. BasicNeeds has helped 79% of participants obtain either paid employment or productive, non-remunerative work.	symptom reduction, creation of self-help groups, and training and mobilizing participants and staff to increase program reach.
4 Youth by Youth (4YBY)	Nigerian youth are at the epicenter of an expanding HIV crisis, with the second largest number of new youth HIV infections of any country. However, nearly four in five youth aged 15–24 years have ever tested for HIV.	To address the HIV testing gaps among adolescents and young people in Nigeria, 4YBY projects are focused on engaging youth to generate sustainable health solutions. These youth-driven social enterprises enhance youth participation, capabilities, and strength towards driving positive changes in their communities. Specifically, 4YBY engages young people through crowdsourcing and entrepreneurship training to generate social innovations to problems that affect them.	Since its inception in 2018, 4YBY has hosted five youth-participatory contests, engaged over 2000 adolescents and young people in Nigeria, and generated five youth-driven HIV self-testing social enterprises in Nigeria.

Sources: Social Enterprise Websites (*Living Goods*: https://livinggoods.org/; *mothers2mothers*: https://m2m.org/; *Embrace Innovations*: https://www.embraceinnovations.com/; *Last Mile Health*: https://lastmilehealth.org/; *Zipline*: https://flyzipline.com/; *GiftedMom*: http://www.giftedmom.org/index.html; *VisionSpring*: https://visionspring.org/; *Table for Two International*: https://www.tablefor2.org/; *BasicNeeds*: http://www.basicneeds.org/social-entrepreneurship-and-mental-health/; *4 Youth by Youth*: https://4yby.org/).

children (Mothers2Mothers, 2020). M2M operates in Angola, Ghana, Kenya, Lesotho, Malawi, Mozambique, South Africa, Tanzania, Uganda, and Zambia. In the past two-and-a-half decades, 25 million people died from HIV/AIDS. M2M has worked to develop a sustainable platform to combat this issue by identifying mothers living with HIV, recruiting them, and educating them about prenatal health and HIV prevention. These women are then employed as "mentor mothers" who provide community health education about HIV prevention and work alongside doctors and nurses to provide more specialized education and support services for HIV-positive patients. The M2M model improves children's and adolescents' health as well as maternal health while delivering meaningful employment for women living with HIV. As of 2018, M2M has made tremendous strides in ten sub-Saharan African countries, employing over 11,000 HIV-positive women as mentor mothers, and reached more than eleven million women and children in sub-Saharan Africa by providing information and services to improve their health and well-being (2018 Annual Report). Given the reach of M2M, they are poised to assist in delivering the UN's SDGs of ending AIDS, delivering health for all, and ensuring gender equality by 2030 for children and adolescents in sub-Saharan Africa.

The other program *GiftedMom* is a mobile health social enterprise, founded in 2015, aimed at decreasing maternal and infant mortality by providing mothers and pregnant women access to health information and monitoring services provided by health specialists. GiftedMom currently operates in Cameroon. This social enterprise uses a web/mobile platform to sensitize and follow up on pregnant women and guardians of children less than one year. They aim to increase the rate of antenatal care attendance, decrease the rate of HIV transmission from mother-to-child HIV transmission, increase the rate of skilled birth delivery and follow-up of pregnant women, increase child vaccination coverage, and encourage better breastfeeding habits among breastfeeding mothers. By 2018, GiftedMom had over 170,831 subscribers with over 40,000 active users across Cameroon.

Mental Health

One of the social enterprises focused on mental health-*BasicNeeds*. BasicNeeds uses social enterprise techniques to improve access to treatment, reduce symptoms, and provide opportunities for income generation among individuals with mental health conditions. *BasicNeeds* operates in six countries, two in sub-Saharan Africa (Ghana and Kenya). The program targets the challenges faced by individuals with mental health conditions as few developing countries have mental health policies and legislation. Furthermore, many individuals with mental health conditions have difficulty finding regular employment, which prohibits them from obtaining regular health services, including treatment for their mental illness (BasicNeeds, 2017). BasicNeeds uses community engagement to promote awareness of mental illness, trains medical and volunteer workers to treat affected community members to avoid institutionalization, creates peer support and advocacy networks for mentally ill people and caregivers, and provides opportunities for income generation or partic-ipation in productive work to enable sustainable recoveries and reintegration into society. Thus far, BasicNeeds has engaged over 120,000 participants, generated over 100,000 careers, and helped 79% of participants obtain either paid employment or productive, non-remunerative work. Eighty percent of participants were able to work after completion of the program, compared to a baseline rate of 52%. Additionally, following the program, 80% accessed treatment (baseline 58%) and 78% experi-enced a reduction in symptoms (baseline 0%) (BasicNeeds, 2017).

Social Determinants of Health

Two of the social enterprises identified focused on social determinants of health: VisionSpring and Table for Two International. *VisionSpring*, founded in 2001, focuses on providing affordable eyeglasses and vision screenings to communities, including children and adolescents. This social enterprise aims to promote social and economic development and personal well-being through healthy vision. They oper-ate in Kenya, Ghana, Zambia, and Nigeria. For children and adolescents, VisionSpring promotes vision health to increase their ability to succeed in school. They suggest that eyeglasses boost learning outcomes among children and adoles-cents which is equivalent to an additional one-third and up to a full year of schooling. They reach customers using business-to-business (B2B) and business-to-consumer (B2C) approaches, and advance social impact by boosting livelihoods among com-munity members and learning abilities among children and adolescents. Previous research studies have shown a positive association between school attendance and health outcomes among children and adolescents (Chae et al., 2020; Werner et al., 2019). In 2018, VisionSpring provided 176,000 school students with glasses in participating countries.

The other social enterprise that focused on social determinants of health was *Table for Two International* in Malawi, Ethiopia, Uganda, Rwanda, Kenya, and Tanzania. This social enterprise, founded in 2007, focuses on eliminating global hunger to reduce health issues related to unhealthy eating among children and adolescents in resource-constrained settings. They work by partnering with corpo-rations and organizations to provide healthy food options in cafeterias, restaurants, food trucks, and vending machines for an extra $0.25, which is donated to providing school meals in areas of need throughout the world. They currently support schools in Malawi, Ethiopia, Uganda, Rwanda, Kenya, and Tanzania to provide healthy meals for children and adolescents to tackle malnutrition and obesity. In Malawi, Zambia, and Tanzania, Table for Two International built innovative sustainable school gardens with irrigation pumps powered by solar energy to grow food produce. Schools along with community members can grow vegetables and maize and sell the crops to purchase enough maize for school meals. In addition, the students (children and adolescents) and community members can learn about agri-culture practices, food, nutrition education, and environmental conservation. Since

2007, Table for Two International has served meals to over 70 million children and adolescents globally, including the six sub-Saharan African countries (Malawi, Ethiopia, Uganda, Rwanda, Kenya, and Tanzania) in their network. The future goals of this social enterprise are to continue providing healthy food options for children and adolescents while providing sustainable economic generating activities for the community members which include the parents of the children and adolescents.

Health Systems

Embrace Innovations in Somalia and Zipline focuse on addressing health system strengthening. *Embrace Innovations* is a social enterprise that was founded in 2008 to create well-designed baby products and in the process "give 1,000,000 premature and underweight babies in the developing world a better chance at life" (Embrace Innovations, 2020). This social enterprise is focused on reducing infant and maternal deaths in low-resource settings by providing low-cost infant warmers to reduce the incidence of infant mortality in developing countries. The Little Lotus is Embrace's innovative product that costs less than 1% of the cost of a traditional incubator and seeks to help the 15 million preterm and underweight babies born every year (Embrace Innovations, 2020). To date, Embrace Innovations has reached over 300,000 babies in 22 countries including Somalia.

The other social enterprise, *Zipline*, founded in 2011, uses drones known as Zips to deliver medical supplies, vaccines, and blood to health facilities in Rwanda. This cutting-edge technology addresses the issue of infant mortality by delivering medical necessities to healthcare professionals in Rwanda, even in the most remote areas where traditional modes of transportation cannot access. Also, the Zips arrive faster and are cheaper than other modes of transportation, since it utilizes a tracking system that chooses the best route and tracks successful deliveries. Since its inception, Zipline has delivered medical products, such as blood and vaccines for infants and their mothers, to 20 hospitals and health centers in Rwanda.

The reports of these nine social enterprises operating in sub-Saharan Africa show impact and these organizations have made great strides with improving child and adolescent health and well-being in sub-Saharan Africa. Nonetheless, there is room for more rigorous research and assessments to examine the extent to which these social entrepreneurship models influence health outcomes. We, therefore, provide a brief detail of an ongoing research project in Nigeria—4 Youth by Youth (4YBY)— led by the authors that utilizes a social entrepreneurship model to promote the uptake of HIV self-testing among adolescents and young people in Nigeria.

Lastly, 4 Youth by Youth Nigeria, a participatory research project, commenced in 2018 and is aimed at promoting HIV self-testing (HIVST) among adolescents and young people in Nigeria using a crowdsourcing approach and entrepreneurship training (Iwelunmor et al., 2019) to develop new HIVST services. The 4 Youth by Youth model generated five youth-participatory HIVST social enterprises (Nwaozuru et al., 2020). Two of the social enterprises focused on repacking

HIVST kits to increase their appeal among young people; one idea focused on leveraging community engagement platforms (vocational skill training and youth community events) to promote HIVST, and another social enterprise seeks to use a reward-referral system to promote HIVST in young people. Preliminary assessments of 4YBY social enterprises showed a 29% increase in the uptake of HIV self-testing among adolescents and young people in Nigeria between baseline and 3-month follow-up. This research project shows the feasibility of utilizing social enterprises to improve the uptake of preventive sexual and reproductive health services.

State of Social Enterprise and Adolescent and Child Health in Sub-Saharan Africa

This realist evaluation of social enterprises in sub-Saharan Africa demonstrates progress in the utility of social enterprise and health for children and adolescents in the region. This evaluation provides information about the contexts that social enterprises are implemented to provide child and adolescent health in sub-Saharan Africa. The social enterprises reviewed demonstrated positive effects on the health and well-being of children and adolescents in disadvantaged communities. Evidence from the nine programs reviewed from the Schwab Foundation for Social Entrepreneurship suggests that social enterprises can improve health in a variety of ways and increase social capital—which has a positive impact on the health and well-being and the individual and population level (Roy et al., 2014). The social enterprises addressed physical health, mental health, social determinants of health, and health system strengthening for children and adolescents in sub-Saharan Africa. It sheds light on the role of actors beyond formal health providers who play a critical role in strengthening health systems and improving the health outcomes of children and adolescents in sub-Saharan Africa (Roy et al., 2018). The impact of these social enterprise actors and the reach of their solutions can be expanded through partnerships within the academic research community to maximize the gains.

Unfortunately, academic researchers and social entrepreneurs usually operate in different sectors. While social entrepreneurs are business savvy, they may not be equipped to evaluate the large body of literature to identify best practices and update current practices based on the most recent evidence (Smith et al., 2015). Meanwhile, academic researchers may be missing an opportunity to have substantial short- and long-term impacts by partnering with social enterprises to implement, test, and scale up intervention to address health outcomes. It should be noted that we did not conduct rigorous evaluations of each program, and as such we are unable to make assumptions about the effectiveness and generalizability of the enterprises. That notwithstanding, there is compelling evidence that these programs have a positive impact worldwide and could help in the long term with improving health outcomes and reaching SDGs. The relationships between contexts, mechanisms, and outcomes of these social enterprises provide useful starting points for further evaluations to test the scale-up of these strategies to promote sustainable positive health outcomes among children and adolescents in sub-Saharan Africa (Willis et al., 2016).

Overall, one of the central difficulties all health interventions and innovations face is sustainability, or the question of whether the program can be continued beyond its initial implementation (Iwelunmor et al., 2016). Social enterprises, whether focused on health outcomes or otherwise, are advantageous in that they build local capacity to create a sustainable platform that can be continued by individuals and the community. In many cases, individuals are initially given money or supplies, but as they begin, they generate their own income, they can replenish their supply, and they can continue their business, providing vital health products and services to people in the community, while having steady employment. Indeed, many interventions initially incur tremendous resources and ultimately fade away as the externally provided resources diminish (Chambers et al., 2013). The advantage of social enterprises is that, while initially there are start-up costs, individuals eventually become independent entrepreneurs and are able to continue the intervention services through their efforts. For instance, social enterprises such as Living Goods and Zipline are structured to be self-sustaining, such that funds generated from delivering services feed back into the operations of the organizations to provide continued services to individuals in need. This makes such programs much less reliant on external resources and funding once initial resources for implementation have been provided. While the sites in sub-Saharan Africa will continue to bring much-needed health services to hard-to-reach areas, this illustrates that even established programs with long funding histories still face challenges with sustainability.

One notable limitation of this study is that we did not review rigorous, third-party evaluations of each program. This review utilized information from the Schwab Foundation and each program's annual reports. Despite this, we are still able to understand the role of social enterprise models for health in underserved communities, and this review describes certain interventions that have appeared to have success in promoting health in the developing world through this model.

Conclusions

This chapter provides support for the utility of social enterprise models for improving health in disadvantaged communities; it shows them to be an innovative model to achieve SDG 3 to provide good health and well-being for all, alongside SDG 8 which seeks to promote decent work and economic growth. However, future empirical work to help inform and test these initiatives may be an important next step. As we move forward to devise sustainable solutions to address health, researchers, practitioners, and entrepreneurs should consider collaborating to develop and empirically test these interventions, thus providing access to a wider resource body. Research projects such as 4 Youth by Youth in Nigeria set the foundation for the integration of research and entrepreneurial principles to promote health among children and adolescents in SSA. Social enterprises, with their emphasis on reinvesting in communities, could indeed provide a potential sustainable solution, yet one that needs to be backed by rigorous and empirical research. This type of collaboration between the research and enterprise communities could encourage governance structures to provide financial support for social enterprises and foster their sustainability and ultimate success.

References

Addicott, R. (2011). *Social enterprise in health care: Promoting organisational autonomy and staff engagement*. King's Fund.

Agyepong, I. A., Sewankambo, N., Binagwaho, A., Coll-Seck, A. M., Corrah, T., Ezeh, A., … Masiye, F. (2017). The path to longer and healthier lives for all Africans by 2030: The Lancet Commission on the future of health in sub-Saharan Africa. *The Lancet, 390*(10114), 2803–2859.

Akombi, B. J., Agho, K. E., Merom, D., Renzaho, A. M., & Hall, J. J. (2017). Child malnutrition in sub-Saharan Africa: A meta-analysis of demographic and health surveys (2006-2016). *PLoS One, 12*(5), e0177338.

Astbury, B., & Leeuw, F. L. (2010). Unpacking black boxes: Mechanisms and theory building in evaluation. *American Journal of Evaluation, 31*(3), 363–381. https://doi.org/10.1177/1098214010371972

BasicNeeds. (2017). Retrieved from http://www.basicneeds.org/

Berhane, Y., Canavan, C. R., Darling, A. M., Sudfeld, C. R., Vuai, S., Adanu, R., … Guwatudde, D. (2020). The age of opportunity: Prevalence of key risk factors among adolescents 10–19 years of age in nine communities in sub-Saharan Africa. *Tropical Medicine & International Health, 25*(1), 15–32.

Boah, M., Azupogo, F., Amporfro, D. A., & Abada, L. A. (2019). The epidemiology of undernutrition and its determinants in children under five years in Ghana. *PLoS One, 14*(7), e0219665.

Bundy, D. A., de Silva, N., Horton, S., Patton, G. C., Schultz, L., Jamison, D. T., … Allen, N. (2018). Investment in child and adolescent health and development: Key messages from disease control priorities. *The Lancet, 391*(10121), 687–699.

Chae, S., Haberland, N., McCarthy, K. J., Weber, A. M., Darmstadt, G. L., & Ngo, T. D. (2020). The influence of schooling on the stability and mutability of gender attitudes: Findings from a longitudinal study of adolescent girls in Zambia. *Journal of Adolescent Health, 66*(1), S25–S33.

Chambers, D. A., Glasgow, R. E., & Stange, K. C. (2013). The dynamic sustainability framework: Addressing the paradox of sustainment amid ongoing change. *Implementation Science, 8*(1), 117. https://doi.org/10.1186/1748-5908-8-117

Children's Investment Fund Foundation. (2020). *Reducing under-5 mortality in Uganda*. Retrieved from https://ciff.org/impact/uganda-reducing-under-5-mortality/

Clancy, E., & Mayo, A. (2009). Launching a social enterprise see-and-treat service. *Emergency Nurse, 17*(3), 22–24. https://doi.org/10.7748/en2009.06.17.3.22.c7088

Embrace Innovations. (2020). Retrieved from https://www.embraceinnovations.com/

Farmer, J., Kamstra, P., Brennan-Horley, C., De Cotta, T., Roy, M., Barraket, J., … Kilpatrick, S. (2020). Using micro-geography to understand the realisation of wellbeing: A qualitative GIS study of three social enterprises. *Health & Place, 62*. https://doi.org/10.1016/j.healthplace.2020.102293

Gordon, K., Wilson, J., Tonner, A., & Shaw, E. (2018). How can social enterprises impact health and well-being? *International Journal of Entrepreneurial Behavior & Research, 3*, 697–713.

Iwelunmor, J., Blackstone, S., Veira, D., Nwaozuru, U., Airhihenbuwa, C., Munodawafa, D., … Ogedegbe, G. (2016). Toward the sustainability of health interventions implemented in sub-Saharan Africa: A systematic review and conceptual framework. *Implementation Science, 11*(1), 43. https://doi.org/10.1186/s13012-016-0392-8

Iwelunmor, J., Ezechi, O., Obiezu-Umeh, C., Gbajabiamila, T., Nwaozuru, U., Oladele, D., & Tucker, J. (2019). *Crowdsourcing youth-friendly strategies to promote HIV self-testing (HIVST) services in Nigeria.* Paper presented at the APHA's 2019 annual meeting and expo (Nov. 2-Nov. 6).

Jagosh, J. (2019). Realist synthesis for public health: Building an ontologically deep understanding of how programs work, for whom, and in which contexts. *Annual Review of Public Health, 40* (1), 361–372. https://doi.org/10.1146/annurev-publhealth-031816-044451

Kassebaum, N., Kyu, H. H., Zoeckler, L., Olsen, H. E., Thomas, K., Pinho, C., . . . Ghiwot, T. T. (2017). Child and adolescent health from 1990 to 2015: Findings from the global burden of diseases, injuries, and risk factors 2015 study. *JAMA Pediatrics, 171*(6), 573–592.

Kerlin, J. A. (2010). A comparative analysis of the global emergence of social enterprise. *Voluntas: International Journal of Voluntary and Nonprofit Organizations, 21*(2), 162–179. https://doi.org/10.1007/s11266-010-9126-8

Liu, L., Oza, S., Hogan, D., Chu, Y., Perin, J., Zhu, J., . . . Black, R. E. (2016). Global, regional, and national causes of under-5 mortality in 2000–15: An updated systematic analysis with implications for the sustainable development goals. *The Lancet, 388*(10063), 3027–3035.

Living Goods. (2020). Retrieved from https://livinggoods.org/

Macaulay, B., Roy, M. J., Donaldson, C., Teasdale, S., & Kay, A. (2018). Conceptualizing the health and well-being impacts of social enterprise: A UK-based study. *Health Promotion International, 33*(5), 748–759.

Marmot, M., Friel, S., Bell, R., Houweling, T. A. J., Taylor, S., & Commission on Social Determination of Health. (2008). Closing the gap in a generation: Health equity through action on the social determinants of health. *The Lancet, 372*(9650), 1661–1669.

McAllister, D. A., Liu, L., Shi, T., Chu, Y., Reed, C., Burrows, J., . . . Campbell, H. (2019). Global, regional, and national estimates of pneumonia morbidity and mortality in children younger than 5 years between 2000 and 2015: A systematic analysis. *The Lancet Global Health, 7*(1), e47–e57.

McKague, K., & Harrison, S. (2019). Gender and health social enterprises in Africa: A research agenda. *International Journal for Equity in Health, 18*(1), 95.

Mothers2Mothers. (2020). Retrieved from https://www.m2m.org/

Nilsson, M., Griggs, D., & Visbeck, M. (2016). Policy: Map the interactions between sustainable development goals. *Nature, 534*(7607), 320–322.

Nwaozuru, U., Gbajabiamila, T., Obiezu-Umeh, C., Mason, S., Tahlil, K., Oladele, D., . . . Ezechi, O. (2020). An innovation bootcamp model to develop HIV self-testing social enterprise among young people in Nigeria: A youth participatory design approach. *The Lancet Global Health, 8*, S12.

Osgood-Zimmerman, A., Millear, A. I., Stubbs, R. W., Shields, C., Pickering, B. V., Earl, L., . . . Bhatt, S. (2018). Mapping child growth failure in Africa between 2000 and 2015. *Nature, 555* (7694), 41–47.

Pawson, R., & Tilley, N. (1997). *Realistic evaluation.* SAGE Publications.

Roy, M. J., Donaldson, C., Baker, R., & Kay, A. (2013). Social enterprise: New pathways to health and well-being? *Journal of Public Health Policy, 34*(1), 55–68.

Roy, M. J., Donaldson, C., Baker, R., & Kerr, S. (2014). The potential of social enterprise to enhance health and well-being: A model and systematic review. *Social Science & Medicine, 123*, 182–193. https://doi.org/10.1016/j.socscimed.2014.07.031

Schwab Foundation. (2020). *Social entrepreneurships.* Retrieved from http://www.schwabfound.org/entrepreneurs

Smith, T. W., Calancie, L., & Ammerman, A. (2015). Social entrepreneurship for obesity prevention: What are the opportunities? *Current Obesity Reports, 4*(3), 311–318. https://doi.org/10.1007/s13679-015-0162-y

UN. (2015). *United Nations: Transforming our world: The 2030 agenda for sustainable development*. UN.

Van Malderen, C., Amouzou, A., Barros, A. J., Masquelier, B., Van Oyen, H., & Speybroeck, N. (2019). Socioeconomic factors contributing to under-five mortality in sub-Saharan Africa: A decomposition analysis. *BMC Public Health, 19*(1), 760.

Werner, L. K., Jabbarian, J., Kagoné, M., McMahon, S., Lemp, J., Souares, A., ... & De Neve, J. W. (2019). "Because at school, you can become somebody"–The perceived health and economic returns on secondary schooling in rural Burkina Faso. *PloS one, 14*(12), e0226911.

Wilkinson, R. G., & Marmot, M. (2003). *Social determinants of health: The solid facts*. World Health Organization.

Willis, C. D., Riley, B. L., Stockton, L., Abramowicz, A., Zummach, D., Wong, G., ... Best, A. (2016). Scaling up complex interventions: Insights from a realist synthesis. *Health Res Policy Syst, 14*(1), 88.

Index

© Springer Nature Switzerland AG 2022
F. M. Ssewamala et al. (eds.), *Child Behavioral Health in Sub-Saharan Africa*,
https://doi.org/10.1007/978-3-030-83707-5